Marian Zabia

AF881577

# Infectious Diseases of Mice and Rats

Committee on Infectious Diseases of Mice and Rats
Institute of Laboratory Animal Resources
Commission on Life Sciences
National Research Council

NATIONAL ACADEMY PRESS
Washington, D.C. 1991

**NATIONAL ACADEMY PRESS • 2101 Constitution Avenue, NW • Washington, DC 20418**

NOTICE: The project that is the subject of this report was approved by the Governing Board of the National Research Council, whose members are drawn from the councils of the National Academy of Sciences, National Academy of Engineering, and Institute of Medicine. The members of the committee responsible for the report were chosen for their special competences and with regard for appropriate balance.

This report has been reviewed by a group other than the authors according to procedures approved by a Report Review Committee consisting of members of the National Academy of Sciences, National Academy of Engineering, and Institute of Medicine.

The National Academy of Sciences is a private, nonprofit, self-perpetuating society of distinguished scholars engaged in scientific and engineering research, dedicated to the furtherance of science and technology and to their use for the general welfare. Upon the authority of the charter granted to it by the Congress in 1863, the Academy has a mandate that requires it to advise the federal government on scientific and technical matters. Dr. Frank Press is president of the National Academy of Sciences.

The National Academy of Engineering was established in 1964, under the charter of the National Academy of Sciences, as a parallel organization of outstanding engineers. It is autonomous in its administration and in the selection of its members, sharing with the National Academy of Sciences the responsibility for advising the federal government. The National Academy of Engineering also sponsors engineering programs aimed at meeting national needs, encourages education and research, and recognizes the superior achievements of engineers. Dr. Robert M. White is president of the National Academy of Engineering.

The Institute of Medicine was established in 1970 by the National Academy of Sciences to secure the services of eminent members of appropriate professions in the examination of policy matters pertaining to the health of the public. The Institute acts under the responsibility given to the National Academy of Sciences by its congressional charter to be an adviser to the federal government and upon its own initiative to identify issues of medical care, research, and education. Dr. Samuel O. Thier is president of the Institute of Medicine.

The National Research Council was established by the National Academy of Sciences in 1916 to associate the broad community of science and technology with the Academy's purposes of furthering knowledge and advising the federal government. Functioning in accordance with general policies determined by the Academy, the Council has become the principal operating agency of both the National Academy of Sciences and National Academy of Engineering in the conduct of their services to the government, the public, and the scientific and engineering communities. The Council is administered jointly by both Academies and the Institute of Medicine. Dr. Frank Press and Dr. Robert M. White are chairman and vice-chairman, respectively, of the National Research Council.

This project was supported by the National Cancer Institute, National Institutes of Health, under contracts NO1-CM-57644 and NO1-CM-07316, administered by the Division of Cancer Treatment.

Infectious diseases of mice and rats / Committee on Infectious Diseases of Mice and Rats. Institute of Laboratory Animal Resources. Commission on Life Sciences. National Research Council.
p. cm.
Includes bibliographical references.
Includes index.
ISBN 0-309-03794-8
1. Mice—Infections. 2. Rats—Infections. 3. Laboratory animals—Infections. 4. Mice as laboratory animals. 5. Rats as laboratory animals. I. Institute of Laboratory Animal Resources (U.S.) Committee on Infectious Diseases of Mice and Rats.
[DNLM: 1. Animals, Laboratory. 2. Communicable Diseases—veterinary. 3. Mice. 4. Rats.
QY 60.R6 I43]
SF996.5.I54 1990
636'.93233—dc20
DNLM/DLC
for Library of Congress

90-6152
CIP

Copyright ©1991 by the National Academy of Sciences

No part of this book may be reproducerd by any mechanical, photographic, or electronic process, or in the form of a phonographic recording, nor may it be stored in a retrieval system, transmitted, or otherwise copied for public or private use, without written permission from the publisher, except for the purposes of official use by the United States Government.

Printed in the United States of America

## COMMITTEE ON INFECTIOUS DISEASES OF MICE AND RATS

**J. Russell Lindsey**, Department of Comparative Medicine, Schools of Medicine and Dentistry, University of Alabama at Birmingham, Birmingham, Alabama (Chairman)

**Gary A. Boorman**, Chemical Pathology Branch, Toxicological Research and Testing Program, National Institute of Environmental Health Sciences, Research Triangle Park, North Carolina

**Michael J. Collins**, Jr., Animal Health Diagnostic Laboratory, NCI, Frederick Cancer Research Facility, Frederick, Maryland

**Chao-Kuang Hsu,** Smith Kline Animal Health Products, West Chester, Pennsylvania

**Gerald L. Van Hoosier, Jr.**, Division of Animal Medicine, University of Washington, Seattle, Washington

**Joseph E. Wagner,** Veterinary Medical Diagnostic Laboratory, College of Veterinary Medicine, University of Missouri-Columbia, Columbia, Missouri

### Staff

**Dorothy D. Greenhouse**, Senior Program Officer
**Bernadette M. Marriott**, Staff Officer
**Sybil A. Paige**, Administrative Secretary
**Thomas L. Wolfle**, Director

The Institute of Laboratory Animal Resources (ILAR) was founded in 1952 under the auspices of the National Research Council. Its mission is to provide expert counsel to the federal government, the biomedical research community, and the public on the scientific, technological, and ethical use of laboratory animals within the context of the interests and mission of the National Academy of Sciences. ILAR promotes the high-quality humane care of laboratory animals; the appropriate use of laboratory animals; and the exploration of alternatives in research, testing, and teaching.

## INSTITUTE OF LABORATORY ANIMAL RESOURCES COUNCIL

**Steven P. Pakes**, University of Texas Southwestern Medical Center, Dallas, Texas (Chairman)
**June R. Aprille**, Department of Biology, Tufts University, Medford, Massachusetts
**Melvin W. Balk**, Charles River Laboratories, Inc., Wilmington, Massachusetts
**Douglas M. Bowden**, Washington Regional Primate Research Center, University of Washington, Seattle, Washington
**Lester M. Crawford**, Food Safety and Inspection Service, U. S. Department of Agriculture, Washington, D.C.
**Thomas J. Gill III,** University of Pittsburgh School of Medicine, Pittsburgh, Pennsylvania
**Alan M. Goldberg**, School of Hygiene and Public Health, The Johns Hopkins University, Baltimore, Maryland
**Jon W. Gordon**, Department of Obstetrics and Gynecology, Mt. Sinai School of Medicine, New York, New York
**Margaret Z. Jones**, Department of Pathology, Michigan State University, E. Lansing, Michigan
**Michael D. Kastello**, Merck Sharp & Dohme, Rahway, New Jersey
**Robert H. Purcell**, National Institute of Allergy and Infectious Diseases, National Institutes of Health, Bethesda, Maryland
**J. Wesley Robb**, School of Medicine, University of Southern California, Los Angeles, California
**John L. VandeBerg**, Department of Genetics, Southwest Foundation for Biomedical Research, San Antonio, Texas

**Staff**

**Thomas L. Wolfle,** *Director*

## COMMISSION ON LIFE SCIENCES

**Bruce M. Alberts**, University of California, San Francisco, California (Chairman)
**Bruce N. Ames,** University of California, Berkeley, California
**Francisco J. Ayala,** University of California, Irvine, California
**J. Michael Bishop**, University of California Medical Center, San Francisco, California
**Michael T. Clegg,** University of California, Riverside, California
**Glenn A. Crosby,** Washington State University, Pullman, Washington
**Freeman J. Dyson,** The Institute for Advanced Study, Princeton, New Jersey
**Leroy E. Hood**, California Institute of Technology, Pasadena, California
**Donald F. Hornig**, Harvard University School of Public Health, Boston, Massachusetts
**Ernest G. Jaworski**, Monsanto Company, St. Louis, Missouri
**Marian E. Koshland**, University of California, Berkeley, California
**Richard E. Lenski,** University of California, Riverside, California
**Steven P. Pakes**, Southwestern Medical Center, Dallas, Texas
**Emil A. Pfitzer,** Hoffman-LaRoche, Inc., Nutley, New Jersey
**Joseph E. Rall**, National Institutes of Health, Bethesda, Maryland
**Richard D. Remington**, University of Iowa, Iowa City, Iowa
**Paul G. Risser**, University of New Mexico, Albuquerque, New Mexico
**Harold M. Schmeck, Jr.,** Armonk, New York
**Richard B. Setlow**, Brookhaven National Laboratory, Upton, New York
**Carla J. Shatz,** Stanford University School of Medicine, Stanford, California
**Torsten N. Wiesel**, Rockefeller University, New York, New York

**Staff**

**John E. Burris,** *Executive Director*

# Preface

Progress in biomedical science leads inexorably to greater refinements in scientific methodologies. In recent years it has become apparent that further refinement is needed in the quality of laboratory mice and rats. The scientific community has increasingly recognized that infectious diseases in these species significantly alter many research results. Unfortunately, the literature on this subject is voluminous, scattered, and often confusing, with the result that its practical application has been disappointing. Additional material on control of infections in immunodeficient rodents can be found in *Immunodeficient Rodents: A Guide to Their Immunobiology, Husbandry, and Use*, 1989, report of the Institute of Laboratory Animal Resources (ILAR) Committee on Immunologically Compromised Rodents (Washington, D.C.: National Academy Press. 246 pp.).

This text is an expansion of the newly revised second edition of the *Companion Guide to Infectious Diseases of Mice and Rats*. It is intended to serve as a detailed reference of principles, methods, and facts to be applied by biomedical scientists in improving the quality of animals required in individual research settings. The expanded text is written for students of infectious disease and for investigators and veterinarians who want more detail than that contained in the companion guide. There are three main parts. Part I, "Principles of Rodent Disease Prevention," summarizes the basic concepts and practices of infectious disease exclusion and detection, and gives data on the prevalence of infectious agents in contemporary rodent populations. Part II, "Individual Disease Agents and Their Effects on

Research," gives in a synoptic format the factual information deemed most pertinent to understanding the importance, epizootiology, pathogenesis, diagnosis, and control of natural infections due to each agent, complete with a listing of the known instances in which each agent has interfered with research. Part III, "Indexes to Diagnosis and Research Complications of Infectious Agents," contains tabular information intended for use as an aid to diagnostic problem solving.

Many people have contributed to the compilation of the information in this report. The outlines in Part II were patterned after those in the first edition of the handbook, but have been extensively revised by one of us (J. R. L.) through many years of teaching a course on diseases of laboratory animals and have been further revised by this committee. The many contributions of the faculty and students in the Department of Comparative Medicine at the University of Alabama at Birmingham are gratefully acknowledged. In addition, the following gave invaluable advice on specific agents: Drs. Gail H. Cassell and Jerry K. Davis, University of Alabama at Birmingham (mycoplasmal infections); Dr. C. A. Bruggeman, Department of Medical Microbiology, State University of Limburg, Maastricht, The Netherlands (rat cytomegalovirus); Dr. Steven W. Barthold, Yale University (mouse hepatitis virus); Dr. Steven L. Vonderfecht, Johns Hopkins University (rat rotavirus-like agent); Dr. James R. Ganaway, National Institutes of Health, Bethesda, Md. (*Bacillus piliformis*); Dr. Anton M. Allen, National Institutes of Health, Bethesda, Md. (mousepox); and Dr. Lizbeth M. Kraft, National Aeronautics and Space Administration/Ames Research Center, Moffett Field, Calif. (poxviruses of rats). Dr. Kenneth Boschert, formerly a postdoctoral fellow at the University of Alabama at Birmingham, assisted with compiling information for the diagnostic indexes in Part III. Drs. Fred Quimby and Melvin Balk provided review at each stage of preparation for the ILAR Council. Special gratitude is due Ms. Doris Whatley and Ms. Audrey Farrow, who typed the manuscript through numerous revisions.

# Contents

# Part I
# Principles of Rodent Disease Prevention

# 1

# Objectives, Terminology, and Overview of Pathogen Status

## Scientific Objectives

Animal experiments are essential to progress in the biomedical sciences (NRC, 1985; Gay, undated). Like investigations in any field of science, the merit of animal experiments ultimately depends on rigid adherence to principles of the scientific method. Proper practice of these principles yields data that have both reliability and reproducibility, key objectives of all good experiments (Bernard, 1865).

Living systems are remarkably complex and often subject to large deviations in biologic response due to seemingly trivial influences, either endogenous or exogenous. Thus, the biological responsiveness of mice and rats, comprising 90% of the experimental animals used in the United States (ILAR, 1980), can be altered by genetic factors (Kahan et al., 1982; Hedrich, 1983) and numerous environmental influences, including physical, chemical, and microbial factors (Lindsey et al., 1978; Baker et al., 1979; Pakes et al., 1984).

As will be discussed in considerable detail later in this volume, the prevention of many natural infections (microbial factors) in mice and rats is of crucial importance for accomplishing a wide range of scientific objectives for which these rodent species are used.

## Infection Versus Disease

A common misconception, even among senior scientists and laboratory animal specialists, is that infection is synonymous with disease. Bacterial infections of rodents include pathogens, opportunists, and commensals, of which the last two are by far the most numerous as constituents of the normal flora on mucosal and body surfaces (Dubos et al., 1965; Savage, 1971). Similarly, the viral and parasite pathogens of rodents vary considerably in pathogenicity. Also, it is important to distinguish between subclinical (inapparent, covert, or silent) and clinically apparent infections. Two types of subclinical infections are recognized: dormant (the agent can be recovered) and latent (the agent cannot be recovered by direct methods and its presence must be inferred by indirect methods).

Most natural infections due to pathogens in mice and rats are subclinical. Thus, clinical manifestations of pathogen infections in these species have only limited diagnostic value. Also, it cannot be overemphasized that aberrations in research results due to natural infections often occur in the absence of clinical disease. Thus, prevention of infection, not merely prevention of clinical disease, is essential (Lindsey et al., 1986a).

## Terminology of Microbial and Pathogen Status

The development of gnotobiotic methodology in the 1940s and 1950s (Gustafsson, 1948; Reyniers, 1957a,b; Trexler and Reynolds, 1957; Luckey, 1963; Trexler, 1963, 1983; Newton, 1965; ILAR, 1970; Weisbroth, 1972; Myers, 1980) provided the basic technological armamentarium for controlling the microbial and pathogen status of mice and rats. The use of cesarean derivation and gnotobiotic isolator techniques was found to be highly practical in eliminating pathogens from rodent stocks for institutional (Trexler and Barry, 1958; Van Hoosier et al., 1966) and commercial (Cumming and Elias, 1957; Foster, 1958; Foster et al., 1963) purposes. The subsequent widespread application of these methods to the production of mice and rats for research resulted in a bewildering array of terms for the designation of microbial and pathogen status (Table 1). Some of the terms have etymological clarity and consistently convey clear meanings. However, many of the terms have proved unfortunate; they convey imprecise meanings that lead to confusion about animal quality. The resulting state of affairs has been detrimental to the continuing quest for improvement in the quality of rodents for research.

Six terminology systems for laboratory rodent microbiological status, representing the major systems in use in the Western world, are shown in Table 1. Based on the microbial exclusion method(s) required, the different types of animals in Table 1 are separable into three major groupings:

a. *Isolator maintained.* An isolator is a sterilizable life-support chamber, usually constructed of stainless steel or plastic, in which gnotobiotes may be housed and maintained free from contamination (ILAR, 1970). "Isolator maintained" as used here means continuous, uninterrupted maintenance of animals in an isolator so as to prevent any microbial contamination.

TABLE 1 Terminology for Microbiological Status of Laboratory Rodents[a]

| Country | Terminology Systems: Isolator Maintained | | | Barrier Maintained | | | | No Containment | Reference |
|---|---|---|---|---|---|---|---|---|---|
| United States (ILAR)[b] | Axenic → | Gnotobiotic → | Defined microbially associated → | | Barrier maintained → | | Monitored → | Conventional | ILAR, 1976 |
| (Common usage) | Germfree → | | Defined flora → | Pathogen free → | Specific pathogen free → | Virus antibody free → | | Conventional | Lindsey et al., 1986a |
| Holland | Germfree → | | Defined flora → | | Specific pathogen free → | | Clean conventional → | Conventional | Solleveld, 1978 |
| West Germany | Keimfrei → | | Gnotobiotisch assozliert → | | Specific pathogen free → | | | Konventionell | Bonath, 1983 |
| France | Axenique → | | Gnotoxenique → | | EOPS[c] → | | Heteroxenique → | Holoxenique | Bonath, 1983 |
| United Kingdom | Category:[d] ***** → | | **** → | | *** → | | ** → | * | MRC-LAC, 1974 |

[a]See text for definition of terms; table is modified from Bonath (1983).
[b]Institute of Laboratory Animal Resources.
[c]Animaux exempts d'organismes pathogenes specifiques = specific pathogen free.
[d]Categories are defined on the basis of designated microbial agents and parasites absent/present for each category. Categories ****, ***, and ** do not have direct equivalences in the other systems.

b. *Barrier maintained.* A barrier is a housing "system that combines construction features, equipment, and operating methods to stabilize the enclosed environment to minimize the probability that pathogens or other undesirable organisms will contact or infect the enclosed animal population" (ILAR, 1976a). Barriers may be provided at the facility, room, rack, and/or cage levels. "Barrier maintained" as used here means continuous, uninterrupted maintenance of animals in one or more barriers so as to prevent contamination by any pathogen.

c. *No containment.* The term no containment means the housing of animals without measures to prevent pathogen contamination. Animals housed in this manner are generally designated conventional (see below).

The individual types of animals included in Table 1 are defined as follows:

a. *Germfree (or axenic, keimfrei, axenique) animal.* Derived by hysterectomy, reared and maintained in an isolator by germfree techniques, and demonstrably free of associated forms of life including viruses, bacteria, fungi, protozoa, and other saprophytic or parasitic forms (ILAR, 1970,1976a; Bonath, 1983). Endogenous viruses, e.g., leukemia viruses that occur in all mice, are present (ILAR, 1970).

b. *Gnotobiotic animal.* Derived by hysterectomy, reared and maintained in an isolator by germfree techniques, and has one or more associated nonpathogenic agent(s), all of which are known (ILAR, 1970, 1976).

c. *Defined flora* (or defined microbially associated, gnotobiotisch assozliert, gnotoxenique) animal. A germfree animal that has been intentionally associated with one or more microorganisms (e.g., the "Schaedler cocktail," consisting of eight nonpathogenic bacteria) and maintained continuously in an isolator to prevent contamination by other agents (ILAR, 1976a; Bonath, 1983). This term may be used synonymously with gnotobiote.

d. *Pathogen-free (PF) animal.* Free of all demonstrable pathogens (Sacquet, 1965). This term is frequently abused because there is no universal agreement on which agents are pathogens, which tests should be done for them, how the animal populations should be sampled, or how frequently testing should be done. A pathogen (in the context of laboratory animal quality) may be defined as an infectious agent that can cause overt disease and/or alter biologic response(s) during experimentation (Lindsey et al., 1986a). Proper usage of the term pathogen-free requires that the pathogen-free status of a given subpopulation of animals be supported by current test results from a battery of tests appropriate for all pathogens of the rodent species in question. In actual practice, a list of pathogens must be specified. Thus, this term differs very little from specific pathogen free (Lindsey et al., 1986a).

e. *Specific pathogen free (SPF)* (or barrier maintained, EOPS) animal. Free of a specified list of pathogens. This term also is frequently abused.

TABLE 2 Prevalence of Murine Virus Infections in Mouse Colonies[a]

| Virus | United States | | Canada | United Kingdom | West Germany and Others | Japan | | |
|---|---|---|---|---|---|---|---|---|
| | Commercial Breeders[b] | Commercial Breeders and Research Institutions[c] | Breeders and Research Institutions[d] | Breeders and Research Institutions[e] | Breeders and Research Institutions[f] | Commercial Breeders and Research Institutions[g] | Breeders[h] | Research Institutions[i] |
| PVM | 36 | 95 | 83 | 42 | 14 | | | |
| Sendai | 73 | 86 | 47 | 34 | 23 | 52 | 46 | 54 |
| Mouse hepatitis | 83 | 81 | 73 | 40 | 60 | 26 | 19 | 36 |
| Minute | 73 | 81 | 50 | 0 | 33 | | | |
| Theiler's | 5 | 62 | 40 | 0 | 33 | | | |
| Reovirus-3 | 14 | 52 | 33 | 4 | 13 | 8 | | |
| Adenovirus | 19[j] | 0 | 0 | 0 | | 0 | | |
| Polyoma | 0 | 5 | 14 | 0 | 0 | | | |
| Mousepox | 0 | 0 | 14 | 0 | 0 | | | |
| LCMV[k] | 0 | 0 | 0 | 0 | 0 | | | |
| No. of colonies | 77 | 21 | 12-18/agent | 1-35/agent | 2-60/agent | 89 | 196 | 61 |

[a]Data are percentages of colonies found to be infected. Serologic methods were used except where specified otherwise.
[b]From Lindsey et al., 1986a.
[c]From Parker, 1980.
[d]From Lussier and Descoteaux, 1986.
[e]From Gannon and Carthew, 1980.
[f]From Kraft and Meyer, 1986.
[g]From Nakagawa et al., 1984.
[h]From Suzuki et al., 1982.
[i]From Fujiwara, 1980.
[j]Diagnosis was based on the finding of typical intranuclear inclusions in intestinal epithelium (Luethans and Wagner, 1983). All animals were serologically negative for adenovirus.
[k]Lymphocytic choriomeningitis virus.

TABLE 3 Prevalence of Murine Virus Infections in Rat Colonies[a]

| | United States | | Canada | United Kingdom | West Germany and Others | Japan | | |
|---|---|---|---|---|---|---|---|---|
| Virus | Commercial Breeders[b] | Commercial Breeders and Research Institutions[c] | Breeders and Research Institutions[d] | Breeders and Research Institutions[e] | Breeders and Research Institutions[f] | Commercial Breeders and Research Institutions[g] | Breeders[h] | Research Institutions[h] |
| PVM | 44 | 64 | 70 | 72 | 40 | | | |
| Sendai | 61 | 52 | 55 | 30 | 30 | 28 | 3 | 6 |
| SDAV[i] | 44 | 68 | 75 | 45 | 41 | 8 | 41 | 43 |
| KRV[i] | 44 | 71 | 74 | 60 | 32 | | | |
| Toolan H-1 | 11 | 52 | 71 | 0 | 27 | | | |
| Reovirus-3 | 6 | 44 | 44 | 0 | | 16 | | |
| Adenovirus | 6[j] | 36 | 17 | | | 8 | | |
| Theiler's | | 44 | 58 | | | | | |
| LCMV[i] | | | 7 | 0 | | | | |
| No. of colonies | 18 | 25 | 15-24/agent | 1-33/agent | 36-45/agent | 71 | 34 | 49 |

[a]Data are percentages of colonies found to be infected. Serologic methods were used except where specified otherwise.
[b]From Lindsey et al., 1986a.
[c]From Parker, 1980.
[d]From Lussier and Descoteaux, 1986.
[e]From Gannon and Carthew, 1980.
[f]From Kraft and Meyer, 1986.
[g]From Suzuki et al., 1982.
[h]From Fujiwara, 1980.
[i]SDAV = Sialodacryoadenitus virus
KRV = Kilham rat virus
LCMV = Lymphocytic choriomeningitus virus
[j]Diagnosis was based on the finding of typical intranuclear inclusions in intestinal epithelium (Luethans and Wagner, 1983). All animals were serologically negative for adenovirus.

Proper usage requires that the absence of certain specified pathogens from a given subpopulation of animals be supported by current test results from a battery of tests appropriate for those pathogens (Lindsey et al., 1986a).

f. *Virus antibody-free animal.* Free of antibodies to viral pathogens. Proper usage requires that the absence of viral pathogens for a given subpopulation of animals be supported by current test results from a battery of appropriate serologic tests for a list of specified pathogens (Lindsey et al., 1986a).

g. *Monitored (or clean conventional, heteroxenique) animal.* Housed in a low-security barrier and demonstrated by sequential monitoring to be free of major pathogens (ILAR, 1976a; Bonath, 1983). These terms are even less specific than pathogen-free and specific pathogen free. They imply a standard of quality without defining the standard, and their usage is to be discouraged.

h. *Conventional (or konventionell, holoxenique) animal.* Microbial burden is unknown and uncontrolled, and housing is generally in open rooms that have unrestricted access (ILAR, 1976a; Bonath, 1983).

Based on the foregoing information, it should be apparent that the terms used in defining rodent microbial status vary greatly in precision of meaning. Four terms (germfree, gnotobiotic, defined flora, and conventional), representing the extremes of microbial status, have clear definitions that are generally accepted and understood by scientists as well as technical personnel. However, major confusion is encountered in the definition and use of terms representing the middle ground of pathogen status. Herein lies a problem of major proportions. Pathogen-free, specific pathogen free, virus antibody free, and clean conventional are relative terms that require explicit definition every time they are used. Their definitions must include the background of the rodent subpopulation in question (e.g., hysterectomy derived?, isolator maintained?, barrier maintained?); details of current housing (e.g., isolator, barrier); and data from laboratory tests, including the specific tests done for pathogens, the number of tests, the frequency of testing, and the results of all tests to date (Lindsey et al., 1986a).

## Pathogen Status of Contemporary Rodents

The conceptual approaches and technological advances necessary for the prevention of pathogen infections in laboratory mice and rats have been available since the 1950s (Cumming and Elias, 1957; Reyniers, 1957a,b; Trexler and Reynolds, 1957; Foster, 1958; Trexler and Barry, 1958; Luckey, 1963). The prevalence of pathogens in contemporary rodent populations (colonies) provides an indication of the degree to which these concepts and methods have found practical application in the prevention of pathogen infections.

Tables 2 and 3 give the prevalence of virus infections in laboratory mice and rat populations in the United States, Canada, the United Kingdom, West

Germany, and Japan. [Additional prevalence data have been reported from the United States by Casebolt et al. (1988) and from Europe by Van Der Logt (1986)]. In mice, infections of pneumonia virus of mice (PVM), Sendai virus, mouse hepatitis virus, and minute virus of mice were commonly present in 50% or more of the colonies surveyed. Theiler's virus and reovirus-3 were not uncommon, and a few colonies had adenovirus, polyomavirus, or ectromelia virus. In rats, PVM, Sendai virus, SDA/RCV, Kilham rat virus (KRV), and Toolan H-1 virus were frequently found in more than 50% of colonies. Reovirus-3 and adenovirus were fairly common. LCMV was reported in 7% of rat colonies in Canada. Although antibodies to Theiler's virus were reported in 44% of rat colonies in one survey in the

TABLE 4 Prevalence of Bacterial Infections in Mouse Colonies[a]

| | United States | United Kingdom | West Germany and Others | Japan | | |
|---|---|---|---|---|---|---|
| Bacterium | Commercial Breeders[b] | Accredited Institutions[c] | Breeders and Research Institutions[d] | SPF Breeders[e] | Conventional Breeders[f] | Research Institutions[f] |
| *Mycoplasma pulmonis* | 19 | 17 | | 0 | 24 | 20[g] |
| *Mycoplasma arthritidis* | 3 | | | | | |
| *Pseudomonas* sp. | 57 | | | 33 | 32 | |
| *Pasteurella pneumotropica* | 18 | 66 | | 0 | 74 | |
| *Salmonella enteritidis* | 6 | | | 0 | 5 | |
| *Mycobacterium avium* | 1 | | | | | |
| *Citrobacter freundii* (4280) | 1 | | | | | |
| *Streptococcus moniliformis* | 0 | | | | | |
| *Corynebacterium kutscheri* | 0 | | | 0 | 2 | 0[g] |
| *Bacillus piliformis* | 0[h] | | 0[g] | 0 | 6[g] | 5[g] |
| No. of colonies | 77 | 96 | 8 | 33 | 89 | 61 |

[a]Data are percentages of colonies found to be infected.
[b]From Lindsey et al., 1986a.
[c]From Sparrow, 1976.
[d]From Kraft and Meyer, 1986.
[e]From Nakagawa et al., 1984.
[f]From Fujiwara, 1980.
[g]Results based on serologic methods.
[h]Results based on absence of lesions, as determined by necropsy and histopathology.

TABLE 5 Prevalence of Bacterial Infections in Rat Colonies[a]

| | United States | United Kingdom | West Germany and Others | Japan | | |
|---|---|---|---|---|---|---|
| Bacterium | Commercial Breeders[b] | Accredited Institutions[c] | Breeders and Research Institutions[d] | SPF Breeders[e] | Conventional Breeders[f] | Research Institutions[f] |
| *Mycoplasma pulmonis* | 17 | 24 | 23[g] | 0 | 38 | 18[g] |
| *Mycoplasma arthritidis* | 6 | | | | | |
| *Pseudomonas* sp. | 50 | | | 36 | 39 | |
| *Pasteurella pneumotropica* | 33 | 58 | | 10 | 70 | |
| *Salmonella enteritidis* | 0 | | | 0 | 0 | |
| *Streptococcus moniliformis* | 0 | | | | | |
| *Corynebacterium kutscheri* | 0 | | | 0 | 8 | 6[g] |
| *Bacillus piliformis* | 0[h] | | 41[g] | 0 | 17[g] | 47[g] |
| No. of colonies | 18 | 67 | 34-40/agent | 31 | 64 | 49 |

[a]Data are percentages of colonies found to be infected.
[b]From Lindsey et al., 1986a.
[c]From Sparrow, 1976.
[d]From Kraft and Meyer, 1986.
[e]From Nakagawa et al., 1984.
[f]From Fujiwara, 1980.
[g]Results based on serologic methods.
[h]Results based on absence of lesions, as determined by necropsy and histopathology.

United States (Parker, 1980) and 58% of rat colonies in Canada (Lussier and Descoteaux, 1986), the significance of these findings appears uncertain.

The reported prevalences of bacterial infections in laboratory mouse and rat populations are given in Tables 4 and 5. Infections of *Pseudomonas* sp. and *Pasteurella pneumotropica* are quite common. The data for *Mycoplasma pulmonis* and *Mycoplasma arthritidis* are very deceiving. Most of the reported data were obtained by culture methods that are insensitive. Thus, the true prevalence of *M. pulmonis* is probably at least 5 to 10% greater than the percentage reported for each survey that used culture methods. The situation for *M. arthritidis* is far worse in that subclinical infections due to this agent are extremely difficult to demonstrate through cultures and are presently thought to be extremely common in contemporary mouse and rat populations (Cassell et al., 1986; Lindsey et al., 1986b). Similarly, the known insensitivity of culture methods for *Salmonella enteritidis* and *Corynebacterium kutscheri*

TABLE 6 Prevalence of Parasitic Infections and Infestations in Mice and Rats[a]

| | United States: Commercial Breeders[b] | | United Kingdom: Accredited Breeders[c] | |
|---|---|---|---|---|
| Parasite | Mice | Rats | Mice | Rats |
| *Entamoeba muris* | 51 | 24 | 27 | 28 |
| *Spironucleus muris* | 42 | 17 | 29 | 28 |
| Pinworms | 38 | 17 | 35 | 39 |
| *Tritrichomonas muris* | 26 | 17 | 24 | 27 |
| *Giardia muris* | 12 | 11 | 8 | 10 |
| *Hymenolepis* sp. | 4 | 0 | 2 | |
| *Eimeria* sp. | 1 | 0 | 3 | |
| Mites | 29 | 0 | 26 | 8 |
| *Polyplax* sp. | | 0 | | 5 |
| No. of colonies | 77 | 18 | 96 | 67 |

[a]Data are percentages of colonies found to be infected.
[b]From Lindsey et al., 1986a.
[c]From Sparrow, 1976.

suggests that the data given in Tables 4 and 5 for these agents are very conservative estimates of the true prevalence. The true prevalence of *Bacillus piliformis* is unknown, but recent surveys by serologic methods in Japan (Fujiwara, 1980), Scandinavia (Fries, 1980), and West Germany (Kraft and Meyer, 1986) suggest that infection by this agent may be common in mice and rats.

The data from two surveys of parasitic infections and infestations in mice and rats are given in Table 6. *Entamoeba muris*, *Spironucleus muris*, pinworms, *Tritrichomonas muris*, *Giardia muris*, and mites were all fairly common.

Based on the data in Tables 2 through 6, it must be concluded that only very modest success has been achieved in the prevention of microbial infections and parasitic infections and infestations of contemporary mice and rats.

# 2

# Breeding, Transportation, and Use of Pathogen-free Rodents

Past experience has taught that the use of pathogen-free rodents in research is possible only when breeding, transportation, and maintenance programs specifically designed for the exclusion of pathogens are followed. Genuine commitments must be made to preventing infections throughout the life of the rodent. Some of the essential commitments are as follow:*

a. The investigator must be strongly committed.

b. The investigator and the support personnel must understand the terminology and principles involved.

c. Appropriate facilities and equipment must be available.

d. Housing practices must ensure physical separation and avoidance of cross-contamination between different animal subpopulations throughout their lives.

e. Reliable health monitoring must be maintained to identify breeding populations free of pathogens and to redefine the microbiological status of the animals at regular intervals after receipt in the user facility until completion of each study.

f. Written standard operating practices must be developed and followed

*From a consensus developed during a seminar entitled "Barrier Maintenance of Rodents in Multipurpose Facilities," held at the Thirty-Sixth Annual Session of the American Association of Laboratory Animal Science on November 3-8, 1985 in Baltimore, Md. Seminar participants were J.R. Lindsey (leader); G.L. Van Hoosier, Jr.; D.B. Casebolt; J.G. Fox; R.O. Jacoby, and T.E. Hamm, Jr.

without interruption; clear objectives must be defined in advance along with detailed procedures for reaching those objectives.

A range of optional approaches should be considered in the design of specific programs of pathogen exclusion for each investigator or institution. Inasmuch as 65% of the mice and 80% of the rats used for research purposes in the United States are produced by commercial breeding facilities (ILAR, 1980), such programs usually consist of breeding facility, transportation, and user facility components. However, some investigators choose to breed their own animals, eliminating or reducing the transportation component. The following are the range of options within which most investigator or institutional needs can be met (Lindsey et al., 1986a):

Option 1:

| | | | | |
|---|---|---|---|---|
| Animals are unmonitored and obtained from many breeding facilities | ➡ | Transported in open cartons | ➡ | Housed in a conventional multi-purpose breeding facility |

Option 1 is the least effective. Rodents are purchased, transported, and used with little or no regard for pathogen status. They usually harbor many subclinical infections but appear normal. Although such animals may be acceptable for selected research projects, they serve as an important source of contamination for other rodent stocks and, therefore, pose a risk for other research programs in the user facility. Thus, for a variety of reasons this option cannot be recommended.

Option 2:

| | | | | |
|---|---|---|---|---|
| Animals are unmonitored and obtained from barrier breeding facilities | ➡ | Transported in filter-protected cartons | ➡ | Housed in a barrier room in a multi-purpose research facility |

In Option 2 the animals are obtained from a so-called barrier breeding facility, but no health monitoring is done to determine pathogen status. The term barrier is meaningless unless it is supported by current health surveillance data. Such barrier breeding facilities often have rooms containing pathogen-free animals and others that are contaminated with pathogens. Also, they may use a common shipping room where cross-contamination between groups can occur prior to shipping. Thus, the animals may have active infections due to some agents and be incubating other infections upon arrival at the user facility. Filter-protected cartons provide containment transport, but their purpose is largely negated by the infections accumulated prior to shipping. Since the research facility is multipurpose (i.e., houses animals of different pathogen status, from different sources, and for different research purposes), there are risks of cross-contamination between animal subpopulations, despite the fact that they are housed in a room operated by a barrier program. In essence, this option represents a partial commitment to prevention of pathogen infections, and it is only partially effective.

Option 3:

| | | | | |
|---|---|---|---|---|
| Animals are user and vendor monitored and are from a vendor protected barrier breeding facility | → | Transported in filter-protected cartons | → | Quarantined in remote facility until tested and shown free of pathogens; then moved to a barrier facility or barrier room |

Option 3 incorporates the principles necessary for a high degree of success in preventing pathogen infections. The breeding facility is operated by strict barrier protocol. All subpopulations are pathogen free and are monitored regularly by the vendor for pathogens. The vendor has made a commitment to protecting all subpopulations by promptly eliminating any subpopulation found to be infected by a pathogen (vendor protected facility). The user also regularly monitors subpopulations of the breeding facility to confirm pathogen-free status. All animals are shipped in filter-protected cartons. The user initially quarantines the animals for 4-6 weeks in a separate barrier room at a quarantine facility remote from the research facility (Hoag, 1964; Parker and Richter, 1982). The stock is monitored and found to be free of pathogens and then transferred in filter-protected cartons to a barrier room in the research facility where the experimentation is accomplished.

Option 4:

| | | | | |
|---|---|---|---|---|
| Animals are user maintained, controlled, and monitored and are from protected barrier breeding facility | → | Transported in filter-protected cartons | → | Housed in barrier facility, barrier room, barrier room with filter cages and laminar flow change station, or Trexler isolators |

Option 4 offers maximum effectiveness in preventing pathogen contamination. The user of the animals (or an entire institution) has complete control of the barrier breeding program, containment transfer, housing in the user facility, health surveillance program, and decision making for corrective action if needed. Breeding stocks are preferably gnotobiotic or defined flora animals and are held in isolators in a remote quarantine facility and monitored repeatedly before they are entered into the barrier breeding facility. Animals in both the barrier breeding facility and those involved in experiments are monitored regularly for pathogens. Any breeding subpopulation in the barrier breeding facility found to have any of the predetermined list of pathogens is immediately eliminated, and health monitoring of other nearby subpopulations is intensified to prevent the spread of infection.

Options 1 through 4 are not intended to be separate and distinct systems for preventing pathogen infections. Instead, they are presented here to illustrate general approaches of increasing effectiveness by which individual investigators or institutions can develop those programs most appropriate for their particular needs and resources (Lindsey et al., 1986a).

# 3

# Barrier Programs

The term barrier (used as either an adjective or noun), like some of the terms for pathogen status, identifies a general concept rather than a definitive qualitative standard. In essence, the concept requires beginning with formerly germfree or defined flora animals and maintaining them as a breeding or experimental population under conditions that exclude pathogens. A barrier is not merely a facility of a certain design. A barrier is a systematic, comprehensive program for the prevention of pathogen contamination. Facility design is one aspect of such a program (Jonas, 1965; Brick et al., 1969; Serrano, 1971). An effective or true barrier cannot exist in the absence of a systematic, comprehensive program.

Barrier programs consist of several essential elements: stocking with animals known to be free of pathogens, appropriate design of housing environments, rigorous management of the physical plant and caging environments, regular monitoring of pathogen status, and corrective action (e.g., elimination of pathogen-contaminated subpopulations) to ensure program effectiveness.

The barrier concept can be applied at different levels: an entire facility, part of a facility, room(s), groups of cages, or a single cage. As indicated above in Option 4, these alternative approaches can be used singly or in combination in accordance with the specific needs and research objectives of individual investigators or entire institutions.

### Barrier Facilities

An entire facility or part of a facility can be designed and operated as a barrier. However, this is only practical when a facility or part of a facility is fully committed to a specific objective (e.g., breeding pathogen-free animals) or a community of investigators has agreed to conduct their research under the constraints of a single barrier program.

Barrier facilities are classified on the basis of operational criteria and the degree of security provided (ILAR, 1976a): type I (maximum-security barrier), type II (high-security barrier), type III (moderate-security barrier), and type IV (minimal-security barrier). The criteria for classification include the following (ILAR, 1976a):

a. quality, quantity, and source of animals;
b. frequency and method of introducing animals and animal-derived biologic materials into the barrier;
c. processing of materials into the barrier;
d. entry of animal technicians into the barrier;
e. entry of investigators and laboratory technicians into the barrier;
f. method of housing and handling animals;
g. the environmental systems, particularly heating and air-conditioning; and
h. monitoring practices.

The effective operation of a barrier facility generally requires that written standard operating procedures be followed to maintain each of the criteria (from the list above) established for that facility. In addition, a written statement of key objectives and principles of operation should be prepared and posted in conspicuous locations accessible to all personnel. It is essential that all personnel know and support the objectives and principles of operation of a barrier facility.

### Barrier Rooms

Most animal research facilities are multipurpose, i.e., they must house animals of variable pathogen status, from many sources, and for many different research purposes. The principles of barrier maintenance can be successfully applied to individual rooms or groups of rooms within a multipurpose facility; however, even if appropriate operating procedures are followed, the risk of pathogen contamination is greater than it would be in a properly managed barrier facility. Emphasis is given to protecting the room population(s) from known or potential pathogens in all other rodent populations in the facility. As with barrier facilities, written standard operating procedures, based on the criteria listed above, should be prepared and followed for each barrier room.

### Isolators as Barriers

In addition to their usefulness in the maintenance of germfree or defined flora animals, isolators can be used as absolute barriers for populations of pathogen-free rodents consisting of one to many cages. Isolators made of clear plastic are the most versatile and economical (Trexler and Reynolds, 1957) and can be fabricated in varying dimensions up to room size (Lattuada et al., 1981). They may be used as barriers for breeding or experimental populations. By comparison with most other housing systems, they tend to be expensive and labor intensive. For these reasons, many laboratories use isolators primarily for maintaining small numbers of "seed stock" of their most valuable strains in reserve for use in the eventuality that their regular breeding stocks become contaminated. The isolators are serviced by standard gnotobiotic methods, and the animals are monitored regularly (Newton, 1965; ILAR, 1970). Again, written standard operating procedures are essential.

### Airflow Systems as Barriers

A number of different systems have been developed that use airflow to prevent or control airborne infection of laboratory animals. Incoming air is passed through high-efficiency particulate air (HEPA) filters that remove 99.9% of 0.3 μm particles. Laminar airflow (LAF) rooms or cabinets move the filtered air vertically or horizontally over the animal cages at an average velocity of 30.5 m/min (100 ft/min). Mass airflow (MAF) involves the flow of the filtered air through orifices in the ceilings of entire rooms and vertical flow of the air at average velocities of only 6.1-10.7 m/min (20-35 ft/min) (McGarrity and Coriell, 1976).

Limited data are available on the effectiveness of these systems. LAF has been demonstrated to be effective in the prevention of cage-to-cage transmission of the intestinal bacterial flora of rodents (van der Waaij and Andreas, 1971) but has been tested only superficially for the prevention of rodent pathogen transmission (Beall et al., 1971; Coriell and McGarrity, 1973). MAF has been shown to be effective in reducing or preventing the transmission of the bacterial flora (McGarrity et al., 1969; McGarrity and Coriell, 1976), reovirus-3 (McGarrity and Coriell, 1973), and polyomavirus (McGarrity et al., 1976). In one study, MAF was found to be ineffective in preventing cage-to-cage and rack-to-rack transmission of indigenous virus infections in rats, particularly sialodacryoadenitis virus/rat coronavirus, Sendai virus, and Kilham rat virus (Thigpen and Ross, 1983).

Based on the currently available evidence, LAF and MAF may serve as useful barrier systems for selected research objectives. Animals of known pathogen status should be used, and written standard operating procedures should be followed. Disadvantages of LAF and MAF are the added costs of the purchase, maintenance, and operation of the equipment.

### Barrier Cages

Filter cage systems provide barriers at the level of the individual cage. Factors that influence cage-to-cage transmission of airborne infection include type of cage used, use of bedding, distance between cages, number of animals per cage, relative humidity, and the generation of airborne dust particles during cage changing and cleaning (McGarrity et al., 1969; van der Veen et al., 1972). Filter cage systems, if properly used, act as barriers by preventing the transmission of contaminated particulates and aerosols between cages.

In order to be effective, filter cage systems must be used according to the following principles. Each cage within a room is fitted with a filter, usually made of fiberglass. The filter is removed from only one cage in the room at any given time, and filter removal is permitted only in a transfer hood. The animals and inner surfaces of each cage are handled only with disinfected forceps or sterile gloves. Changing of cages is accomplished by transferring animals to autoclaved cages supplied with autoclaved bedding, food, and water. After the filter on each cage is replaced, the inner surfaces of the transfer hood are disinfected before the next cage is serviced (Kraft, 1958; Kraft et al., 1964).

Kraft (1958) originally introduced the filter cage system for the control of mouse rotavirus and mouse hepatitis virus infections. Subsequently, this methodology has been tested extensively and found to be effective in preventing transmission of mouse diarrheal diseases (Jennings and Rumpf, 1965; Schneider and Collins, 1966), pinworm infection (Wescott et al., 1976), normal intestinal bacterial flora (Sedlacek and Mason, 1977; Sedlacek et al., 1981), and various pathogens (Simmons et al., 1967). In addition to being highly effective, filter cage systems are relatively inexpensive, simple to use, and readily adapted to a wide range of research needs and objectives. As with other barrier systems, written standard operating procedures for their use should be prepared and followed.

# 4

# Health Surveillance Programs

Health surveillance (or health monitoring) is the term usually applied to the testing of laboratory animals to determine their pathogen status and general state of health. Health surveillance programs are systematic laboratory investigations that employ batteries of tests for the purpose of defining the pathogen and health status of an animal population. Health surveillance programs are crucially important in rodent disease prevention—they provide data, the only reliable basis for rodent pathogen status or health quality assurance.

Although the need for health surveillance programs is generally accepted, there is a great diversity of opinion about the design of individual programs (Hsu et al., 1980; Iwai et al., 1980; Thigpen and Tortorich, 1980; Jacoby and Barthold, 1981; Hamm, 1983; Loew and Fox, 1983; Small, 1984). No two programs are identical. Some are limited in scope, while others are very comprehensive. Numerous factors should be considered in designing individual programs, with special emphasis placed on objectivity in testing rather than merely the adoption of customary practices. Some of those factors are listed in the following sections.

### Scientific Objectives

Health surveillance efforts should, to the fullest extent possible, be matched qualitatively and quantitatively with the requirements to meet the specific scientific objectives of individual research programs. Clearly, the requirements for a study of transmissible leukemia will differ from those of a study of chemical carcinogenesis of the respiratory tract in mice. Similarly, an elaborate program may be required to ensure the validity of research results from a project comparing the immune responses of immunodeficient mouse strains to challenge with an infectious agent, whereas a modest program might suffice for a study concerned with inheritance of a coat color gene in mice. Just as research objectives can differ greatly, health surveillance requirements also may vary over a wide range.

### Agent Detection Objectives

Indigenous infections of laboratory rodents include strong pathogens, weak pathogens, opportunists, and commensals. Therefore, in designing health surveillance programs, decisions must be made as to which agents are to be covered in the test battery. For practical reasons, it is impossible to test for all known infectious agents of rodents, or even all infectious agents that theoretically could interfere with a particular study. Therefore, testing is, of necessity, always selective. Specific justification based on pathogen significance and likelihood of interference with research is needed to include an agent in the test battery. Such information is given in Part II of this volume.

### Test Procedures

The procedures used in health surveillance generally include serologic tests, bacterial cultures, parasitologic examinations, and histopathology. Each of these may include very few or many procedures to detect different infectious agents or disease processes. Some health surveillance programs are limited to only one of these types of procedures, e.g., serologic testing.

Serologic tests are the main procedures used for detecting virus infections in rodents, but they also have been found useful for some bacterial and protozoan infections (Table 7). In recent years the enzyme-linked immunosorbent assay (ELISA) and the indirect immunofluorescent antibody (IFA) test have largely replaced the complement fixation (CF) test, and the hemagglutination inhibition (HAI) test. The ELISA and IFA tests have much greater sensitivity than the CF and HAI tests, and they give much fewer false positives than the HAI test (Smith, 1986b). False positive HAI tests have been particularly troublesome in the diagnosis of reovirus-3 and Theiler's virus infections (Kraft and Meyer, 1986; Van Der Logt, 1986). Serologic tests have the advantages of being relatively inexpensive and quickly performed in comparison to virus isolation (Balk, 1983; Smith, 1986b).

TABLE 7 Serologic Tests for Detection of Infectious Agents in Mice and Rats[a]

| Agent | Recommended Rests[b] | Tests Not Recom-mended | Species[c] | Comments |
|---|---|---|---|---|
| A. Viruses[d] | | | | |
| Adenoviruses | ELISA, CF | | M, R | Test should include both FL and K87 antigens. |
| Cytomegalovirus | ELISA | | M, R | |
| Hantaviruses | IFA, NT, HAI | | R | |
| Kilham rat virus | ELISA, HAI | | R | |
| K virus | HAI | | M | Value of test for rats is uncertain. |
| Lactic dehydrogenase virus | Lactic dehydrogenase assay | | M | Serum must be kept frozen to preserve enzyme activity. |
| LCMV | IFA, ELISA | CF | M, R | |
| Mousepox virus | ELISA, IFA | CF, HAI | M | |
| Minute virus of mice | ELISA, IFA | | M | |
| Mouse hepatitis virus | ELISA, IFA | CF | M | Tests have only coronavirus specificity. |
| Mouse rotavirus | ELISA | | M | |
| Mouse thymic virus | IFA | | M | Test not available commercially. |
| Pneumonia virus of mice | ELISA, HAI, IFA | | M, R | |
| Polyomavirus | ELISA, HAI | | M | |
| Reovirus-3 | ELISA, IFA | | M | |
| Sendai virus | ELISA, HAI, CF, IFA | | M, R | |
| SDA/RCV | ELISA, IFA | CF | R | Tests have only coronavirus specificity. |
| Theiler's virus | ELISA, NT | HAI | M | Value of tests for rats is uncertain. |
| Toolan H-1 virus | ELISA, HAI | | R | |
| B. Bacteria | | | | |
| CAR Bacillus | ELISA | | R | |
| *Corynebacterium kutscheri* | ELISA | | M, R | |
| *Bacillus piliformis* | CF, IFA | | M, R | Tests not available commercially. |
| *Leptospira interrogans* | IFA | | M, R | Test available through state animal diagnostic laboratories. |
| *Mycoplasma arthritidis* | ELISA | CF | M, R | Test has only *Mycoplasma* genus specificity. |
| *Mycoplasma pulmonis* | ELISA | CF | M, R | Test has only *Mycoplasma* genus specificity. |
| C. Protozoa | | | | |
| *Encephalitozoon cuniculi* | IFA and others | | M, R | |

[a]For further information and references, refer to summaries of individual agents in Part II of this volume.
[b]Abbreviations used for tests: ELISA = enzyme-linked immunosorbent assay, CF = complement fixation, IFA = indirect immunofluorescence, NT = neutralization test, HAI = hemagglutination inhibition.
[c]M = mouse; R = rat.
[d]Modified from information originally compiled by P.N. Bhatt (Section of Comparative Medicine, Yale University, New Haven, Conn.).

Serologic tests also have certain disadvantages. They require special technical competence to assure rigorous standardization of reagents, the inclusion of appropriate controls in each test run and accurate interpretation of results (Smith, 1986b). They are indirect tests that rely on humoral antibody responses, and they vary in specificity and sensitivity, depending on the test and the agent. Therefore, positive results based on a single serologic procedure are far less definitive in diagnostic value than positive results of a direct test such as isolation and identification of an agent. For this reason, serologic testing should rely on a primary test for each agent and one or more tests to confirm the positive results of any primary test (Smith, 1986b). False-positive test results can occur on serum from young animals due to passively acquired antibody. False-negative results may be obtained on serum from young animals infected prior to the age of immunocompetence or on serum from animals infected for too brief a time for an antibody response to be mounted (Jacoby and Barthold, 1981).

One of the most useful applications of serologic testing in rodent health surveillance is the mouse antibody production (MAP) test. Although originally developed as a method for broadly screening mouse tissues for viruses (Rowe et al., 1959a, 1962), it can be used to test transplantable tumors, hybridomas, cell lines, and other biologic materials for contaminating infectious agents of different types. As originally performed by Rowe et al. (1959a, 1962), test material is injected intraperitoneally into a group of five pathogen-free mice; they are maintained in a caging system that excludes pathogen contamination for five weeks, then killed and individually tested serologically for a range of agents. Uninoculated, separately housed control mice must be used (Rowe et al., 1959a, 1962). An equivalent test procedure, the rat antibody production (RAP) test, can be done using rats (Johnson, 1988). In general the MAP or RAP test is considered more sensitive than virus isolation (de Souza and Smith, 1989).

The isolation of bacteria by cultural methods and the demonstration and identification of parasites are the standard procedures for the detection of these agents. However, these methods also have limitations that depend on the agent. In general, causative agents are more difficult to isolate or demonstrate in subclinical infections than in clinically apparent infections. Some bacterial infections of mice and rats, e.g., *Corynebacterium kutscheri* or *Mycoplasma arthritidis*, commonly occur as subclinical infections in which cultural isolation is extremely difficult. With each of the bacteria and parasites it is imperative that specimens be collected from the most appropriate site(s) and processed expeditiously by methods known to maximize the chances of successful recovery or demonstration of the agent.

Gross and microscopic evaluations of tissues for lesions are also invaluable in health surveillance. In the more comprehensive health surveillance programs, histopathologic examination of all major organs by a qualified pathologist is standard practice. Lesions due to pathogen infections can occur before seroconversion in viral infections. Some histopathologic changes are diagnostic, and others provide clues of disease processes for further investigations (Jacoby and Barthold, 1981).

The foregoing discussion has presented the major methodological approaches presently in use in rodent diagnostic laboratories. It must be recognized, however, that diagnostic methodology currently is in transition. Refinements continue to be made in existing methods and newer methods employing molecular biology, e.g., nucleic acid hybridization and specific gene product detection, are being developed at a rapid pace (Sklar, 1985; Edberg, 1986; Smith, 1986a,c; DeLellis and Wolfe, 1987; Grody et al., 1987; Howanitz, 1988).

## Sampling Strategies

The purpose of health surveillance is to detect at least one animal with each of the infections or diseases present in the population. The purpose is not to determine prevalence of infection or disease.

The number of animals (sample size) to be tested is of critical importance and can be determined mathematically with two important assumptions: rates of infection and randomness in sampling (ILAR, 1976a; Hsu et al., 1980; Small, 1984; DiGiacomo and Koepsell, 1986). As shown in Table 8, if one assumes that 40% of the animals in a population are infected with an agent, there is a 99% probability that one infected animal will be detected in a randomly selected sample of 10 animals. At a 50% infection rate, a sample size of only five is required for a 97% probability of detecting infection in at least one animal.

It should be recognized that although the sample size required to detect a single agent can be determined with reasonable precision (Table 8), it is virtually impossible to maintain the same degree of precision for all agents to be included in a large test battery. Different agents typically have very different infection rates within rodent colonies. For example, typical rates for established infections in mouse colonies are greater than 90% for Sendai virus, approximately 25% for pneumonia virus of mice, and less than 5% for *Salmonella enteritidis*. A health surveillance test battery for these three agents, then, would be required to use the lower assumed infection rate (i.e., 5%); a 95% confidence limit would require a sample size of at least 60 animals. This is entirely appropriate in instances where subclinical *S. enteritidis* infection is suspected. However, for routine health surveillance sample sizes are usually based on assumed infection rates of 40-50% in order to keep sample sizes reasonable.

Proper sampling also requires random sampling of the entire population. This means taking animals from different cages, shelves, and racks. Attention

TABLE 8 Confidence Limits for Detecting Infection Using Different Sample Sizes and Assumed Rates of Infection[a]

| Sample Size (N)[b] | Assumed Infection Rate (%) 1 | 2 | 3 | 4 | 5 | 10 | 15 | 20 | 25 | 30 | 40 | 50 |
|---|---|---|---|---|---|---|---|---|---|---|---|---|
| 5 | 0.05 | 0.10 | 0.14 | 0.18 | 0.23 | 0.41 | 0.56 | 0.67 | 0.76 | 0.83 | 0.92 | 0.97 |
| 10 | 0.10 | 0.18 | 0.26 | 0.34 | 0.40 | 0.65 | 0.80 | 0.89 | 0.94 | 0.97 | 0.99 | |
| 15 | 0.14 | 0.26 | 0.37 | 0.46 | 0.54 | 0.79 | 0.91 | 0.95 | 0.99 | | | |
| 20 | 0.18 | 0.33 | 0.46 | 0.56 | 0.64 | 0.88 | 0.95 | 0.99 | | | | |
| 25 | 0.22 | 0.40 | 0.53 | 0.64 | 0.72 | 0.93 | 0.98 | | | | | |
| 30 | 0.25 | 0.45 | 0.60 | 0.71 | 0.79 | 0.96 | 0.99 | | | | | |
| 35 | 0.30 | 0.51 | 0.66 | 0.76 | 0.83 | 0.97 | | | | | | |
| 40 | 0.33 | 0.55 | 0.70 | 0.80 | 0.87 | 0.99 | | | | | | |
| 45 | 0.36 | 0.69 | 0.75 | 0.84 | 0.90 | 0.99 | | | | | | |
| 50 | 0.39 | 0.64 | 0.78 | 0.87 | 0.92 | 0.99 | | | | | | |
| 60 | 0.45 | 0.70 | 0.84 | 0.91 | 0.95 | | | | | | | |
| 70 | 0.51 | 0.76 | 0.88 | 0.94 | 0.97 | | | | | | | |
| 80 | 0.55 | 0.80 | 0.91 | 0.96 | 0.98 | | | | | | | |
| 90 | 0.60 | 0.84 | 0.94 | 0.97 | 0.99 | | | | | | | |
| 100 | 0.63 | 0.87 | 0.95 | 0.98 | 0.99 | | | | | | | |
| 120 | 0.70 | 0.91 | 0.97 | 0.99 | | | | | | | | |
| 140 | 0.76 | 0.94 | 0.99 | | | | | | | | | |
| 160 | 0.80 | 0.96 | 0.99 | | | | | | | | | |
| 180 | 0.84 | 0.97 | | | | | | | | | | |
| 200 | 0.87 | 0.98 | | | | | | | | | | |

[a]From ILAR (1976a), Hsu et al. (1980), and Small (1984).

[b]$N = \frac{\log(1 - \text{probability of detecting infection})}{\log(1 - \text{assumed infection rate})}$

also should be given to sampling animals of both sexes and of different ages. Sampling of two age groups is desirable. Young animals tend to have greater parasite burdens. For serologic testing, sampling of young adults (approximately 90 days old) and retired breeders is recommended. Young adults are best for detecting recent viral infections (without interference from passive antibody), and retired breeders give an indication of the infection history of the colony (Jacoby and Barthold, 1981).

### Test Frequency

One of the most difficult questions to be answered in designing health surveillance programs is how frequently should a given rodent population be tested? There are no established guidelines, but the problem seems to revolve around four central issues: the specific purpose of the population in question, the potential or real importance a pathogen or other contamination is to the use of the population, the level of risk of pathogen contamination from other nearby rodent populations, and economic considerations. After evaluating these basic questions, one should have a basis for deciding whether testing should be monthly, quarterly, biannually, or annually. However, the frequency of testing may be different for different agents. For example, if the greatest risks are deemed to be from mouse hepatitis virus and Sendai virus, tests for these agents could be performed monthly and the larger battery could be done biannually.

### Sentinel Animals

Rodents for health surveillance purposes are sometimes introduced into a rodent population, housed in open cages placed systematically throughout the colony, and designated as sentinels for use in periodic testing. Pathogen transmission from the principal population to the sentinels may be increased by transferring the sentinels into dirty cages from the principal population at each cage change. Sentinel animals preferably should be of the same stock as the principal population and should be subjected to any experimental treatments given the principal population. The introduction of a second stock as sentinels, although tested and found to be free of pathogens, may pose an unnecessary risk for contaminating the principal population.

### Rodent Diagnostic Laboratories

Rodent diagnostic laboratories are indispensable to the production and maintenance of mice and rats for high quality research. Such laboratories specialize in health-surveillance testing, investigations of clinical diseases, and other quality control methods specifically designed for laboratory rodents. Depending on the breadth of their activities, these laboratories most often include competence in serology, bacteriology, parasitology, and pathology. Virology and hematology expertise may also be required in some instances. Many of the larger research institutions have well-equipped and -staffed institutional diagnostic laboratories. Testing services also can be obtained through commercial laboratories.

Traditionally, rodent diagnostic laboratories have tended to give highest priority to the investigation of clinical illnesses and necropsy evaluations of dead animals. That approach is no longer acceptable. While those services are certainly necessary, the needs of modern research and the principles of the scientific method demand that diagnostic laboratories give greater priority to rodent disease prevention. Most of the pathogen infections and pathogen-induced diseases of laboratory rodents are preventable.

# Part II
# Individual Disease Agents and Their Effects on Research

# 5

# Introduction

In Part II information on the infectious agents of mice and rats is presented by using an organ system approach. This approach was chosen for pragmatic reasons. For most individuals (although not for erudite specialists) concerned with the whole animal, it is easier to organize thoughts around organ system presentations of clinical, pathological, etiological, and other data sets than approaches such as taxonomic groupings of agents. We hasten to add, however, that the organ system approach also has its disadvantages. Many agents do not affect a single organ system by infection or disease expression. Thus, final decisions in deciding groupings sometimes became very arbitrary.

Within the organ system groupings, information on each agent is presented, as much as is feasible, in a standard outline format. The intent has been to provide objective, reliable data applicable to contemporary rodent populations. Data collected 20 or more years ago often are out of date and misleading (except possibly for those few stocks that have never been rederived by cesarean section).

The standard outlines for information on each agent include subheadings with the following definitions and contents:

*Significance.* An overall appraisal of the real or potential importance of each agent as a research complication for the general biomedical community that uses the host species (mouse or rat). In instances where an agent poses risks unique to research results in one or more specialized disciplines, this is emphasized.

*Perspective.* Key developments in evolution of knowledge concerning infection with each agent including its natural history, host effects, diagnosis, control, and significance.

*Agent.* A listing of those characteristics important to recognition, laboratory manipulation, and control of each agent. Includes taxonomy, strains, morphology, cultural requirements, biochemical reactions (bacteria), stability (viruses), and inactivation (viruses).

*Hosts.* Does the infection occur in mice, rats, or both? Are they the natural, reservoir, or incidental hosts? What other laboratory animals can serve as hosts? Are there reservoir hosts for mice and rats?

*Epizootiology.* Epizootiology of the infection plus consideration of specific ecological niches inhabited by the agent inside and outside of the host(s).

*Clinical.* Clinical signs of infection, if any. The majority of natural infections in mice and rats are subclinical or have only transient clinical signs.

*Pathology.* Strain differences in susceptibility (if known), pathogenesis, gross pathology, histopathology, pathology of infection in immunodeficient or immunosuppressed hosts (if different from that in immunocompetent hosts), and immune response(s).

*Diagnosis.* Direct and indirect methods for agent detection, including serology, culture, and immunofluorescence, with comments on sampling and interpretation of results, as appropriate. Guidelines are given for pathologic workups on diseased animals.

*Control.* Methods most likely to succeed in prevention of infection are emphasized. Approaches to eradicating or limiting spread of established existing infections are also presented. Medications usually are not given as their use may impose additional variables on experiments.

*Interference with research.* A compilation from the literature of specific examples in which the agent was found to complicate research results or alter host responses.

# 6

# Respiratory System

## Overview

Diseases of the respiratory tract are among the most common health problems encountered in mice and rats. Numerous reports have dealt with inapparent respiratory infections as well as the respiratory diseases due to infectious agents in these animals. Nevertheless, the subject is large and tends to be confusing to persons not intimately involved in the study of these infections.

At present there are 14 specific agents that have been recognized as respiratory pathogens in laboratory mice and rats (at some point in history and under some set of circumstances). They are extremely varied in pathogenicity and importance as research complications (which are not always directly related). Subclinical infection is far more common than overt disease for all of the agents. Synergistic interactions in which combined infections have more than an additive effect in producing disease are common (probably far more common than currently recognized). Dual or multiple infections usually are responsible when severe respiratory disease occurs (thus, diagnostic efforts must test for multiple agents and must obtain positive evidence for incriminating some and negative evidence for excluding others).

Table 9 gives a perspective to the relative importance of respiratory infections as causes of clinical and morphologic disease. Agents are listed in order of descending importance (this is a rough approximation) for mice and rats. Those agents listed in group I are by far the major causes of overt respiratory disease in the species indicated. *Mycoplasma pulmonis* is deemed

TABLE 9 Agents Grouped According to Importance as Causes of Natural Respiratory Disease

| Group[a] | Mouse[b] | Rat[b] |
|---|---|---|
| I | Sendai virus<br>*Mycoplasma pulmonis* | *Mycoplasma pulmonis*<br>Sendai virus<br>CAR bacillus<br>*Streptococcus pneumoniae*<br>*Corynebacterium kutscheri* |
| II | Pneumonia virus of mice<br>*Pneumocystis carinii*<br>*Mycobaterium avium-intracellulare*<br>*Chlamydia trachomatis*<br>*Klebsiella pneumoniae*<br>*Streptococcus pyogenes*<br>*Mycoplasma neurolyticum*<br>*Mycoplasma collis*<br>K virus | Rat coronavirus<br>Sialodacryoadenitis virus<br>Pneumonia virus of mice<br>*Pneumocystis carinii*<br>*Klebsiella pneumoniae*<br>*Mycoplasma collis* |
| III | *Corynebacterium kutscheri*<br>*Chlamydia psittaci*<br>*Pasteurella pneumotropica*<br>*Bordetella bronchiseptica*<br>Adenovirus | *Pasteurella pneumotropica*<br>*Bordetella bronchiseptica*<br>Adenovirus |

[a]Group Key:
I = Agents that are unquestionably important respiratory tract pathogens.
II = Agents of questionable importance or pathogenicity as respiratory tract pathogens, except in special circumstances.
III = Agents that are not primary respiratory tract pathogens in the species indicated.
[b]Reading down each list of agents for the mouse or rat, agents are listed apprroximately in descending order of importance as respiratory pathogens for that rodent species.

the most important in the rat and Sendai virus the most important in the mouse. In actual practice, however, severe natural respiratory disease in the rat usually is due to *M. pulmonis* in combination with Sendai virus and/or the cilia-associated respiratory (CAR) bacillus. In the mouse, combined infections of Sendai virus and *M. pulmonis* are responsible for the most severe outbreaks of natural respiratory disease, although Sendai virus infection alone also can cause severe disease when first introduced into a naive population of genetically susceptible mice. *Streptococcus pneumoniae* and *Corynebacterium kutscheri* are potent respiratory pathogens in the rat but seldom in the absence of some combination involving *M. pulmonis,* Sendai virus, and/or CAR bacillus.

The agents listed in group II of Table 9 are relatively unimportant as natural respiratory pathogens in comparison to those of group I. Some of them (*Mycobacterium avium-intracellulare*, *Chlamydia trachomatis*, *Klebsiella pneumoniae ozaenae*, and *Streptococcus pyogenes*) have been reported to cause natural disease in only a few instances. Under natural conditions current evidence indicates that pneumonia virus of mice causes minimal upper respiratory tract disease and very mild transient lung disease (the rodent equivalent of man's common cold?). Sialodacryoadenitis virus (see "Digestive System" later in this volume) is listed here as some strains are also mild respiratory pathogens.

Disease expression due to *Pneumocystis carinii* requires immunodeficiency or immunosuppression. Active disease due to *Chlamydia psittaci* and K virus are laboratory-induced occurrences. *Mycoplasma neurolyticum* and *Mycoplasma collis* are probably commensals.

The agents included in group III of Table 9 are not primarily respiratory tract pathogens in the species indicated (*Corynebacterium kutscheri* in the mouse, *Pasteurella pneumotropica*, and adenovirus) or are not conclusively demonstrated to be natural pathogens of mice or rats (*Bordetella bronchiseptica*).

## Sendai Virus

### *Significance*

Very high.

### *Perspective*

*1950s*: The early history of Sendai virus (SV) is confusing. The original isolations of the virus were made in the 1950s from mice that had been inoculated for diagnostic purposes using specimens from: (a) human infants with "newborn pneumonitis" in Japan, (b) swine with an influenza-like disease in Japan, or (c) humans with influenza in Russia. In subsequent years, evidence accumulated to show that an indigenous virus of the mice had been isolated (rodents are the exclusive natural hosts of SV). The seropositives among the human patients probably were due to a closely related, serologically cross reactive virus, parainfluenza 1, hemadsorption type 2, for which man is the natural host (Parker and Richter, 1982).

*1968:* Degre and Glasgow (1968) published the first in a series (Degre and Solberg, 1971) of papers from their laboratory demonstrating that SV infection increases susceptibility of mice to bacterial infection of the respiratory tract. Subsequently, major contributions in that area were made by Jakab and his colleagues (Jakab, 1981).

*1975*: Fukumi and Takeuchi (1975) reported development of a formalin killed SV vaccine.

*1976*: Ward et al. (1976) reported that athymic (*nu/nu*) mice had increased susceptibility to the virus, resulting in chronic infection with progressive emaciation. Increased susceptibility to SV infection was later reported to occur in athymic (*rnu/rnu*) rats (Carthew and Sparrow, 1980c).

*1978*: Parker et al. (1978) demonstrated an extremely wide range of susceptibility to SV among 24 strains of mice, and also reported that two-thirds or more of the mouse, rat, and hamster colonies in the United States were infected. Their work attracted great interest in SV infection and probably helped to stimulate the flurry of papers since 1978 that have documented the great importance of this agent as a complication of research.

*1978*: Howard et al. (1978) presented evidence that SV infection exacerbates *Mycoplasma pulmonis* infection in mice. Their findings in mice were confirmed by Saito et al. (1981). Schoeb et al. (1985) reported similar findings for rats.

### *Agent*

An RNA virus, family Paramyxoviridae, genus *Paramyxovirus*, species *parainfluenza* 1 (Sendai). All known strains of SV are antigenically homologous. Some of the more common laboratory strains are: 52 (ATCC VR-105), Fushimi, Akitsugu, MN, and Z (Parker and Richter, 1982).

The virus particles are spherical, 150-250 nm in diameter, and have a helical nucleocapsid and a continuous single stranded RNA genome. The virus contains HN glycoprotein with hemagglutinating and neuraminidase activities that are responsible for adsorption to host cells, and F glycoprotein with cell fusion and hemolytic activities that mediate virus entry into host cells. Entry of wild type Sendai virus into host cells requires conversion of the F glycoprotein to the biologically active form by host proteases. The HN glycoprotein also has been shown to be an inducer of type I interferon. The HN and F glycoproteins also are T cell-dependent B cell mitogens. The virus agglutinates erythrocytes of many species (Parker and Richter, 1982; Ito and Hosaka, 1983; Kizaka et al., 1983; Tashiro and Homma, 1983, 1985; Brownstein, 1986).

SV is commonly grown in embryonated hen's eggs, and BHK-21 and primary monkey kidney cell cultures. It is inactivated by UV light, temperatures above 37°C, and lipid solvents (Parker and Richter, 1982).

### *Hosts*

Laboratory mice, rats, and hamsters. Possibly, guinea pigs (based on serological evidence only, not confirmed by virus isolation).

*Epizootiology*

SV is EXTREMELY CONTAGIOUS, one of the most contagious infections of laboratory rodents. First time infections usually are epizootic within rooms, but can become epizootic throughout entire facilities or institutions (Zurcher et al., 1977)! The virus is highly prevalent (≈70% of colonies) in laboratory mice and rats worldwide (Parker and Richter, 1982).

Natural infection occurs via the respiratory tract. Contact and airborne transmission are born highly efficient (Parker and Reynolds 1968; van der Veen et al., 1970, 1972; Iida, 1972). Airborne transmission can occur over a distance of 5-6 feet (van der Veen et al., 1970, 1972). Viral replication is thought to be limited to the respiratory tract and occurs for only about 1 week post infection under usual circumstances. Viremia probably is a seldom occurrence. Transfer of embryos from infected mice to noninfected recipient mothers has been used successfully in eliminating the virus (Carthew et al., 1983; Parker and Richter, 1982).

*Clinical*

Natural infections of SV alone (i.e., not complicated by other agents) in rats are usually inapparent or cause only small reductions in litter size and growth rate of pups (Makino et al., 1972). Experimental infections of pregnant females have been reported to cause prolonged gestation, fetal resorptions, retarded embryonic development, and mortality of neonates (Coid and Wardman, 1971, 1972).

Natural SV infections alone in mice usually follow one of two clinical patterns:

a. *Enzootic (subclinical) infection.* This is the common pattern occurring in breeding populations. Adults have active immunity due to prior infection, and do not carry the virus. Newborn mice are passively protected by maternal antibody until around 4 to 8 weeks of age when they become infected. Recovery is prompt without morbidity or mortality. Infection is maintained by continuous supply of young susceptible mice (Iida et al., 1973; Fujiwara et al., 1976; Goto and Shimizu, 1978; Parker and Richter, 1982).

b. *Epizootic (clinically apparent) infection.* This is the pattern that occurs when a population is first infected by the virus. Infection spreads through the entire population within a short time. Signs are variable but may include chattering, mild respiratory distress, and prolonged gestation in adults, deaths (even whole litters) in neonates and sucklings, and poor growth in weanling and young adult mice. Breeding colonies return to normal productivity in 2 months, and thereafter maintain the enzootic pattern of infection (Fukumi et al., 1962; Parker and Reynolds, 1968; Bhatt and Jonas,

1974; Fujiwara et al., 1976; Zurcher et al., 1977; Itoh et al., 1978; Parker and Richter, 1982).

Epizootics of disease involving SV virus infection in mice and rats which exceed the above general patterns in clinical severity should arouse suspicion of complication by other agent(s), particularly concurrent *M. pulmonis* and/or CAR bacillus infection (Lindsey et al., 1985a; Schoeb et al., 1985).

*Pathology*

Strains of mice vary markedly in susceptibility to SV. The more susceptible stocks include 129/ReJ, 129/J, S-*nu/nu* (Swiss nude), DBA/1J, and DBA/2J. Stocks of intermediate susceptibility are A/HeJ, A/J, SWR/J, C57BL/10Sn and BALB/c. The most resistant stocks include SJL/J, RF/J, C57BL/6J and S. Strain 129/J is 25,000 times as susceptible to lethal infection as SJL/J (Parker et al., 1978). The mode of inheritance and mechanisms of host resistance are poorly understood (Brownstein, 1983, 1986, 1987a,b; Brownstein and Winkler, 1986, 1987).

SV infections have been studied most in mice of the resistant stocks. In resistant stocks of mice and in rats, pathogenesis is approximately as follows. After intranasal infection, descending infection follows with virus replication occurring in respiratory epithelium of the nasal passages, trachea, bronchi, bronchioles, and in type I and II pneumocytes and macrophages of the alveoli. Virus titer peaks in tracheobronchial epithelium at 5 to 6 days, then decreases to undetectable levels throughout the respiratory tract around day 14 post infection. Serum antibody appears at 6 to 8 days and remains detectable for approximately 1 year depending on sensitivity of the test used. Secretory antibody may appear as early as day 3, but is usually difficult to demonstrate before days 6 to 10 post infection (Sawicki, 1962; Parker and Reynolds, 1968; Robinson et al., 1968; van der Veen et al., 1970; Appell et al., 1971; Blandford and Heath, 1972; Charlton and Blandford, 1977; Parker et al., 1978; Brownstein et al., 1981; Castleman, 1983, 1984; Castleman et al., 1987; Garlinghouse et al., 1987 ).

Morphogenesis of lesions in SV infection of mice and rats proceeds by the following general pattern. Following intranasal infection, there is descending infection with transient hypertrophy, necrosis, and repair of airway epithelium occurring in rapid succession. Necrosis of respiratory epithelium is mild and focal in nasal passages beginning at 2-3 days, becomes progressively more severe distally with peak severity in the distal trachea and major bronchi around day 5. Regeneration of airway epithelium becomes evident by day 9, with epithelial hyperplasia, squamous metaplasia, and occasional syncytial giant cell formation. Focal interstitial pneumonia occurs with alveolar septal thickening by edema, mononuclear cell infiltration, alveolar epithelial hypertrophy and hyperplasia, and atelectasis. Resolution is in progress well before 21 days, although residual inflammatory lesions may persist up to 1 year or longer. These most often consist of lymphocytes around airways and vessels, always in loose concentration rather than dense cuffs. Some reports mention vasculitis. Despite these impressive histologic changes, few gross lesions are seen in uncomplicated SV infections. The lungs may appear focally reddened or atelectatic and serous fluid may be visible in the pleural and pericardial cavities (Sawicki, 1961, 1962; Fukumi et al., 1962; Robinson et al., 1968; Appell et al., 1971; Degre and Midtvedt, 1971; Blandford and Heath, 1972; Richter, 1973; Ward, 1974; Brownstein et al., 1981; Parker and Richter, 1982; Castleman, 1983, 1984; Hall et al., 1985; Schoeb et al., 1985; Castleman et al., 1987; Giddens et al., 1987).

The most severe lesions due to SV are seen in fully susceptible mice infected while very young (as sucklings or weanlings) and in mice of the more susceptible stocks (such as DBA/2J and 129/ReJ). The terminal bronchioles are particularly susceptible to severe injury. During the period of severe necrotizing bronchitis and bronchiolitis, there may be intense inflammatory injury to terminal bronchioles. This may result in scarring with severe distortion of the smaller airways and formation of polypoid outgrowths into the bronchiole lumens. Also, there may be pronounced hyperplasia of airway epithelium resulting in peribronchiolar "adenomatous hyperplasia" (also called "adenomatoid change" and "alveolar bronchiolization") that may persist throughout life of the animal. In aged mice the air spaces in these lesions may be filled with mucus, large macrophages, and cellular debris. There may be large eosinophilic crystals in the air spaces, and in the cytoplasm of the macrophages and cells forming the "adenomatoid" structures (Yang and Campbell, 1964; Richter, 1970, 1973; Parker and Richter, 1982; Zurcher et al., 1977). The terminal bronchioles of rats also may be scarred and distorted but do not show the hyperplastic peribronchiolar changes seen in mice (Castleman, 1983, 1984).

Athymic (*nu*/*nu*) mice have increased susceptibility to SV. They develop chronic pneumonia similar to that in immunocompetent mice but have abundant intranuclear and intracytoplasmic inclusions in laryngeal, tracheal, bronchial, and bronchiolar epithelium, as well as in type I and II pneumocytes and alveolar macrophages. The virus persists for 10 weeks or longer (Ward et al., 1976; Ueda et al., 1977b; Iwasaki, 1978; Iwai et al., 1979). Nude (*rnu*/*rnu*) rats also have increased susceptibility to SV and develop a similar chronic lung disease (Carthew and Sparrow, 1980c).

The immune responses to SV that confer protection have not been completely defined. However, it appears that both T and B cells have important roles (Kizaka et al., 1983; Ertl and Finberg, 1984a,b). Passive immunization of mice using monoclonal antibodies against specific subgroup antigens of the viral F and HN glycoproteins has given protection against experimental SV challenge (Orvell and Grandien, 1982; Mazanec et al., 1987). In mice, L3T4$^+$ (and Lyt-1$^+$) and Lyt-2$^+$ subsets of T cells may be important in clearing the virus from infected lungs (Iwai et al., 1988).

Some reports of SV infection in the literature include lesions that are not attributable to SV alone (Burek et al., 1977). Lesions such as suppurative bronchitis, pulmonary abscesses, and dense peribronchial and perivascular lymphoid cuffs are suggestive of *M. pulmonis* infection, possibly superimposed on SV infection. SV is a strong promoter of murine respiratory mycoplasmosis due to *M. pulmonis* in mice (Howard et al., 1978; Saito et al., 1981) and rats (Schoeb et al., 1985).

### *Diagnosis*

The enzyme-linked immunosorbent assay (ELISA) is the test of choice for routine serologic monitoring. It is 100 times more sensitive than the complement fixation (CF) test and 300 times more sensitive than the hemagglutination inhibition (HI) test. Because of the high contagiousness of the virus, typically about 90% of animals in infected populations will be positive by the ELISA (Parker et al., 1978, 1979; Ertl et al., 1979; Parker, 1980). The ELISA successfully detects anti-SV antibody in infected athymic (*nu/nu*) mice (Iwai et al., 1984), compared to the CF test that is sometimes positive at low titer (Ward et al., 1976; Iwai et al., 1977), and the HI and neutralization tests that usually do not detect antibody to SV in infected nude mice (Iwai et al., 1977). A quantitative immunofluorescence test for detection of serum antibody to SV has been reported (Lucas et al., 1987).

In instances where natural SV infection is associated with clinical disease or gross lung lesions, other intercurrent infection(s), e.g., *M. pulmonis*, often have a contributory role. Definitive diagnosis of such disease states requires detection of each of the agents involved, demonstration of the characteristic lesions due to each agent, and exclusion of other agents and disease processes. An avidin-biotin-peroxidase complex method has been used successfully for demonstrating SV antigen in histologic sections (Hall and Ward, 1984).

Isolation of SV may be achieved using BHK-21 or primary monkey kidney cell cultures, or 8 to 10 day embryonated hen's eggs inoculated into the amniotic or allantoic sac (Parker and Richter, 1982). The mouse antibody production (MAP) test may be used in testing transplantable tumors and other biologic materials for contamination by SV (Rowe et al., 1962).

### *Control*

Exclusion of SV is EXTREMELY DIFFICULT in most institutions that receive rodents from outside sources. Ordinarily, exclusion requires very strict adherence to systematic measures for preventing entrance of the infection into an entire facility or institution. SV free subpopulations of rodents must be identified by regular health surveillance of a supplier, transported to the user facility in containers which prevent contamination en route, quarantined by barrier system at the receiving institution until tested and shown to be free of infection, and subsequently maintained by strict barrier protocol. In addition, all biological materials such as transplantable tumors coming into the institution must be pre-tested and shown to be free of the virus before experimental use (Collins and Parker, 1972; Parker and Richter, 1982).

Once infection has been diagnosed in a facility, prompt elimination of infected subpopulation(s) is essential to prevent spread of the infection to other rodents on the premises. A less effective alternative is to place the infected animals under strict quarantine, remove all young and pregnant females, suspend all breeding, and prevent addition of other susceptible animals for a period of 6-8 weeks until the infection has run its course and the virus has been eliminated naturally. Because of this alternative, cesarean derivation of infected stocks usually is not justified.

Vaccination may prove useful in some situations (Parker, 1980; Eaton et al., 1982). A number of killed vaccines (Fukumi and Takeuchi, 1975; Nedrud et al., 1987; Tsukui et al., 1982), a temperature sensitive mutant strain vaccine (Kimura et al., 1979), and a trypsin-resistant mutant strain vaccine (Tashiro and Homma, 1985; Tashiro et al., 1988) have been tested experimentally. A formalin-killed SV vaccine is available commercially in the United States (Microbiological Associates, Bethesda, Md.).

### *Interference with Research*

Experimental infection of mice with SV decreases pulmonary bacterial clearance (Degre and Glasgow, 1968; Degre and Solberg, 1971), probably through a variety of mechanisms including altered phagocytic function. Altered functions in pulmonary macrophages that have been identified include: decreased Fc receptor and non-Fc receptor mediated attachment, decreased Fc receptor and non-Fc receptor mediated ingestion, inhibited phagosome-lysosome fusion, decreased intracellular killing, decreased degradation of ingested bacteria, and decreased lysosomal enzyme content (Jakab, 1981; Jakab and Warr, 1981).

Concurrent SV and *M. pulmonis* infections are synergistic in mice (Howard et al., 1978; Saito et al., 1981) and rats (Schoeb et al., 1985), causing disease of far greater severity than either alone.

SV infected mice have been reported to have deficiencies in T and B cell function that persist throughout life (Kay, 1978, 1979; Kay et al., 1979). (Unfortunately, these results have not been confirmed by other investigators).

SV infection transiently increased splenic IgM and IgG plaque forming cell responses to sheep red blood cells in mice (Brownstein and Weir, 1987).

SV infection inhibited in vitro mitogenesis of lymphocytes (Wainberg and Israel, 1980; Roberts, 1982).

In rats, infection altered the mitogenic responses of T cells, reduced severity of adjuvant arthritis, and decreased antibody response to sheep erythrocytes (Garlinghouse and Van Hoosier, 1978).

Mice naturally infected with SV have been found to have increased natural killer cell mediated cytotoxicity (Clark et al., 1979), and increased cytotoxic lymphocyte responses after stimulation with SV-coated syngeneic cells (Finberg et al., 1980).

SV infection altered isograft rejection in mice (Streilein, et al., 1981).

SV infection altered host responses to transplantable tumors (Wheelock, 1966, 1967; Collins and Parker, 1972; Matsuya et al., 1978; Takeyama et al., 1979).

Previous or concurrent infection in mice may increase or decrease neoplastic response to respiratory carcinogens (Nettesheim et al., 1974, 1981; Parker, 1980; Peck et al., 1983; Hall et al., 1985).

SV infection delayed wound healing in mice (Kenyon, 1983).

Athymic (*nu*/*nu*) mice (Ueda et al., 1977b; Iwasaki, 1978; Iwai et al., 1979) and nude (*rnu*/*rnu*) rats (Carthew and Sparrow, 1980c) had increased susceptibility and developed chronic lung disease when infected with SV.

Cyclophosphamide increased clinical and pathological severity of SV infection in mice (Robinson et al., 1969; Blandford, 1975; Anderson et al., 1980).

SV infection can cause deaths and retarded growth of young mice (Parker and Reynolds, 1968; Bhatt and Jonas, 1974) and rats (Makino et al., 1972).

### *Mycoplasma pulmonis*

#### *Significance*

Very high, particularly in long term studies.

#### *Perspective*

*1937*: Nelson (1937a,b,c) described the proximal airway disease called "infectious catarrh" in mice and attributed it to "coccobacilliform bodies" (later identified as *M. pulmonis*).

*1937*: Klieneberger and Steabben (1937) described pulmonary "bronchiectasis" in rats, and subsequently (Klieneberger and Steabben, 1940) recognized the association of their "L3" organism (later identified as *M. pulmonis*) with this lesion.

*1957*: Nelson (1957) advanced the term "chronic respiratory disease" and proposed that it was due to two agents: *M. pulmonis* which caused "infectious catarrh" (proximal airway disease), and "enzootic bronchiectasis virus" alleged to cause the bronchopulmonary (distal airway) disease. (This putative virus still has not been identified.)

*1966*: Lutsky and Organick (1966) fulfilled Koch's postulates (for both proximal and distal airway disease) by the inoculation of *M. pulmonis* into pathogen free mice; their work was confirmed by Lindsey and Cassell (1973).

*1969*: Kohn and Kirk (1969) fulfilled Koch's postulates (for proximal and distal airway disease) by inoculation of *M. pulmonis* into pathogen free rats. Their work was confirmed by Lindsey et al. (1971), Whittlestone et al. (1972), and Jersey et al. (1973).

*1976*: Broderson et al. (1976a) demonstrated that intracage ammonia promotes respiratory disease due to *M. pulmonis* in rats. The work was confirmed in rats by Schoeb et al. (1982), and in rats and mice by Saito et al. (1982).

*1978*: Howard et al. (1978) showed that Sendai virus infection promotes respiratory disease due to *M. pulmonis* in mice; this was confirmed in mice by Saito et al. (1981) and in rats by Schoeb et al. (1985).

*1978*: Horowitz and Cassell (1978) developed an enzyme-linked immunosorbent assay (ELISA) for detection of rodent mycoplasma infections. The test was extensively field tested by Cassell et al. (1981, 1983b).

*1984*: Minion et al. (1984) introduced the immunoblot method for discriminating between infections due to *M. pulmonis* and *Mycoplasma arthritidis* using mycoplasma ELISA positive sera.

*1987*: Schoeb and Lindsey (1987) demonstrated that sialodacryoadenitis virus infection exacerbates respiratory disease due to *M. pulmonis* in rats.

### *Agent*

This is a bacterium, class Mollicutes, order Mycoplasmatales, family Mycoplasmataceae (sterol-requiring mycoplasmas). Gram negative, lacks a cell wall, pleomorphic but usually spherical to pear-shaped, 0.3 to 0.8 μm in diameter. Grows on conventional horse serum-yeast extract mycoplasma medium, usually under facultatively anaerobic conditions at pH 7.8, 37°C, and 95% relative humidity. Ferments glucose. Rarely produces "fried egg" appearance when grown on solid medium (Razin and Freundt, 1984). For details of methodology for cultural isolation, see Cassell et al. (1983a).

Speciation of mycoplasmas is based on biochemical and serological tests (Razin and Freundt, 1984). Rapid presumptive identification of *M. pulmonis* can be made by the hemadsorption test (Manchee and Taylor-Robinson, 1968), but some strains do not hemadsorb (Tamura et al., 1981).

Type strain is ATCC 19612 [NCTC 10139; Ash (PG34)]. Other well known strains include: Peter C, Negroni, WRAIR, JB and Ogata T. All strains are currently considered members of a single serotype. Different strains vary greatly in virulence (Davidson et al., 1988a), but virulence factors of *M. pulmonis* have not been defined (Razin and Freundt, 1984; Davidson et al., 1988b).

*M. pulmonis* can be preserved indefinitely by lyophilization or freezing at –70°C (Razin and Freundt, 1984).

### *Hosts*

Rats and mice are considered the natural hosts. Isolated on occasion from wild rats, cotton rats, rabbits, Syrian hamsters and guinea pigs (Lindsey et al., 1982).

### *Epizootiology*

*M. pulmonis* infection and disease are common in conventionally reared rats and mice. Subclinical (often noncultivable) infection occurs in some cesarean derived, barrier maintained stocks (Cassell et al., 1981, 1983a,b; 1986).

Sites of predilection for the organism in the host are nasopharynx and middle ears (Davidson et al., 1981). *M. pulmonis* also has been reported from up to 40% of genital tracts in conventionally reared LEW rats (Cassell et al., 1979; Cassell, 1982).

Transmission is thought to be by the intrauterine route and by aerosol between cagemates, including from dam to offspring, and between adjacent cages (Hill, 1972; Lindsey et al., 1982).

*M. pulmonis* poorly resists environmental conditions outside the host, particularly drying (Vogelzang, 1975).

### *Clinical*

Infection occurs most commonly without clinical signs (as is true of most indigenous pathogens of rats and mice). Signs are nonspecific, but may include: "snuffling" in rats, "chattering" in mice, rales, polypnea, weight loss, hunched posture, ruffled coat, inactivity, "head tilt" and in rats, accumulation of porphyrin pigment around the eyes and external nares (Lindsey et al., 1971, 1982).

### *Pathology*

*M. pulmonis* is an extracellular parasite that preferentially colonizes the luminal surface of respiratory epithelium. Organisms (and lesions if present) tend to decrease from proximal to distal airways. Under ideal conditions for the host, the organism probably is a commensal (Cassell, 1982; Lindsey et al., 1986b).

Murine respiratory mycoplasmosis (MRM) is the disease of laboratory rats and mice which is caused by *M. pulmonis* but varies greatly in expression because of environmental, host, and organismal factors that influence this host-parasite relationship (Lindsey et al., 1985, 1986b). Intracage ammonia concentrations of 19 μg/liter of air or greater (Broderson et al., 1976a; Saito et al., 1982; Schoeb et al., 1982), concurrent Sendai virus infection (Howard et al., 1978; Saito et al., 1981; Schoeb et al., 1985), or concurrent sialodacryoadenitis virus infection (Schoeb and Lindsey, 1987) promote MRM by increasing growth of *M. pulmonis* in the respiratory tract. Other factors that influence expression of MRM include: concurrent infection with the CAR bacillus (see page 48); administration of hexamethylphosphoramide (Overcash et al., 1976; K. T. Lee and Trochimowicz, 1982a,b) or cyclophosphamide (Singer et al., 1972); vitamin A or E deficiency (Tvedten et al., 1973); inhalation of tobacco smoke (Wynder et al., 1968); genetic susceptibility of the host [e.g., LEW rats are more susceptible than F344 rats (Davis and Cassell, 1982; Davis et al., 1982); and C3H/HeN mice are more susceptible than C57BL/6N mice (Davis et al., 1985)]; and virulence of the *M. pulmonis* strain (Lindsey et al., 1971; Whittlestone et al., 1972; Howard and Taylor, 1979; Davidson et al., 1988a).

Characteristic microscopic lesions of MRM at any level in the respiratory tract include: neutrophils in the airways, hyperplasia of mucosal epithelium, and a lymphoid response in the submucosa. Lesions may be acute or chronic, and include: rhinitis, otitis media, laryngitis, tracheitis, bronchitis, bronchiectasis, pulmonary abscesses, and alveolitis (Lindsey et al., 1978b, 1982). Pleuritis and emphysema are rare. The dramatic hyperplasia of bronchus associated lymphoid tissue (BALT) characteristic of MRM in the rat has been related to the finding that *M. pulmonis* is a potent non-specific mitogen for rat lymphocytes (Naot et al., 1979a,b). Syncytial epithelial giant cells may occur in nasal and bronchial mucosa in mice (Lindsey and Cassell, 1973).

Athymic mice are no more susceptible to pneumonia and death due to *M. pulmonis* than immunocompetent mice. However, they often develop arthritis after intranasal inoculation of the organism (Cassell, 1982).

Natural infections of *M. pulmonis* also occur in the genital tract of female rats (Graham, 1963; Juhr and Obi, 1970; Casillo and Blackmore, 1972; Ganaway et al., 1973; Cassell et al., 1979; Davidson et al., 1981). LEW rats are highly susceptible to severe genital (as well as respiratory) disease due to *M. pulmonis*, and this is characterized by purulent endometritis or pyometra, salpingitis and perioophoritis (Cassell et al., 1979; Cassell, 1982). Similar genital lesions attributable to *M. pulmonis* are rare in rats of other strains.

In mice, humoral antibody is protective and can be passively transferred. In the rat, little metabolic inhibiting, complement fixing, or hemaglutinating antibody is produced and BALT may be a nonspecific response. Cellular immunity appears to be more important in rats than in mice (Cassell, 1982).

### *Diagnosis*

Cultural isolation of *M. pulmonis* from rats or mice with clinical MRM usually is readily accomplished by culturing lavage or swab samples from the respiratory tract using medium which has been pretested and shown to support growth (Cassell et al., 1983a). The nasopharynx is considered the best single site for culture (Davidson et al., 1981), but culturing multiple sites increases the isolation rate (Davidson et al., 1981). Diagnostic workups should include a battery of procedures (bacterial, viral, and histopathologic) designed to identify the responsible agent(s) and exclude other possible causes or contributors. Efforts should be made to identify all promoters (e.g., Sendai virus infection, intracage ammonia, etc.) that contribute to expression of MRM within the affected rodent population. Cultural isolation also is effective in diagnosing *M. pulmonis* infection of the genital tract in rats (Cassell, 1982, 1983a).

The ELISA is the method of choice for rodent health surveillance as it is far more sensitive and cost effective than culture. However, since the mycoplasma ELISAs currently in use are only genus specific (Horowitz and Cassell, 1978; Cassell et al., 1981, 1983a,b), ELISA positive sera should be tested by immunoblot (Davis et al., 1987; Minion et al., 1984) in order to differentiate between *M. pulmonis* and other mycoplasma infections. The detection of subclinical infection often is a major problem as ELISA seropositivity may occur only sporadically, the percentage of ELISA positive animals may be very small, and animals once seropositive may become negative again (Cassell et al., 1986; Cox et al., 1988). Animals with subclinical infections usually have so few mycoplasmas that they cannot be detected by routine culture (Davidson et al., 1981; Cox et al., 1988). These problems may be counteracted to some extent by testing only adults (weanlings with subclinical infection usually are ELISA negative), increasing the sample size, and testing repeatedly. Once a subclinically infected stock is shown to be ELISA positive, immunoblot and culture methods should be helpful in making decisions about suitability of the stock for research purposes (Cassell et al., 1983a; Lindsey, et al., 1986b; Davis et al., 1987).

### *Control*

Cesarean derivation and barrier maintenance programs appear to have reduced the prevalence of *M. pulmonis* disease but may not have been as successful in reducing the prevalence of *M. pulmonis* infection (i.e., subclinical infection) in contemporary rodent stocks (Cassell et al., 1981, 1983a,b; Lindsey et al., 1986b; Cox et al., 1988). Thus, major emphasis must be given to selection of mycoplasma free breeding stocks. This probably can be achieved in some instances by housing small groups of young adult breeders (known to be free of non-mycoplasmal pathogens) in plastic film isolators and repeatedly testing them by the ELISA over many months (e.g., monthly until 12 months of age). Stocks found to be consistently negative could then be used for establishment of breeder production populations under barrier programs.

Definitive information on the elimination of *M. pulmonis* from clinically or subclinically infected stocks is lacking but the following suggestions might prove useful. For cesarean derivations, use only dams that are several months old and have been repeatedly found to be ELISA negative. Candidate stocks for rederivation may be maintained for a few months on tetracycline or other antibiotics for the purpose of suppressing the mycoplasma flora as much as possible prior to cesarean operation. A separate isolator should be used for the pups of each donor female and a single foster female (from a stock known to be free of mycoplasmas and other pathogens). The placental membranes from each donor female should be cultured for mycoplasmas using a variety of media (Tram et al., 1970; Cassell et al., 1983a).

Control of environmental factors that favor MRM may be helpful in preventing clinical disease or ameliorating outbreaks (e.g., more frequent cage sanitation and reduction of cage population density to reduce intracage ammonia concentrations, and prevention of Sendai and sialodacryoadenitis virus infections). While administration of antimicrobials such as tetracyclines may help to control clinical signs, such agents are not curative and may introduce variables if animals on experiment are treated.

### *Interference with Research*

MRM can cause morbidity and mortality, particularly in long term studies (Lindsey et al., 1971, 1982).

*M. pulmonis* respiratory infection can alter results of many experimental responses of the respiratory tract, including: carcinogenesis (Schrieber et al., 1972), ciliary function (Irvani and van As, 1972; Westerberg et al., 1972), cell kinetics (Wells, 1970), and immunity (Cole et al., 1975; Naot et al., 1979a,b; Davis et al., 1982).

*M. pulmonis* infection of the genital tract can alter histology (Cassell et al., 1979) and reproductive efficiency (Leader et al., 1970; Goeth and Appel, 1974; Fraser and Taylor-Robinson, 1977; Lal et al., 1980; Cassell, 1982).

*M. pulmonis* infection in LEW rats has been found to delay onset and reduce the severity of adjuvant arthritis, reduce the incidence of experimental collagen-induced arthritis, and reduce antibody response to collagen (Taurog et al., 1984).

*M. pulmonis* infection has been found to increase natural killer cell activity in mice (Lai et al., 1987), and suppress humoral antibody response to sheep red blood cells in rats (Aguila et al., 1988).

*M. pulmonis* can contaminate transplantable tumors and cause arthritis in recipient mice (Barden and Tully, 1969).

Subclinical *M. pulmonis* infection can be exacerbated by known experimental procedures (e.g., deficiencies of vitamin A or E, administration of hexamethylphosphoramide, etc.), and probably by many others yet to be identified (Lindsey et al., 1986b).

*M. pulmonis* has been a frequent contaminant of rodent cell cultures (Barile, 1973).

Mycoplasmas have been shown to produce "lymphokine-like" substances that are mitogenic for B and T lymphocytes in vitro (Proust et al., 1985).

## Cilia-Associated Respiratory Bacillus

### *Significance*

Uncertain.

### *Perspective*

*1980*: van Zwieten et al. (1980a) in The Netherlands reported this organism in a colony of aged laboratory rats with severe murine respiratory mycoplasmosis (MRM). Morphologically similar organisms had been observed previously in the U.S. in *Mystromys albicaudatus* with chronic pulmonary lesions (A. E. McKee, Naval Medical Research Institute, Naval Medical Center, Bethesda, Md., personal communication, 1977), and as an apparent incidental finding in laboratory rats in Sweden (Afzelius, 1979).

*1981*: Mackenzie et al. (1981) reported that they found the organism in wild rats with an MRM-like disease, and in rabbits and a mouse in the United States.

*1985*: Ganaway et al. (1985) named the organism the "cilia-associated respiratory (CAR) bacillus". They also reported success in propagating the bacillus in embryonated hen's eggs and in experimentally infecting gnotobiotic rats with the organism to produce severe respiratory disease.

*1986*: Matsushita (1986) and Matsushita et al. (1987) reported natural infections of CAR bacillus in rats in Japan.

### *Agent*

A Gram-negative, argyrophilic, filamentous, rod-shaped bacillus, measuring approximately 0.2 μm × 6.0 μm. Presently it is not classified, but it possibly belongs to the group called gliding bacteria (Ganaway et al., 1985). It has been cultivated in embryonated hen's eggs but has not been grown in cell free media (Ganaway et al., 1985; van Zwieten et al., 1980a). The organism withstands freezing and thawing, and has been stored at –70°C and 23°C for short periods (Ganaway et al., 1985).

*Hosts*

Laboratory and wild rats (*Rattus norvegicus*), African white-tailed rats (*Mystromys albicaudatus*), laboratory rabbits, and laboratory mice (Mackenzie et al., 1981; Waggie et al., 1987; Griffith et al., 1988). However, the assumption that morphologically similar bacteria observed in different hosts are all the same organism may or may not be true.

*Epizootiology*

Unknown.

*Clinical*

The clinical manisfestations are those of severe MRM. Signs are nonspecific, but may include: hunched posture, ruffled coat, inactivity, "head tilt," and accumulation of porphyrin pigment around the eyes and external nares in rats (Lindsey et al., 1978b; van Zwieten et al., 1980a,b; Ganaway et al., 1985). No description of clinical disease in mice has been published.

*Pathology*

The pathology of natural CAR bacillus infection has been described only for rats and mice. The predominant lesions are those of advanced MRM (see "Pathology" of *Mycoplasma pulmonis* infection, pp. 44) with added distinctive features, as follows. Severe bronchiectasis and bronchiolectasis, pulmonary abscesses, and atelectasis of entire lung lobes are common and may be seen in rats only one month old. Severe bronchiectasis and bronchiolectasis are associated with accumulation of purulent or mucopurulent exudate in airways. An abundance of mucus often is present in peribronchiolar alveoli. Multifocal necrosis of bronchiolar and bronchial epithelia with an acute inflammatory response occurs and often progresses to severe granulomatous inflammation in walls of airways and abscess formation in airway lumens. Disordered repair may result in distorted, scarred bronchioles and bronchiolitis obliterans. The ciliated border of respiratory epithelium in affected airways often appears quite dense in hematoxylin and eosin stained sections because of the large numbers of CAR bacilli present between the cilia. The CAR bacillus also may be found on epithelial surfaces associated with lesions of MRM in nasal passages, larynx, trachea, and middle ears (van Zwieten et al., 1980a,b; Mackenzie et al., 1981; Griffith et al., 1988; J. R. Lindsey, Department of Comparative Medicine, University of Alabama at Birmingham, personal communication).

In instances where the CAR bacillus has been found in rats with natural disease the predominant lesions have been those of MRM and mycoplasmas compatible with *M. pulmonis* have been present (van Zwieten et al., 1980a,b; Mackenzie et al. 1981; J. R. Lindsey, Department of Comparative Medicine, University of Alabama at Birmingham). An epizootic of Sendai virus infection preceeded one outbreak (van Zwieten et al., 1980a,b). It may be that in rats *M. pulmonis* is the primary pathogen and the CAR bacillus is a promotor of MRM. Whether the CAR bacillus can cause natural disease in rats in the absence of *M. pulmonis* is unknown.

CAR bacillus-associated respiratory lesions similar to those in rats were recently reported in C57BL/6J–*ob/ob* mice (Griffith et al., 1988). These mice also had Sendai virus and pneumonia virus of mice infections, and *ob/ob* mice are known to have impaired cell mediated immunity (Sheena and Meade, 1978).

### *Diagnosis*

At present, diagnosis is dependent upon recognition of the argyrophilic CAR bacillus on respiratory epithelium in lesions of the respiratory tract. The Warthin-Starry silver stain gives by far the best results, and should be used as a standard procedure in pathologic evaluation of rat lungs with the characteristic lesions described above. Also, the organism can be demonstrated by transmission electron microscopy (van Zwieten et al., 1980a,b).

Enzyme-linked immunosorbent assays for CAR bacillus infection are under development, but their specificity and sensitivity have not been reported (Ganaway et al., 1985; Lukas et al., 1987). An indirect immunofluorescence test for CAR bacillus infection has been developed in Japan (Matsushita et al., 1987).

### *Control*

Uncertain. The infection probably can be eliminated by cesarean derivation but definitive studies have not been done.

### *Interference with Research*

Uncertain. The organism may be an important contributor to the morbidity and mortality due to MRM in rats and mice.

### *Streptococcus pneumoniae*

*Significance*

Low.

*Perspective*

*1950*: Recognition of *S. pneumoniae* as a natural pathogen of laboratory rats was a relatively recent development as the first reported outbreak was by Mirick et al. (1950). Only an occasional report has appeared since that time, bringing the present total to only about seven papers (Mirick et al., 1950; Ford, 1965; Baer, 1967; Baer and Preiser, 1969; Weisbroth and Freimer, 1969; Tucek, 1971; Fallon et al., 1988).

*1969*: Weisbroth and Freimer (1969) found the organism to be present in 19 of 22 breeding colonies of conventionally reared rats in seven states in the United States, but none of five pathogen free (cesarean derived, barrier maintained) colonies in four states.

*1988*: Fallon et al. (1988) reported *S. pneumoniae* infections not associated with disease in rats and mice free of other pathogens at a large commercial breeding facility. This was the first report of natural *S. pneumoniae* infection in mice.

*Agent*

*Streptococcus pneumoniae* is a bacterium with the following synonyms: *Diplococcus pneumoniae*, *Pneumococcus pneumoniae*. An encapsulated, Gram positive, lancet-shaped diplococcus. Although found mainly in pairs, the organism may occur in short chains or singly. As cultures age they become Gram negative (Deibel and Seeley, 1974).

It grows on blood agar producing $\alpha$-hemolysis. Growth may be facilitated by 10% $CO_2$. Some isolates require microaerophilic environments. On solid medium the organism forms round, glistening, unpigmented colonies that reach 0.5-1.5 mm in diameter after 24-36 hours. It differs from other streptococci of the viridans group in being bile soluble, sensitive to optochin (ethylhydrocupreine), and virulent for mice (Deibel and Seeley, 1974).

More than 80 different capsular types are known. Typing is by the Quellung reaction (swelling of carbohydrate capsules of individual organisms in the presence of type-specific antiserum). The most common capsular types reported from rats have been 2, 3, and 19; types 8, 16 and 35 have been encountered less frequently (Weisbroth, 1979; Fallon et al., 1988).

### *Hosts*

Humans are the main natural host. Between 40% and 70% of normal human adults carry one or more serologic types of pneumococci in their throats. Severe epizootics have been reported occasionally in rats, guinea pigs, and monkeys (Deibel and Seeley, 1974; Quie et al., 1981).

### *Epizootiology*

The agent is rarely seen in rats except in some conventionally reared stocks. Within colonies, isolates are usually monotypic, i.e., one capsular type (Weisbroth and Freimer, 1969).

Host sites of greatest predilection for the infection are nasal passages and middle ears. The carrier state is common in infected colonies.

Transmission is mainly by aerosol. The organism can remain viable for days on fomites, but fomites are of doubtful importance in transmission.

### *Clinical*

Signs are non-specific. Dyspnea, weight loss, hunched posture, snuffling respiratory sounds, and abdominal breathing have been reported. Clinical onset can appear to be sudden. Young rats are affected most often (Weisbroth and Freimer, 1969).

### *Pathology*

Pneumococcal capsules consist of large polysaccharide polymers that form hydrophilic gels on the surface of the microorganisms. Only encapsulated strains are pathogenic.

Very little is known about mechanisms by which the organism spreads from nasopharynx to lungs in rats or man. Infection becomes established in a bronchopulmonary segment and spreads centrifugally. As shown by Wood (1941) in his classic studies using rats, affected alveoli at the front of the spreading infection form an edema zone; an influx of polymorphonuclear leukocytes gives rise to consolidation; the organisms are removed by phagocytes leading to resolution; and the persistence of macrophages characterizes the macrophage reaction, the final healing stage of the local lesion. The infection readily spreads from the lung to the pleural space and pericardium, and into the blood stream.

Host defense is dependent in large part on efficient phagocytosis, with type-specific antibody (Wood, 1941; Wood and Smith, 1950) and complement opsonization (Coonrod and Yoneda, 1982) playing key roles. Evidence also has been advanced to suggest a nonphagocytic mechanism for pulmonary clearance of *S. pneumoniae* (Coonrod et al., 1983), perhaps mediated by surfactant (O'Neill et al., 1984). C-reactive protein may have a protective role against pneumococcal septicemia (Horowitz et al., 1987). Athymic (*nu*/*nu*) mice do not have increased susceptibility (Winkelstein and Swift, 1975). Organisms often persist in the nasopharynx long after recovery from disease.

Susceptibility to *S. pneumoniae* is influenced by splenectomy (Biggar et al., 1972; Bogart et al., 1972; Leung et al., 1972; Cooney et al., 1979a,b; Cohn and Schiffman, 1987; Harding et al., 1987), pulmonary edema (Johanson et al., 1974), and iron deficiency (Shu-heh et al., 1976).

A circadian periodicity of susceptibility to experimental infection with *S. pneumoniae* has been observed in mice (Feigin et al., 1969; Wongwiwat et al., 1972; Shackelford and Feigin, 1973). Hyperthermia has been reported to protect mice against the experimental infection (Liddle et al., 1987).

The predominant lesions in affected rats are suppurative rhinitis and otitis media. With extension of infection into distal airways, there is acute tracheitis and fibrinous lobar pneumonia. Extension to organs adjacent to the lungs is common, resulting in fibrinous pleuritis or empyema, fibrinous pericarditis, and/or acute mediastinitis. In some cases, these pleural and pericardial lesions occur in the absence of identifiable pulmonary lesions and thus, may result from bacteremia rather than direct spread of infection from the lungs (Mirick et al., 1950; Baer, 1967; Baer and Preiser, 1969; Weisbroth and Freimer, 1969; Tucek, 1971).

Severe bacteremia is an important part of advanced disease due to *S. pneumoniae* in the rat. One or more of the following may occur: suppurative arthritis, meningitis, hepatitis, splenitis, peritonitis, and orchitis. There may be multiple infarcts in the spleen or infarction of entire testicles. Enormous numbers of organisms can be demonstrated in such lesions by Gram stain. In some cases, the primary cause of death is one of these abdominal lesions (Weisbroth and Freimer, 1969; J. R. Lindsey, Department of Comparative Medicine, University of Alabama at Birmingham).

### *Diagnosis*

Cultural isolation of *S. pneumoniae* from the respiratory tract is diagnostic of infection but, because of the common carrier state, is not necessarily diagnostic of disease. Isolation of the organism from blood, body cavity, or a diseased organ is much stronger evidence to implicate the organism as a cause of disease.

Necropsy diagnosis must correlate presence of the organism at a given site with characteristic lesions, while excluding other possible causes and contributors to the disease process. This is of critical importance. Many of the reported outbreaks attributed to *S. pneumoniae* in the literature documented lesions more characteristic of murine respiratory mycoplasmosis than pneumococcal infection, but failed to exclude the possibility of *M. pulmonis* infection. Similarly, possible concurrent viral infections were not excluded.

Imprints of diseased organs and exudates due to *S. pneumoniae* often contain myriads of the organisms that are readily demonstrated by Gram stain. These methods can provide strong evidence for a preliminary necropsy diagnosis.

Several serologic tests, including enzyme-linked immunosorbent assays and a radioimmunoassay, have been developed for human patients (Schiffman et al., 1980) but have not been used in testing rats.

### *Control*

Cesarean derivation and barrier maintenance have been extremely effective. The high rate of carriers in man suggests the need for personnel working with rats to wear masks, but this has not been borne out by practical experience. Vaccines are available for people and conceivably could prove useful for animals in special situations.

### *Interference with Research*

Septicemia due to *S. pneumoniae* in the rat has been shown to alter hepatic metabolism (Powanda et al., 1972; Canonico et al., 1975; DeRubertis and Woeber, 1972; Thompson and Wannemacher, 1980), serum biochemistries (Mitruka, 1971), blood pH and electrolytes (Elwell et al., 1975), and thyroid function (Shambaugh and Beisel, 1966).

Infection with *S. pneumoniae* can jeopardize studies in rats involving the respiratory tract.

## ***Corynebacterium kutscheri***

### *Significance*

Uncertain; subclinical infections may be common in conventionally reared mice and rats.

### *Perspective*

*1894*: The organism was first isolated from mice in Germany by Kutscher (1894) who called the disease it causes, "pseudotuberculosis."

*1964*: Pierce-Chase et al. (1964) and Fauve et al. (1964) studied mice from 21 conventionally reared colonies and demonstrated that 9 of these colonies had "latent" *C. kutscheri* infection. Latency was explained on the basis of two forms of the organism, avirulent and virulent. They proposed that "latent" infections were due to the avirulent form, and that administration of cortisone provoked reversion to the virulent form which was responsible for disease expression.

*1978*: Hirst and Olds (1978a,b) refuted the claims of Pierce-Chase et al. (1964) and Fauve et al. (1964), and presented evidence that the avirulent organism was a group N streptococcus, not *C. kutscheri*.

*1984*: Ackerman et al. (1984) reported development of an enzyme-linked immunosorbent assay (ELISA) for *C. kutscheri*, and compared its efficacy with that of the tube agglutination test for detection of experimental infections in rats.

*1986*: Saltzgaber-Muller and Stone (1986) developed and tested a number of *C. kutscheri* DNA probes for detection of early infections due to this organism in rats.

### *Agent*

*Corynebacterium kutscheri* is a Gram positive, metachromatic, diphtheroid bacillus. Synonyms are *Corynebacterium murium*, *Bacillus pseudotuberculosis murium*, *Corynethrix pseudotuberculosis murium*, and *Bacterium kutscheri*. Colonies on blood agar are 1 to 2 mm in diameter after 24 hours; they appear circular, entire, dome-shaped, yellow or gray, smooth, and nonhemolytic.

The organism reduces potassium tellurite and produces acid from glucose, fructose, maltose, mannose, salicin, and sucrose. Does not produce acid from dulcitol, lactose, or mannitol. Usually hydrolyzes urea, does not produce indole or grow on MacConkey agar, and is catalase positive (Weisbroth, 1979; Coyle et al., 1985).

### *Hosts*

Mice, rats, and rarely, guinea pigs.

### *Epizootiology*

Natural infections of *C. kutscheri* are usually subclinical, occur in conventionally reared mice and rats, and result in disease expression only after severe immunosuppression of hosts by experimental regimens, dietary deficiencies, or concurrent infections of other agents (Weisbroth, 1979). A few epizootics have occurred in which the provoking factors could not be identified (Giddens et al., 1968). The infection is rare in cesarean-derived, barrier-maintained stocks.

The host-parasite relationships in naturally infected colonies (with inapparent, subclinical infection) are poorly understood. Infected animals presumably become chronic carriers but the natural habitat(s) of the organism remain uncertain. The oropharynx, submaxillary lymph nodes, and large intestine may be the main sites of predilection (Brownstein et al., 1985; Barthold and Brownstein, 1988; Suzuki et al., 1988), with transmission being mainly by the fecal-oral route. Other sites of infection include the respiratory tract, middle ears and preputial glands (Weisbroth, 1979). Whether naturally infected colonies have dormant or latent infections remains unresolved (Fox et al., 1987; Suzuki et al., 1988).

In rats experimentally infected by the oronasal route, the organism has been isolated from the oral cavity and submaxillary lymph nodes for at least eight weeks post infection (Brownstein et al., 1985). Whether this simulates the natural subclinical infection is unknown.

*Clinical*

Signs are not present in animals with the inapparent infection. In active infection of rats, signs are most often those of respiratory disease: dyspnea, rales, weight loss, humped posture, and anorexia. In mice, findings are usually those of a severe septicemia, particularly dead and moribund animals. In either species, arthritis or abscesses (in most any organ) may occur (Weisbroth, 1979).

*Pathology*

Inbred C57BL/6 mice are much more resistant to infection than are outbred S (Swiss) mice. Resistance reportedly is due to greater efficiency of C57BL/6 mononuclear phagocytes and is controlled by a single autosomal dominant gene (Hirst and Wallace, 1976; Hirst and Campbell, 1977).

Active disease characteristically begins as a septicemia which results in lodgement of septic emboli in many organs, most notably:

a. *In mice*, kidney and liver, less frequently in lungs, skin and joints (Weisbroth and Scher, 1968a).

b. *In rats*, the lungs. Subsequent expansion from the initial embolic foci in the lungs explains the characteristic pneumonia (i.e., parenchymal infection which spreads by contiguity, not a broncho-pneumonia) due to this agent in rats (J. R. Lindsey, Department of Comparative Medicine, University of Alabama at Birmingham).

In mice, during the septicemic phase large bacterial emboli are trapped in capillary beds, particularly in kidney and liver. Embolic glomerulitis is characteristic. If the animal survives the acute episode, each focus of infection may enlarge forming an abscess (Weisbroth and Scher, 1968a).

In rats, bacterial emboli lodge in capillaries of the lungs, break out and enlarge, often coalescing with adjacent foci. Along each advancing front alveoli contain edema fluid and a few polymorphonuclear leukocytes (PMNs), along with a high concentration of the organism. As this front expands, the alveoli behind become packed with PMNs and eventually may form large necropurulent centers. The expanding infection often involves the pleura resulting in fibrinous to fibrous pleuritis. The lungs usually have gross lesions of varying size (0.25 mm to 1 cm), indicating lesions of different ages related to repetitive showers of emboli, perhaps arising in part from active lesions in the lungs. Occasionally, abscesses may occur in the liver, kidneys, subcutis, peritoneal cavity, and other sites (Ford and Joiner, 1968; Giddens et al., 1968; J. R. Lindsey, Department of Comparative Medicine, University of Alabama at Birmingham).

The term "pseudotuberculosis" usually is inappropriate for the infection in mice and rats as septicemia and acute inflammation tend to predominate without formation of tubercle-like lesions. However, this term may be applicable to occasional focal lesions (e.g., abscesses) which reach chronicity (Giddens et al., 1968).

### *Diagnosis*

Detection of the infection in subclinically infected colonies is a major problem. Culture methods give inconsistent results and are not reliable for routine purposes (Fujiwara, 1971; Suzuki et al., 1988). The agglutination reaction, indirect fluorescent antibody technique, and agar-gel immunodiffusion methods are unsatisfactory for the detection of subclinical infections (Weisbroth and Sher, 1968b). The *C. kutscheri* ELISA holds great promise for detection of antibodies in subclinical infections (Ackerman et al., 1984; Fox et al., 1987). Similarly, a *C. kutscheri* DNA probe method for the diagnosis of *C. kutscheri* infection has been reported (Saltzgaber-Muller and Stone, 1986), but whether it has the specificity and sensitivity required to detect subclinical infections has not been determined.

In Japan, cortisone provocation followed in 6 days by the tube agglutination test for an anamestic rise in titer has been used as a routine diagnostic test (Takagaki et al., 1967; Fujiwara, 1971). In persistently infected mice, a single dose of 10 mg of cortisone acetate given intraperitoneally is sufficient to provoke active disease (Fauve et al., 1964). In rats, 10 mg cortisone acetate daily for 28 days, given by subcutaneous injection, has been successful in activating the subclinical, persistent infection (LeMaistre and Tompsett, 1952).

The diagnosis of active disease is made by culture of the organism, demonstration of characteristic lesions, and exclusion of other infectious agents and disease processes (Giddens et al., 1968; Fox et al., 1987). Efforts should be made to identify those factors responsible for provocation of natural epizootics.

Primary isolation of the organism from mucosal sites such as nasopharynx can be very difficult because colonies of *C. kutscheri* on blood agar have the same appearance as colonies of *Staphylococcus epidermidis* (M. Davidson, Department of Comparative Medicine, University of Alabama at Birmingham).

Presumptive diagnosis of active disease due to *C. kutscheri* can be made at necropsy by identifying the characteristic lesions and demonstrating typical colonies of the organism in Gram or Giemsa stained tissue imprints. In tissue sections the organism often can be demonstrated in greater numbers by the methenamine silver method than by Gram stain methods (J. R. Lindsey, Department of Comparative Medicine, University of Alabama at Birmingham).

### *Control*

Cesarean derivation and barrier maintenance have proved very successful. There is one report of possible vertical transmission (Juhr and Horn, 1975).

### *Interference with Research*

Experimental procedures which immunocompromise mice or rats can be complicated by *C. kutscheri* unless stocks free of this agent are used. Latent infection has been provoked to active disease:

a. *In mice*, by cortisone as a single dose of 10 mg cortisone acetate given intraperitoneally (Antopol, 1950; Antopol et al., 1951, 1953; Fauve et al., 1964), x-irradiation (Shechmeister and Adler, 1953), concurrent ectromelia (Lawrence, 1957), or concurrent salmonellosis (Topley and Wilson, 1920; Wolff, 1950).

b. *In rats*, by cortisone (LeMaistre and Tompsett, 1952) or deficiency of pantothenic acid (Seronde, 1954; Zucker, 1954, 1956, 1957; Seronde et al., 1955; Seronde et al., 1956; Zucker and Zucker, 1956).

In one study, experimental infections of rats with Sendai virus, sialodacryoadenitis virus or Kilham rat virus were unsuccessful in causing disease expression due to prior *C. kutscheri* infection (Barthold and Brownstein, 1988).

## Rat Coronavirus

The virus originally reported as "Rat Coronavirus" by Parker et al. (Arch. Ges. Virusforsch. 31:239-302, 1970c) is now considered a strain of sialodacryoadenitis virus (see page 97, this volume).

## Pneumonia Virus of Mice

*Significance*

Low.

*Perspective*

Two laboratory groups (Horsfall and Hahn, 1939, 1940; Mills and Dochez, 1944, 1945) independently discovered this virus during attempts to isolate influenza virus and other agents from human patients with respiratory infections. Nasopharyngeal washings or homogenates of diseased lung were serially passaged in mice resulting in high rates of "pulmonary consolidation" and mortality in the mice. As of this date, confirmation is lacking that pneumonia virus of mice (PVM) is a significant pathogen for immunocompetent rodents under natural conditions.

*Agent*

PVM is an RNA virus, family Paramyxoviridae, genus *Pneumovirus.* It is antigenically distinct from other members of the paramyxoviridae. All known strains of PVM have antigenic homology (Parker and Richter, 1982).

The virus particles are pleomorphic, occurring either as filaments 100 nm in diameter and up to 3,000 nm in length or as spheres 80-200 nm in diameter. The virus is labile under environmental conditions such as room temperature and heating to 56°C for 30 minutes. It agglutinates erythrocytes of mice, rats, and hamsters at room temperature or 5°C (Parker and Richter, 1982).

*Hosts*

Mice, rats, and hamsters. Possibly, guinea pigs and rabbits based on serologic evidence without virus isolations (Jacoby et al., 1979; Parker and Richter, 1982).

*Epizootiology*

PVM is a very common infection of laboratory rodents worldwide, the general prevalence rates being >50% of colonies of mice, rats, and hamsters. Prevalence rates within colonies vary greatly but tend to be higher (≈50%) in rats and hamsters than in mice (≈20%). Thus, the virus has relatively low infectivity for mice and tends to cause focal enzootics of infection within mouse colonies. Hemagglutination inhibition antibody titers also tend to be lower in mice (Parker and Richter, 1982).

Active infection in mice (and presumably rats and hamsters) is short lived, lasting only up to about 9 days (Horsfall and Ginsberg, 1951; Carthew and Sparrow, 1980a; Smith et al., 1984). Persistent infections do not occur in euthymic mice. Transmission is exclusively horizontal via the respiratory tract, mainly by direct contact and aerosol. Fomites are probably not important in transmission (Tennant et al., 1966; Parker and Richter, 1982).

Athymic (*nu/nu*) mice infected with PVM develop chronic pneumonia with terminal emaciation and death (Richter et al., 1988; Weir et al., 1988).

*Clinical*

Natural infections are subclinical in euthymic rodents. Athymic (*nu/nu*) mice infected with PVM have chronic illness with emaciation and deaths (Richter et al., 1988.

*Pathology*

Very little useful information is available on pathogenesis and morphologic expression of natural PVM infection. There are no reports of lesions demonstrated to be due to PVM alone in naturally infected mice or rats.

The pathologic description of Horsfall and Hahn (1940) is generally cited as the prototype for PVM infection in the mouse. However, the severe lung disease which they observed was produced only after serial passage of lung tissue in mice. Furthermore, their description of dense peribronchial and perivascular cuffs of mononuclear cells, purulent bronchitis, hyperplasia of bronchial epithelium, and a mononuclear response in alveoli, plus the isolation of mycoplasmas from consolidated lungs provide the essential criteria for a diagnosis of murine respiratory mycoplasmosis due to *Mycoplasma pulmonis* (see pp. 232, Horsfall and Hahn, 1940)! In sharp contrast, later investigators (Tennant et al., 1965, 1966) using cultures of the virus as inocula found it necessary to use ether anesthesia to increase host susceptibility in their standard experimental model using mice.

It may be that natural infections in mice are due to relatively small intranasal doses of virus with viral replication (and mild lesions) occurring principally in the nasal passages. Experimental infections of PVM in mice have given different results that appear to relate to the dose of virus given. In one study (Smith et al., 1984), 25 day old Crl:CF1® mice were given $2.5 \times 10^2$ median tissue culture infectious doses ($TCID_{50}$) of PVM intranasally and they developed only mild rhinitis. In another study (Carthew and Sparrow, 1980a), NMRI mice (age not specified) given either $10^4$ or $10^5$ $TCID_{50}$ of PVM intranasally developed severe interstitial pneumonia. The latter authors stated that similar lung lesions due to PVM had been seen in naturally infected mice, but they gave no details.

Chronic pneumonia, emaciation, and deaths have been reported in athymic (*nu/nu*) mice naturally infected with PVM (Richter et al., 1988; Weir et al.,

1988). Athymic (*nu/nu*) mice given $10^5$ $TCID_{50}$ of PVM intranasally have been reported to have interstitial pneumonia that persisted at least until 20 days post infection (Carthew and Sparrow, 1980b). Susceptibility to PVM may be increased by ether anesthesia (Tennant et al., 1966), urethane administration (Mirick et al., 1952), and pyridoxine deficiency (Leftwich and Mirick, 1949; Mirick and Leftwich, 1949). Susceptibility to the virus has been decreased by the intranasal administration of polysaccharides from a variety of bacterial and nonbacterial sources (Horsfall and McCarty, 1947; Ginsberg and Horsfall, 1951).

### *Diagnosis*

For routine monitoring purposes, the enzyme-linked immunosorbent assay is the most sensitive (Payment and Descoteaux, 1978; Descoteaux et al., 1980; Descoteaux and Payment, 1981; London et al., 1983), but the hemagglutination inhibition test is highly reliable and has served as the standard for PVM for many years (Parker and Richter, 1982). With either of these tests, serum antibody is first detected around day 9 post infection (Parker and Richter, 1982; Smith et al., 1984). The complement fixation (CF) test is useful in detection of recent infections as CF antibody appears about 9 days post infection, begins to decline after 2 weeks post infection, and disappears altogether by 3 months post infection (Tennant et al., 1966). The antibody response to PVM infection may be delayed and reduced in mice previously infected with mouse hepatitis virus (Carrano et al., 1984).

The mouse antibody production (MAP) test may be used for testing biologic specimens for presence of the virus (Rowe et al., 1962). PVM may be isolated using primary hamster kidney, BHK-21, Vero, and hamster embryo cells (Parker and Richter, 1982).

### *Control*

Cesarean derivation and barrier maintenance have given excellent results. Since the normal pattern of infection within mouse populations is focal enzootics and active infection is present in the individual mouse for only about 9 days, it may be possible to remove a few breeding pairs to individual gnotobiotic isolators and select those that are free of the infection by serologic testing. Alternatively, pairs which are serologically positive but produce only seronegative young while being maintained under gnotobiotic conditions can provide large numbers of breeders.

### *Interference with Research*

PVM conceivably could alter the experimental results of some studies involving the respiratory tract in euthymic mice but, no examples have been reported. Athymic (*nu/nu*) mice with natural infections of PVM develop chronic pneumonia and emaciation with deaths (Richter et al., 1988; Weir et al., 1988).

### *Mycobacterium avium-intracellulare*

#### *Significance*

Very low.

#### *Perspective*

Natural infection and disease due to this agent have been observed only in breeder C57BL/6N mice housed in a single room at a commercial breeding facility (Waggie et al., 1983a). Koch's postulates were fulfilled by oral and subcutaneous inoculation of the organism into pathogen free C57BL/6N mice (Waggie et al., 1983b).

#### *Agent*

A bacterium, family Mycobacteriaceae, *Mycobacterium avium-intracellulare*. *Mycobacterium avium* and *Mycobacterium intracellulare* are virtually indistinguishable organisms that belong to the "*M. avium* complex" within the "Runyon Group III" of the "nontuberculous" (or, "atypical") mycobacteria (i.e., mycobacteria other than *Mycobacterium tuberculosis* and *Mycobacterium bovis*). Thus, the species designation is *avium-intracellulare*. However, *avium* is frequently used as the species name because identification beyond the complex level usually is not practical (Sommers and Good, 1985).

Mycobacteria are aerobic, acid fast, nonsporeforming, nonmotile bacilli. Growth in artificial medium is usually slow. For methods of cultivation and identification of *M. avium-intracellulare*, see Sommers and Good (1985).

The nontuberculous (atypical) mycobacteria generally are considered normal inhabitants of soil and water (Chapman, 1982).

#### *Hosts*

Birds, man, swine, and rarely, mice (reported only in the C57BL/6N strain).

#### *Epizootiology*

The source of infection for the C57BL/6N mice was thought to be contaminated drinking water. The affected C57BL/6N population received chlorinated (9 ppm) water while an unaffected population of C57BL/6N mice elsewhere in the same facility had been given acidified (pH 2.5) water. *M. avium-intracellulare* is known to be resistant to sodium hypochlorite Waggie et al., 1983a).

*M. avium-intracellulare* has been isolated from public water supplies (Goslee and Wolinsky, 1976; Saito and Tsukamura, 1976; DuMoulin and Stottmeier, 1978).

*Clinical*

Clinical signs have not been reported to occur in naturally infected mice (Waggie et al., 1983a).

*Pathology*

Approximately 8% of 5 month old C57BL/6N females had gross lung lesions consisting of raised, tan, subpleural foci 1 to 5 mm in diameter. Sixty-three percent had microscopic lung lesions. These were foci in which large foamy macrophages and multinucleate giant cells filled the alveoli, particularly in the vicinity of terminal bronchioles but sometimes extending out to the pleura. Rarely, a few small nests of polymorphonuclear neutrophils were seen among the macrophages. Alveolar septae in affected foci often were widened and sometimes the interstitium was infiltrated by lymphocytes. Microgranulomas also occurred in livers, spleens, and mesenteric lymph nodes of a few mice. Acid fast bacilli were demonstrated in 37% of lung lesions using the Ziehl-Neelson method (Waggie et al., 1983a).

Sixty-seven percent of the breeder C57BL/6N females from the affected population also had either unilateral or bilateral chronic suppurative otitis media in addition to lesions in other organs. Acid fast bacilli were demonstrated in these ear lesions using the Fite Faraco method (J. R. Lindsey, Department of Comparative Medicine, University of Alabama at Birmingham).

C3H/HeN and (C57BL/6 × C3H) $F_1$ mice, and F344/N rats housed in the same room with affected C57BL/6N mice did not have lesions attributable to the mycobacterial organism, nor was the organism isolated from these animals by culture. This suggests that they were less susceptible to the disease and possibly, to the infection (Waggie et al., 1983a).

Other investigators (Gangadharam et al., 1981) also have found C57BL/6 to be one of the more susceptible mouse strains. Also, an experimental model has been established using beige (C57BL/6J-*bg*/*bg*) mice (Gangadharam et al., 1983; Bertram et al., 1986). Athymic (*nu*/*nu*) mice are no more susceptible than immunocompetent mice (Ueda et al., 1976).

### *Diagnosis*

Diagnosis of the disease in C57BL/6N mice is made by demonstration of typical lesions and cultural isolation of the organism. In tissue sections stained by acid fast methods the organisms are often beaded in appearance and measure 0.5 μm × 2.0 μm (Waggie et al., 1983a).

Cultural isolations of *M. avium-intracellulare* from C57BL/6N mice were made as follows. The left lobe of the lung was removed aseptically and ground in 5 ml of sterile saline using a tissue grinder. A loopful of the suspension was transferred to 10 mm deep blood agar plates and these were incubated in a humidified atmosphere with 10% carbon dioxide. Small (<1 mm) translucent colonies appeared after one week of incubation (Waggie et al., 1983a).

For purposes of differential histologic diagnosis, it is instructive to compare the lung lesions due to *M. avium-intracellulare* in C57BL/6N mice with the idiopathic lung lesion known as "alveolar histiocytosis" that has been reported to occur in both germfree as well as conventional rats (Beaver et al., 1963; Yang et al., 1966; Flodh et al., 1974). The latter condition is characterized by focal subpleural accumulations of foamy macrophages in alveoli immediately beneath the pleura, especially over the dorsal surfaces of the right caudal lobe and the posterior half of the left lobe. Grossly, these lesions appear as slightly raised, 1 to 2 mm, pale foci with discrete margins. Their characteristic location subpleurally distinguishes them from the mycobacterial lesions in C57BL/6N mice which primarily are located around the terminal airways.

### *Control*

Uncertain, probably by acidification or ultrafiltration of water supply.

### *Interference with Research*

Infection of susceptible mice such as C57BL/6N could complicate studies of the respiratory tract. Immunosuppression probably could result in active disease in less susceptible mice and possibly, in rats.

## ***Pneumocystis carinii***

### *Significance*

Low, except in immunodeficient and immunosuppressed animals.

*Perspective*

*1966*: Although small numbers of *Pneumocystis carinii* had been described in the lungs of rats as early as 1912, it was not until the development and experimental use of cortisone in rats that this infection began to take on significance (Frenkel et al., 1966). Following the administration of cortisone, Frenkel et al. (1966) demonstrated latent *P. carinii* in six of eight rat stocks from different commercial breeders in the U.S.

*1977*: Ueda et al. (1977a) reported natural disease due to *P. carinii* in athymic (*nu*/*nu*) mice. Walzer et al. (1977) transmitted rat- and human-derived organisms to athymic (*nu*/*nu*) mice.

*1979*: Walzer et al. (1979) demonstrated widespread natural infections in mice by giving cortisone, low (8%) protein diet, and tetracycline. Using a similar immunosuppressive regimen, Walzer et al. (1980) demonstrated a high prevalence of natural infection in rats.

*1989*: Walzer et al. (1989) reported natural outbreaks of *P. carinii* pneumonia in colonies of athymic (*nu*/*nu*) and severe combined immunodeficient (*scid*/*scid*) mice at four institutions.

*Agent*

Unclassified, but generally regarded as a protozoan or fungus, with the consensus favoring classification as a protozoan (Long et al., 1986). The recent ultrastructural demonstration of membrane surface rosettes during endocytosis and exocytosis is more supportive of classification as a protozoan (Yoneda et al., 1982). *P. carinii* of human, mouse, and rat origin have been found to have shared as well as host species-specific antigenic determinants (Walzer and Linke, 1987; Walzer et al., 1989).

The life cycle consists of four morphologically distinct stages, and occurs entirely within alveoli of the lung (Barton and Campbell, 1967; Campbell, 1972; Vossen et al., 1978; Yoneda et al., 1982).

a. *Trophozoite*—1.5 to 2.0 µm diameter. Uninucleate, pleomorphic (round, oval, or crescent shaped), limited by a double-layered membrane or pellicle. May have filopodia extending from the surface. The filopodia often intermesh with the filopodia of other organisms forming an intra-alveolar cluster or aggregate. Thought to be an obligate parasite of the type 1 pneumocyte (Long et al., 1986).

b. *Precyst*—2 to 4 µm diameter. Uninucleate, oval, thick cell wall, smooth surface without pseudopodial tubular extensions.

c. *Cyst*—5 to 7 µm diameter. Thick (three layered) cyst wall. Filopodial extensions may be present (but are not as prominent as those in trophozoites). The cytoplasm contains up to 8 nuclei, each representing a sporozoite.

d. *Sporozoite*—1.0 to 1.7 μm diameter. Undergoes development in the cyst and transforms into extracystic trophozoites that escape from the cyst and multiply (? asexually), or can develop into precysts or cysts.

Limited success has been achieved in growing the organism in cell cultures, including the A549 and WI-38 VA 13 cell lines (Pifer et al., 1977; Bartlett et al., 1979; Cushion and Walzer 1984a,b; Cushion et al., 1985).

### *Hosts*

Natural hosts include man, mice, rats, rabbits, ferrets, and numerous other mammals.

### *Epizootiology*

*P. carinii* is an ubiquitous opportunistic pathogen that inhabits pulmonary alveoli. Active pulmonary infection and disease are practically always manifestations of deficiency or compromise in host resistance.

The organism is extremely prevalent as a persistent, subclinical infection in mice and rats (Walzer et al., 1979, 1980, 1983; Walzer and Rutledge, 1981, 1982; Pifer, 1983).

Transmission is thought to be mainly by inhalation of infective cysts expelled during exhalation or coughing. Vertical transmission has been suggested (Pifer, 1983, 1984; Pifer et al., 1984), but has not been proved.

### *Clinical*

Immunocompetent rats and mice have subclinical infection (unless immunosuppressed). Immunodeficient and immunocompromized animals with *P. carinii* infection have chronic wasting and respiratory insufficiency that may persist for months. Clinical signs can include rough hair coat, dyspnea, cyanosis, severe weight loss and death (Ueda et al., 1977a; Tamura et al., 1978a; Walzer et al., 1979, 1980, 1983, 1989; Weir et al., 1986).

### *Pathology*

Active infections may occur or be produced as follows:

a. *Athymic* (nu/nu) *mice*—natural (Ueda et al., 1977a; Tamura et al., 1978a; Weir et al., 1986; Walzer et al., 1989) or experimental (Walzer et al., 1979) infections.

b. *Severe combined immunodeficient (*scid/scid*) mice*—natural infections (Walzer et al., 1989).

c. *C3H/HeJ mice*—when C3H/HeJ (lipopolysaccharide unresponsive) mice and C3HeB/FeJ (lipopolysaccharide responsive) mice with persistent infection are given 1 mg cortisone acetate subcutaneously (s.q.) twice weekly, with or without low (8%) protein diet, the C3H/HeJ mice develop more severe *P. carinii* infections and lung lesions than the immunologically normal C3HeB/FeJ mice (Walzer et al., 1983).

d. *Adult immunocompetent mice*—To produce lesions in persistently infected animals, give: 1 mg cortisone acetate s.q. twice weekly (or dexamethasone, 1 mg/1,000 ml in the drinking water), low (8%) protein diet, and tetracycline (1 mg/ml tap water) in drinking water for 8 weeks (Walzer et al., 1979).

e. *Adult immunocompetent rats*—To produce lesions in persistently infected animals, give: 25 mg cortisone acetate (for rats weighing 200 gm or less, 40 mg for rats weighing over 200 gm) s.q. twice weekly, low (8%) protein diet, and tetracycline (0.5 to 1.0 mg/ml) in drinking water for 8 to 10 weeks. The organism usually can be found in the lungs after 6 to 8 weeks of immunosuppression (Walzer et al., 1980; Bartlett et al., 1987b). The development of large numbers of trophozoites in alveoli and their attachment to the type I pneumocytes lining the alveoli appear to be central events in pathogenesis. The attachment mechanism is unknown, but probably is not by filopodia as has been suggested (Barton and Campbell, 1969). Attachment of large numbers of trophozoites to type I pneumocytes apparently alters alveolar capillary membrane permeability resulting in fluid accumulation along the basement membrane beneath type I pneumocytes leading to death of these pneumocytes (Lanken et al., 1980; Yoneda and Walzer, 1980, 1981, 1983).

Host defense mechanisms are poorly understood. The increased susceptibility of nude mice (Walzer et al., 1977), the protective effect of spleen T cells from previously infected immunocompetent mice (Furuta et al., 1985), evidence that specific antibody is required to opsonize the organism for phagocytosis by alveolar macrophages (Masur and Jones, 1978), and the protective effect of specific monoclonal antibody against *P. carinii* pneumonitis in animal models (Gigliotti and Hughes, 1988), indicate roles for both cellular and humoral immunity. Polymorphonuclear leukocytes also may have an important role (Pesanti, 1982).

Animals with active disease usually become progressively emaciated. The lungs are enlarged, rubbery in consistency, plum colored, and heavier than normal. On histopathology, the alveolar septae are variably thickened and there is a meager inflammatory response of lymphoid cells. Many alveoli are distended by homogeneous, foamy, eosinophilic material characteristic of *P. carinii* pneumonia. Ultrastructural studies have demonstrated that this material consists of serum protein, myelin figures consistent with pulmonary surfactant, degenerate host cells and organisms, and viable organisms (Yoneda and Walzer, 1980; Walzer et al., 1989).

In imprints or histologic sections of lung, definitive identification of *P. carinii* depends on demonstration of cysts (characteristically containing 8 sporozoites) and trophozoites. The cysts measure 5 to 7 μm in diameter and have a thick wall that stains with methenamine silver, cresyl violet, periodic acid-Schiff, or toluidine blue–0 (Shiota, 1986). Giemsa stain traditionally has been preferred for demonstration of trophozoites and sporozoites in imprints (Frenkel et al., 1966). Indirect fluorescent antibody (IFA) methods also have been used (Milder et al., 1980; Kovacs et al., 1986). An immunoperoxidase method using a monoclonal antibody has been reported (C.-H. Lee et al., 1986). Acridine orange has been proposed for rapid screening of imprints; the trophozoites stain yellow to orange while the cyst walls do not stain (Thompson and Smith, 1982).

### *Diagnosis*

For rats or mice with active infection and disease, the most reliable method is necropsy and demonstration of typical organisms in diseased lungs by the use of special staining methods, e.g., methenamine silver. Athymic (*nu/nu*) and severe combined immunodeficient (*scid/scid*) mice are unable to mount a significant antibody response to *P. carinii* and thus, serologic tests are of no value (Walzer et al., 1989).

Diagnosis of latent infection in mouse and rat stocks is a major problem. Two different approaches have been used:

a. *An immunosuppressive regimen followed by attempts to demonstrate organisms in diseased lung tissue* (Barton and Campbell, 1969; Ogino, 1978; Walzer et al., 1979, 1980; Bartlett et al., 1987a,b). Use of this method to test a given immunocompetent rodent population for latent *P. carinii* infection requires either (i) testing representative animals within the confines of the domiciliary space occupied by that population, or (ii) if removed to another location, animals must be transported and maintained in a containment device such as a gnotobiotic isolator to avoid contamination during transportation and the period of immunosuppression.

b. *Serologic testing*. This approach is possible but may be of limited usefulness because of the high prevalence of serum antibodies due to persistent infection in contemporary rat and mouse stocks. By IFA technique, young rats from two commercial sources were found to be negative and retired breeders were usually positive for serum antibodies to *P. carinii*. Serum antibodies were detected in five of six strains of immunocompetent mice up to 3 months of age. In both rats and mice the predominant serum antibody class was IgG. Nude mice rarely produced serum antibodies to *P. carinii* (Walzer and Rutledge, 1981, 1982).

Several serologic tests including IFA (Walzer et al., 1987) and enzyme-linked immunosorbent assay (Maddison et al., 1982) have been developed for detection of *P. carinii* infection but have not been shown to be useful for health surveillance or diagnostic purposes in laboratory rodents.

#### *Control*

Subclinical infection is probably common in conventionally reared and "pathogen free" colonies (Bartlett et al., 1987a). Gnotobiotic methods probably are useful in excluding the infection but, even this approach may not be completely effective because of possible vertical transmission (Pifer, 1983, 1984; Pifer et al., 1984). Cesarean derivation followed by maintenance under gnotobiotic methods has been found to exclude the infection in rats Wagner, 1985).

Prolonged treatment with trimethoprim-sulfamethoxazole or dapsone, may be useful in controlling disease but does not eradicate the infection (Hughes, 1979, 1988).

#### *Interference with Research*

Animals for use in studies involving long term, severe immunosuppression require careful selection and maintenance to avoid complication by *P. carinii* (Bartlett et al., 1987a). Gnotobiotic conditions are preferred for this purpose. Athymic (*nu/nu*) mice and mice with severe combined immunodeficiency (*scid/scid*) may develop active infection under natural conditions (Ueda et al., 1977a; Walzer et al., 1989).

### ***Chlamydia trachomatis***

#### *Significance*

Low.

#### *Perspective*

This latent pathogen of the mouse was discovered at Yale University in 1939 by Dr. Clara Nigg during attempts to isolate influenza virus by intranasally inoculating throat washings from human patients into mice (Nigg, 1942; Nigg and Eaton, 1944). It was subsequently reported as a cause of pneumonia after serial passages of tissues in mice in Australia (DeBurgh et al., 1945), Germany (Gonnert, 1941, 1942), and Chicago (Gordon et al., 1938; Karr, 1943).

### *Agent*

A bacterium, order Chlamydiales, family Chlamydiaceae, *C. trachomatis* biovar mouse. The mouse biovar does not share type-specific antigens with the two human strains of *C. trachomatis* (biovars trachoma and lymphogranuloma venereum), and has only 30-60% DNA homology with them. The type strain is ATCC VR-123 (Nigg II). Synonyms are Nigg agent and mouse pneumonitis agent (Moulder, 1984).

Members of the genus *Chlamydia* are nonmotile, Gram-negative, coccoid organisms that measure 0.2-1.5 μ in diameter and are obligate intracellular parasites. They multiply within membrane-bound vacuoles in the cytoplasm of host cells. The life cycle consists of elementary bodies (0.2-0.4 μ in diameter) and reticulate bodies (0.6-1.5 μ in diameter). They can be propagated in cell cultures, particularly in McCoy and HeLa 220 cells, and in the yolk sac of chick embryos (Moulder, 1984). *C. trachomatis* has compact or oval glycogen-positive inclusions. Growth in the chick embryo yolk sac is inhibited by sulfadiazine (Moulder, 1984).

### *Host*

Mice.

### *Epizootiology*

Natural infections are persistent and subclinical. All reported instances of disease have been the result of passaging infected mouse tissues, particularly lung, in mice (Gonnert, 1941, 1942; Nigg, 1942; Karr, 1943; Nigg and Eaton, 1944; DeBurgh et al., 1945).

Natural transmission is thought to be by inhalation and, possibly, cannibalism (Genest, 1959). There is no information available on the prevalence of this agent in contemporary mouse stocks.

### *Clinical*

Natural infections are persistent and subclinical. The clinical signs seen in mice with active disease during serial passage of mouse tissues have been nonspecific. They have included chattering, dyspnea, cyanosis, reluctance to move, humped posture, and weight loss. The interval from inoculation to death is dose dependent, ranging from 1 to 20 days (Gonnert, 1941, 1942; Nigg, 1942; Karr, 1943; Nigg and Eaton, 1944; DeBurgh et al., 1945).

### *Pathology*

The major lesion is multifocal to diffuse interstitial pneumonia. Following intranasal inoculation of the organism, alveolar macrophages are the predominant responding cell until about 30 hours post infection, when the first *C. trachomatis* developmental cycle in macrophages and bronchial epithelium is completed. Death of these infected cells is associated with edema and infiltration of polymorphonuclear neutrophils (PMNs), beginning at about 48 hours after infection. Thereafter, the developmental cycle continues, spreading by contiguity into adjacent lung parenchyma. Macrophages and PMNs are the predominant cell types at the margins of advancing lesions, and lymphohistiocytic cells predominate in the older central zones. Peribronchial lymphoid cuffing is not a prominent feature. The lesions are not completely resolved by 6 weeks post infection. The organism can be demonstrated in alveolar macrophages and bronchial epithelium by using special strains, such as Machiavello, on either tissue sections or imprints of affected tissues (Gonnert, 1941; Weiss, 1949; Gogolak, 1953; Moulder, 1984).

Athymic (*nu/nu*) mice are significantly more susceptible to *C. trachomatis* than their immunocompetent heterozygous littermates. T-cell-dependent cellular immunity is important in host defense (Williams et al., 1984).

Woodland et al. (1983) have summarized the information on animal models that are currently in use for the study of *C. trachomatis* and *C. psittaci* infections.

### *Diagnosis*

Definitive diagnosis requires the isolation and identification of the organism. Isolations are made by using McCoy and HeLa 229 cell cultures, inoculation of the yolk sacs of embryonating eggs, and inoculation of pathogen free mice (Moulder, 1984). The microtiter indirect immunofluorescence method is a practical, sensitive test that is used extensively for the detection of antigens and antibody in man (Wang, 1971). This test has been used experimentally for the detection of antibody to *C. trachomatis* in mice (Williams et al., 1981, 1982).

### *Control*

Mouse stocks for the study of chlamydial infections should be rigorously monitored to ensure that the mice are free of these agents and maintained by a barrier program to exclude contamination. Cesarean derivation should be successful in eliminating the agent from an infected stock of mice.

*Interference with Research*

Probably the greatest risk is the inadvertent use of persistently infected mice for the study of experimental infections of *C. trachomatis*. Also, the infection can be activated in infected mice being used for passage of mouse tissues (Gonnert, 1941, 1942; Nigg, 1942; Karr, 1943; Nigg and Eaton, 1944; DeBurgh et al., 1945).

### *Chlamydia psittaci*

There are two reports in which the serial passage of mouse tissues in conventionally reared mice led to the isolation of *C. psittaci*.

Ata et al. (1971) serially passaged mouse lung tissue intranasally in three strains of mice that had been maintained in their laboratory for 25-38 years. "Small areas of consolidation and hyperemia" were noted in the lungs of mice receiving the second and third passages of lung, and chlamydial elementary bodies were identified in imprints of these lungs stained by the Gimenez method. The *Chlamydia* was isolated from diseased mouse lungs in the yolk sacs of embryonated eggs. The *Chlamydia* was sulfadiazine resistant and negative for glycogen-containing inclusions, thus identified as *C. psittaci*.

Gerloff and Watson (1970) serially passaged liver and spleen suspensions by intraperitoneal inoculation of mice from a stock that had been maintained in their laboratory for 32 years. In mice of the 46th and subsequent passages there was splenomegaly, hepatomegaly, serofibrinous peritonitis, and up to 2 ml of ascitic fluid in the abdomen. A sulfadiazine-resistant *Chlamydia* isolate compatible with *C. psittaci* was established in yolk sacs of chick embryos. The intranasal inoculation of the yolk sac fluid into mice resulted in pneumonia with 50% mortality.

The significance of these reports is unclear. However, they raise the possibility that *C. psittaci* can occur as a persistent infection in some conventionally reared mouse stocks and that serial passage of tissues in such mice can result in activation of the infection. The prevalence of this agent in contemporary mouse stocks is unknown. It is also not known whether the strains of *C. psittaci* isolated from mice were variants peculiar to the mouse.

### *Klebsiella pneumoniae*

*Significance*

Low.

*Perspective*

Organisms of this species are considered part of the normal gastrointestinal flora in humans and animals. Evidence that they may be associated with natural disease in mice and rats is limited to two reports for mice (Flamm, 1957; Schneemilch, 1976) and two for rats (Hartwich and Shouman, 1965; Jackson et al., 1980).

*Agent*

*Klebsiella pneumoniae* is a bacterium, family Enterobacteriaceae, *K. pneumoniae*, subspecies *ozaenae*. Gram-negative, nonmotile, capsulated bacillus, 0.3-1.5 μ × 0.6-6.0 μ, occurs in pairs or short chains. Lacks special growth requirements. Does not utilize malonate. Voges-Proskauer test negative. Produces large mucoid colonies. Four or five capsular types have been identified for *K. pneumoniae ozaenae* (Orskov, 1984).

The taxonomy of the genus *Klebsiella* has been revised recently. *K. pneumoniae* now has three subspecies: *pneumoniae*, *ozaenae*, and *rhinoscleromatis* (replacing the three former species: *K. pneumoniae*, *K. ozaenae*, and *K. rhinoscleromatis*). Capsular types 3, 4, 5, and 6 have been regarded as belonging to *K. pneumoniae ozaenae* (Edwards and Fife, 1952; Orskov, 1957, 1984). Capsular type 5 has been associated with one outbreak of the disease in rats (Jackson et al., 1980), and capsular type 6 has been associated with an outbreak in mice (Schneemilch, 1976). The organisms from two similar outbreaks, one in rats and one in mice, were not typed (Flamm, 1957; Hartwich and Shouman, 1965). Thus, it is possible that *K. pneumoniae ozaenae* was the organism responsible for all four reported outbreaks.

In the past, *K. pneumoniae* included isolates from natural settings such as soil, water, grain, and forest products (Duncan and Razzell, 1972; Newman and Kowalski, 1973). Many of those organisms now belong to two proposed new species: *K. terrigena* and *K. planticola*. Indole-positive *Klebsiella* organisms are now classified as *K. oxytoca* (Orskov, 1984).

*Hosts*

Mice, rats, humans, and others.

*Epizootiology*

The organism is presumably a normal inhabitant of the gastrointestinal tract in man and animals, including mice and rats. It is an opportunistic pathogen. Transmission is by feces, air, and water (Ostrom, 1958).

### *Clinical*

Nonspecific signs of dyspnea, sneezing, cervical lymphadenopathy, inappetence, hunched posture, and rough hair coat have been observed in diseased mice (Flamm, 1957; Schneemilch, 1976). In the reported outbreaks in rats, there were a few deaths, and some rats had abscesses in the cervical and inguinal lymph nodes with fistulous tracts to the adjacent skin surface (Hartwich and Shouman, 1965; Jackson et al., 1980).

### *Pathology*

Mice with natural disease have cervical lymphadenitis; cervical, pharyngeal, renal, and hepatic abscesses; empyema; and granulomatous pneumonia. Experimental inoculation of organisms into the buccal mucosa induced a syndrome identical to that of the naturally occurring disease (Flamm, 1957; Schneemilch, 1976).

Rats with natural disease had submaxillary, parotid, or inguinal lymph node abscesses, often with fistulous tracts draining to the skin; abscesses in mesenteric nodes; and renal abscesses. Respiratory lesions either were not observed or were considered a minor part of the disease (Hartwich and Shouman, 1965; Jackson et al., 1980).

Rats are commonly used for studies of experimental pneumonia induced by the inoculation of capsular type 1 *K. pneumoniae* (Berendt et al., 1977; Coonrod, 1981; Domenico et al., 1982). The extent to which such studies are relevant to the natural disease in rats is uncertain.

### *Diagnosis*

The few reports of natural disease associated with this agent are insufficient to allow firm conclusions about its role as a primary pathogen in mice and rats. Like other opportunistic pathogens, host factors probably are extremely important determinants of disease caused by this organism.

Diagnostic efforts must differentiate between possible roles of *K. pneumoniae*: primary pathogen, secondary pathogen, or coincidental infection. Case studies should include isolation, identification, and serotyping of the organism; serologic and culture procedures to exclude other infectious agents; necropsy with histopathologic examination of all major organs and gross lesions; and efforts to identify possible contributing host factors. Also, efforts should be made to fulfill Koch's postulates through experimental infections of pathogen-free mice or rats by using an isolate of *K. pneumoniae* from a natural lesion.

*Control*

Uncertain. *K. pneumoniae ozaenae* is presumably a part of the normal gastrointestinal flora of mice and rats.

*Interference with Research*

*K. pneumoniae* is an opportunistic pathogen that may complicate studies in which host defenses are compromised.

### *Streptococcus pyogenes*

*Significance*

Very low.

*Perspective*

Nelson (1954) described a natural outbreak of cervical lymphadenitis caused by a group A streptococcus in laboratory mice; the organism was later identified as *S. pyogenes* serotype 50 (Hook et al., 1960). A second occurrence of this disease was reported by Hook et al. (1960), who also obtained evidence that two epizootics of the disease had occurred previously in mice of two additional laboratories in the vicinity of New York City, one in 1935 and the other in 1959.

*Agent*

A bacterium, family Streptococcaceae, *S. pyogenes*, group A, serotype 50. *S. pyogenes* is composed of β-hemolytic, microaerophilic, bacitracin-susceptible, Gram-positive cocci that usually form chains. The species is subdivided into groups on the basis of Lancefield's group antigens and into serotypes based on cell wall M and T antigens. Serotyping is sometimes helpful in tracking common source outbreaks (Lancefield, 1972; Facklam and Carey, 1985).

*Hosts*

Humans are considered the natural host of β-hemolytic group A *S. pyogenes* (Lancefield, 1972). There are only two reports (Nelson, 1954; Hook et al., 1960) of natural infection in laboratory mice.

### Epizootiology

Man is the natural reservoir of β-hemolytic group A streptococci. Transmission is mainly via close contact or contaminated food and usually involves an asymptomatic carrier colonized in the nasopharynx, skin, vagina, or rectum (Facklam and Carey, 1985).

Hook et al. (1960) found that up to 52% of mice from a commercial breeding facility harbored the organism in their throats. One-third of infected mice developed cervical lymphadenitis, and approximately 50% of those observed for 3 months died of the streptococcal infection. The source of infection for the mice studied by Nelson (1954) and Hook et al. (1960) was not determined. The fact that the mice of all epizootics reported by Nelson (1954) and Hook et al. (1960) were in the vicinity of New York City suggests that there could have been a common source of infection. Hook et al. (1960) were unsuccessful in culturing group A streptococci from 40 throat cultures obtained from 15 people who worked with their mice. At least four stocks of mice, S (Swiss), Princeton (the noninbred forerunner of strain PL), C57 (strain designation incompletely given), and A (an unspecified stock designated A by Jacob Furth), have been involved in four spontaneous epizootics (Hook et al., 1960).

### Clinical

Some mice carried the organism in their throats for more than 90 days without developing clinical signs of infection. Affected mice showed ruffled hair coats and inactivity for a few days before death. In the more advanced cases the cervical lymph nodes were enlarged and often had purulent exudate draining through fistulous tracts to the skin (Nelson, 1954; Hook et al., 1960).

### Pathology

Only gross descriptions of the pathology in this disease have been published. The lesions reported included suppurative cervical lymphadenitis (with or without drainage to the skin), otitis media, rhinitis, and pneumonia. Myriads of organisms were demonstrated in exudates from cervical nodes. Septicemia caused by *S. pyogenes* was considered an important cause of death because the organism was often cultured from heart blood of animals that died (Nelson, 1954; Hook et al., 1960).

Wildfeuer et al. (1978) carried out experimental studies in which mice were infected intranasally with the organism. Suppurative cervical lymphadenitis was produced regularly, and the infection in mice was proposed as an experimental model of human streptococcal pharyngitis.

### *Diagnosis*

The diagnosis is based on demonstration of characteristic lesions, isolation and identification of the organism, and exclusion of other possible causes.

### *Control*

Uncertain. Cesarean derivation and barrier maintenance should be effective in eliminating the organism from an infected stock of mice.

### *Interference with Research*

Mortality due to this organism reached 50% during one epizootic in mice (Hook et al., 1960). Hook et al. (1960) observed increased numbers of deaths in naturally infected mice injected intracerebrally with either sterile saline or sublethal doses of bacterial endotoxin.

## ***Mycoplasma neurolyticum***

### *Significance*

Uncertain, probably very low.

### *Perspective*

*M. neurolyticum* has been isolated occasionally from mice and rats since 1938 (Findlay et al., 1938; Sabin, 1938a,b), but there is only one instance in which it has been thought to be a natural pathogen. Nelson (1950a,b) described a colony of mice in which he associated the occurrence of conjunctivitis with presence of this organism. However, that alleged association has not been confirmed in the intervening 35 years since Nelson's reports; and experimental inoculations of *M. neurolyticum* into mice by the conjunctival, intranasal, or intravenous route have consistently failed to cause conjunctivitis (Cassell and Hill, 1979). Thus, this organism is not considered a natural pathogen.

### *Agent*

*Mycoplasma neurolyticum* is a bacterium, class Mollicutes, order Mycoplasmatales, family Mycoplasmataceae (sterol-requiring mycoplasmas). It is Gram negative, lacks a cell wall, pleomorphic but usually spherical to pear-shaped, and measures 0.3-0.8 μm in diameter. It may produce filaments up to 160 μm long. *M. neurolyticum* grows on conventional horse serum-yeast extract mycoplasma medium, usually under facultatively anaerobic conditions at pH 7.8, 37°C, and 95% relative humidity. Unlike other rodent mycoplasmas, growth is inhibited by penicillin G (Hottle and Wright, 1966). It ferments glucose. *M. neurolyticum* rarely produces "fried egg" appearance when grown on solid medium. For details of methodology for cultural isolation, see Cassell et al. (1983a). Identification of the species of *Mycoplasma* is based on biochemical and serologic tests (Razin and Freundt, 1984).

The type strain is ATCC 19988 (NCTC 10166). It produces a true exotoxin that is neurotoxic and causes "rolling disease" when injected intravenously into mice or young rats. Neurotoxicity also occurs when washed living organisms are given intravenously, intraperitoneally, or intracerebrally. The exotoxin is a protein with a molecular weight of greater than 200,000. It is thermolabile and is inactivated at 50°C in 10-30 minutes or 45°C in 15-90 minutes (Razin and Freundt, 1984).

### *Hosts*

Laboratory and wild mice and laboratory rats (Cassell and Hill, 1979).

### *Epizootiology*

*M. neurolyticum* has been isolated from the conjunctiva, nasal passages, Harderian glands, and brains of laboratory mice (Findlay et al., 1938; Sabin, 1938a,b, 1939; Sabin and Johnson, 1940; Nelson 1950a,b; Tully and Rask-Nielsen, 1967; Hill, 1974a; Cassell and Hill, 1979) and from the conjunctiva of wild mice and laboratory rats (Hill, 1974a; Cassell and Hill, 1979). Thus, the mucous membranes of the conjunctiva and upper respiratory tract are presumably the main sites of predilection for the organism. Data on the natural history of the infection are lacking.

The prevalence of *M. neurolyticum* infection in contemporary rodent stocks is unknown. However, it appears to be very low because the organism is rarely isolated by those laboratories that routinely culture nasal passages with suitable media for monitoring the health of large numbers of mice and rats (M. K. Davidson, Department of Comparative Medicine, University of Alabama at Birmingham, personal communication).

### *Clinical*

Infections due to *M. neurolyticum* are subclinical.

### *Pathology*

No gross or microscopic lesions are associated with natural *M. neuro-*

*lyticum* infection or experimental inoculation of the organism into the conjunctiva or nasal passages (Cassell and Hill, 1979). In natural infections the organism is apparently a commensal.

The intravenous, intraperitoneal, or intracerebral inoculation of *M. neurolyticum*-infected tissues, broth cultures containing viable organisms, or cell-free filtrates of *M. neurolyticum* cultures into mice or young rats causes severe cerebral edema (spongiform degeneration) manifested clinically by rolling from side to side (Findlay et al., 1938; Tully and Ruchman, 1964; Aleu and Thomas, 1966; Thomas, 1967) and is caused by the exotoxin of *M. neurolyticum* (Tully, 1964; Thomas and Bitensky, 1966; Thomas, 1967; Tully and Rask-Nielsen, 1967). Ultrastructurally, there is extreme distension of astrocytes by fluid with mechanical displacement and compression of myelinated axons, accumulation of extracellular fluid in the white matter, and degeneration of myelin sheaths of axons (Aleu and Thomas, 1966). The neurotoxin is thought to bind to ganglioside receptors on astrocyte podocytes resulting in disruption of normal regulation of fluid transport (Thomas et al., 1966). [This so-called rolling disease experimentally induced by *M. neurolyticum* is not to be confused with the naturally occurring circling or rolling disease in mice that has been associated with inner ear disease caused by *Pseudomonas aeruginosa* (Gorrill, 1956; Ediger et al., 1971; Kohn and Mackenzie, 1980).]

### *Diagnosis*

Cultural isolation of the organism is the only proven method for diagnosing *M. neurolyticum* infection. Lavage or swab samples from nasal passages and conjunctivas should be cultured in mycoplasma media without penicillin, which is inhibitory to some strains of the organism (Hottle and Wright, 1966; Cassell et al., 1983a).

### *Control*

No data are available. Presumably, the organism can be eliminated from infected stocks by cesarean derivation and barrier maintenance techniques.

### *Interference with Research*

The intracerebral passage in mice of *Toxoplasma gondii* (Sabin, 1938a) and lymphocytic choriomeningitis and yellow fever viruses (Findlay et al., 1938) was complicated by contamination of the passaged tissues with *M. neurolyticum* resulting in the occurrence of rolling disease. *M. neurolyticum* may be a common contaminant of transmissible mouse leukemia cell lines (Tully and Rask-Nielsen, 1967).

## Mycoplasma collis

### Significance

Unknown.

### Perspective

This is a recently described species of mycoplasma that appears to be a nonpathogenic inhabitant of the conjunctiva and nasopharynx in mice and rats.

### Agent

*Mycoplasma collis* is a bacterium, class Mollicutes, order Mycoplasmatales, family Mycoplasmataceae (sterol-requiring mycoplasmas). Strains of mycoplasmas provisionally designated Gough from mice (Hill, 1974a) and 58b from rats (Young and Hill, 1974) were later found to be serologically identical and have been assigned to a new species, *M. collis* (Hill, 1983). It grows on standard medium for murine mycoplasmas and utilizes glucose (Cassell et al., 1983a; Hill, 1983).

### Hosts

Mice and rats.

### Epizootiology

The organism has been isolated from one mouse colony and four rat colonies in the United Kingdom. The isolates were from the conjunctiva in mice (Hill, 1974a) and from the conjunctiva, Harderian gland, and nasopharynx in rats (Young and Hill, 1974). The prevalence is unknown (Hill, 1983).

### Clinical

Rats with the natural infection had conjunctivitis (Young and Hill, 1974), but attempts to reproduce the disease experimentally by inoculating pathogen-free rats with cultures of strain 58B failed (Hill, 1974b). Clinical signs have not been observed in infected mice (Hill, 1974a). Thus, *M. collis* infection alone is subclinical.

### *Pathology*

The organism is considered a nonpathogen.

### *Diagnosis*

Diagnosis is by cultural isolation (Hill, 1974a; Young and Hill, 1974; Cassell et al., 1983a). Use of the mycoplasma enzyme-linked immunosorbent assay (Cassell and Brown, 1983) for diagnosing this infection has not been investigated.

### *Control*

No data are available. Presumably, cesarean derivation and barrier maintenance would be effective.

### *Interference with Research*

Unknown.

## ***K Virus***

### *Significance*

Very low.

### *Perspective*

This agent was originally isolated by Kilham (1952) from asymptomatic C3H mice carrying the Bittner agent. Although the virus initially attracted much attention for causing pneumonitis when passaged to infant mice (Fisher and Kilham, 1953; Kilham and Murphy, 1953), it is now mainly of interest as an experimental model of acute and persistent papovavirus infections in mice.

### *Agent*

The agent is a small DNA virus, family Papovaviridae, genus *Polyomavirus*. K virus is taxonomically related to polyomavirus, but the two agents are immunologically distinct (Dalton et al., 1963; Mattern et al., 1963; Bond et al., 1978). Virions are spherical and measure 35-45 nm in diameter. Synonyms for K virus are K papovavirus (Jordan and Doughty, 1969;

Takemoto and Fabisch, 1970), Kilham virus (Kraus et al., 1968), and mouse pneumonitis virus (Parsons, 1963).

K virus is resistant to environmental conditions. In tissue suspensions at room temperature it has been found to remain stable for 11 weeks. It withstands ether, acid pH, repeated freezing and thawing, heating to 70°C for 3 hours, and exposure to 0.5% formalin. It agglutinates sheep erythrocytes (Kilham, 1952, 1961c; Holt, 1959).

Limited success has been achieved in the culture of K virus in vitro using primary mouse embryo cells (Greenlee et al., 1982).

### *Host*

Mice (*Mus musculus*), exclusively. Wild mice are considered the natural hosts.

### *Epizootiology*

K virus is considered to have a worldwide distribution. It occurs as an enzootic, subclinical, persistent infection primarily in feral *Mus musculus*, but it has been found in conventionally reared populations of laboratory mice as well. Prevalence of infection within populations is usually low (about 10%). It is rare in contemporary cesarean-derived, barrier-maintained stocks in the United States (Rowe et al., 1962, 1963; Tennant et al., 1966; Parker and Richter, 1982).

The natural history of infection within mouse populations is poorly understood. The virus is shed in milk, urine, and feces, and natural transmission is thought to be by ingestion. Contaminated food and bedding may be important as the virus is stable for long periods outside the host. The virus persists in the host for at least 8 months and perhaps, for life (Greenlee, 1979, 1981; Greenlee and Dodd, 1984; Parker and Richter, 1982).

### *Clinical*

Natural infections are subclinical. Clinical disease results from experimental inoculation of the virus into infant mice less than 8 days of age (Kilham, 1952; Kilham and Murphy, 1953).

### *Pathology*

In the experimental model of acute K virus infection, 1- to 3-day-old mice are given the virus. The intracerebral route is preferred, but almost any other route (intraperitoneal, intranasal, subcutaneous, or oral) is also satisfactory. After an incubation period of 6-15 days, there is a sudden onset of "chugging" (pumping) respiration followed by death within a few hours. The gross lesions include pulmonary congestion, hemorrhage, atelectasis, and edema, with hydrothorax (Fisher and Kilham, 1953; Kilham and Murphy, 1953; Holt, 1959; Margolis et al., 1976).

The most striking histologic lesions in experimentally infected infant mice occur in the lungs. Characteristically, there is diffuse interstitial pneumonia with numerous prominent amphophilic to basophilic intranuclear inclusions in vascular endothelium throughout the lungs. Because of these findings, it was thought for many years that viral replication and cytopathic effects occurred exclusively in the pulmonary endothelium (Gleiser and Heck, 1972; Margolis et al., 1976). Subsequently, it has been shown that the major sites of K virus replication are the pulmonary endothelium and hepatic sinusoidal lining cells, with less involvement of cells in spleen, lymph nodes, and brain (Greenlee, 1979, 1981).

Susceptibility of infant mice has been related to the inability to mount an antibody response (Mokhtarian and Shah, 1980; Greenlee, 1981). Athymic (*nu/nu*) mice produce low levels of virus-specific IgM and are no more susceptible to infection than immunocompetent mice (Mokhtarian and Shah, 1983).

Persistent K virus infections have been reactivated 8 months post infection by the administration of 8 weekly injections of cyclophosphamide at a dose of 150 mg/kg (Greenlee and Dodd, 1984).

K virus has been reported to transform cells in vitro (Takemoto and Fabisch, 1970; Greenlee and Law, 1984), but unlike polyomavirus, it is not known to be tumorigenic in vivo.

### *Diagnosis*

The hemagglutination inhibition test and the complement fixation test are the most commonly used serologic tests. The intracerebral inoculation of the organism into infant mice and/or the mouse antibody production test may be used for testing biologic materials for K virus contamination (Parker and Richter, 1982).

Even under the best of conditions, the detection of K virus in a population of mice can be difficult, as appropriately emphasized by the following quote from Parker and Richter (1982): "The predominant characteristics of K virus infection are latency, chronicity, low incidence, low antibody titers in recovered mice, and infection in older mice. Thus, testing large numbers of mice at frequent intervals and testing mice of all ages, especially those 7 months and older, may be required to certify a population free of infection."

### *Control*

Cesarean derivation and barrier maintenance have been very successful in eliminating the infection (Parker and Richter, 1982).

### *Interference with Research*

The virus can be a contaminant of transplantable murine tumors causing early deaths in suckling recipient mice (Fisher and Kilham, 1953; Rowe et al., 1962).

K virus infection enhances the severity of hepatic necrosis caused by mouse hepatitis virus (Tisdale, 1963).

K virus has been reported to transform cells in vitro (Takemoto and Fabisch, 1970; Greenlee and Law, 1984).

# 7

# Digestive System

## Overview

Diseases of the digestive system, like those of the respiratory tract, are extremely common in both mice and rats. As a group they clearly rival diseases of the respiratory tract in importance, despite the fact that they possibly tend to be even more subtle clinically. This is explained in part by the fact that many pathogens of the digestive system have their most serious effects in the very young, i.e., neonates and sucklings. Clinical signs may no longer be present when they are delivered to the investigator as weanlings or young adults. In addition, even the more obvious clinical signs of digestive tract disease, such as diarrhea and retarded growth, often go completely undetected in mice and rats.

There are approximately 21 infectious agents of the digestive system in mice and rats. Natural infections are usually due to varying combinations of these agents, and if clinical disease is present, careful judgments may be required in deciding which agent(s) have causative role(s). Additive effects are often suspected but are difficult to prove. Where possible, detection methods should identify all possible causes; and pathologic workups, including histopathology of all organs comprising the digestive system, should be done to make definitive diagnoses. Histologic sections should include the salivary and Harderian glands because they are important target organs of sialodacryoadenitis virus as well as other agents.

Table 10 places in perspective the relative importance of the infections of the digestive system as causes of disease. Agents are listed in descending

TABLE 10 Agents Grouped According to Importance as Causes of Natural Digestive System Disease

| Group[a] | Mouse[b] | Rat[b] |
|---|---|---|
| I | Mouse hepatitis virus<br>*Spironucleus muris*<br>*Bacillus piliformis*<br>*Salmonella enteritidis*<br>*Citrobacter freundii* (biotype 4280)<br>*Giardia muris*<br>Mouse rotavirus | Sialodacryoadenitis virus<br>*Spironucleus muris*<br>*Bacillus piliformis*<br>*Giardia muris* |
| II | Reovirus-3<br>*Pseudomonas aeruginosa*<br>*Hymenolepis nana*<br>*Syphacia* spp.<br>Mouse cytomegalovirus | *Salmonella enteritidis*<br>Rat rotavirus-like agent<br>Pseudomonas aeruginosa<br>*Syphacia* spp. |
| III | Mouse thymic virus<br>*Adenoviruses*<br>*Aspicularis tetraptera*<br>*Entamoeba muris*<br>*Tritrichomonas muris* | Rat cytomegalovirus<br>Reovirus-3<br>Adenoviruses<br>*Entamoeba muris*<br>*Tritrichomonas muris* |

[a]Group Key: I = Agents that are unquestionably important digestive tract pathogens. II = Agents of questionable importance or pathogenicity, except in special circumstances. III = Agents not considered significant, natural pathogens in laboratory animals of the species indicated.
[b]Reading down each list of agents for the mouse or rat, agents are listed approximately in descending order of importance as digestive system pathogens for that rodent species.

order of importance for mice and rats. Agents listed in group I are undisputed important pathogens, but because of their high prevalence and known effects on research, mouse hepatitis virus and *Spironucleus muris* in the mouse and sialodacryoadenitis virus and *S. muris* in the rat are of greatest concern. *Bacillus piliformis*, *Salmonella enteritidis*, and *Citrobacter freundii* (biotype 4280) are important, but far less common, pathogens. *Giardia muris* is common but probably less important. Mouse rotavirus is pathogenic only in neonates.

Those agents listed in group II of Table 10 appear to be of little significance except possibly in rare circumstances. For example, reovirus-3 is a rare contaminant of transplantable tumors, *S. enteritidis* is found very rarely in rats, rat rotavirus-like agent has been found in rats on only one occasion, and mouse cytomegalovirus is probably very rare in laboratory mice (but common in wild mice).

The agents in group III of Table 10 are of doubtful importance as pathogens in laboratory mice and rats. Rat cytomegalovirus has been found only in wild rats.

## Mouse Cytomegalovirus

### *Significance*

Low.

### *Perspective*

Mouse cytomegalovirus (MCMV)* is a common subclinical infection of the submaxillary salivary glands and other tissues in wild mice. Although it has been found in laboratory mice on occasion (Mannini and Medearis, 1961; Rowe et al., 1962), its chief importance is that it provides a variety of laboratory models for the study of phenomena similar to those in human cytomegalovirus infections (Osborn, 1982).

### *Agent*

MCMV is an enveloped, double-stranded DNA virus, family Herpesviridae, subfamily Betaherpesvirinae, cytomegalovirus group. Like other herpesviruses, the virion is 120-200 nm in diameter. The capsid is 100-110 nm in diameter, is icosahedral in symmetry, and has 162 capsomeres (Matthews, 1982).

MCMV differs from most herpesviruses in that it has a larger genome (Misra et al., 1978). Several strains of MCMV are known, but the Smith strain and its substrains have been studied most. All strains are antigenically and biophysically similar and presently are considered the same virus (Mosmann and Hudson, 1973, 1974).

Cytomegaloviruses are relatively unstable, sensitive to freezing and thawing, acid pH, and heating at 56°C for 30 minutes. They can be stored for prolonged periods at –90°C in the presence of 35% sorbitol or dimethyl sulfoxide (Buxton and Fraser, 1977a; Osborn, 1982).

MCMV produces permissive infections in cultures of mouse embryo fibroblasts and 3T3 cells (Osborn, 1982).

### *Hosts*

Wild mice (*Mus musculus*) are considered the natural hosts (Mannini and Medearis, 1961; Rowe et al., 1962; Gardner et al., 1974). A similar virus

*This agent is most often referred to as murine cytomegalovirus in the literature. In this report the designation mouse cytomegalovirus is used to distinguish it from those cytomegaloviruses that have been isolated from rats and other members of the family Muridae.

has been isolated from the field mouse *Apodemus sylvaticus* (Kim et al., 1975), but its relationship to MCMV is uncertain.

### *Epizootiology*

MCMV has been reported to occur in approximately 65% of adult wild mice and in only 0.5-3% of laboratory mice (Mannini and Medearis, 1961; Rowe et al., 1962). More recent surveys of laboratory mice have given conflicting results. One study reported 55% of 256 mice from 9 commercial sources (and mice from 8 of the 9 sources) in the United States to be positive for MCMV by enzyme-linked immunosorbent assay (ELISA), while no positives were found using complement fixation (CF) and immunofluorescent antibody (IFA) test (Anderson et al., 1986) In another study of mice from commercial sources in the United States, no ELISA positive mice were found among mice from 4 commercial sources (Classen et al., 1987). Further studies are needed to clarify the prevalence of MCMV in contemporary laboratory mice.

In natural infections of wild mice, the salivary glands (particularly the submaxillary glands) and possibly the pancreas are persistently infected with MCMV. Virus is transmitted via saliva, and infection can persist for life. Since infection is more frequently seen in adult than in young mice, it appears that infection can be acquired throughout extrauterine life. Latent infections can occur in submaxillary glands, B cells, T cells, the prostate, and the testicles (Osborn, 1982). In spleen the cells that become infected are predominantly sinusoidal-lining cells (Mercer et al., 1988).

Vertical transmission can occur but has not been fully explained. Direct passage of the virus across the placenta to the fetus and/or transmission via germ cells have been suggested (Chantler et al., 1979; Brautigam and Oldstone, 1980; Osborn, 1982).

### *Clinical*

Natural infections of MCMV are subclinical (Osborn, 1982).

### *Pathology*

In naturally infected mice large acidophilic intranuclear inclusions can be seen in salivary gland acinar and duct cells. Affected cells are typically enlarged three or four times their normal size (cytomegaly). The submaxillary glands are affected most, the sublinguals less, and the parotids least (Mims and Gould, 1979; Osborn, 1982);

Pathogenesis of experimental MCMV infection in laboratory mice is very complex because it is markedly influenced by virus strain, passage history, dose, route of inoculation, and mouse strain and age. Newborn mice are most susceptible, and resistance increases greatly at 21-28 days of age. Mice of the *H-2*$^{k}$ haplotype (C3H and CBA) have been found to be relatively more resistant to intraperitoneal inoculation of the virus than are mice of the *H-2*$^{d}$ (BALB/c) and *H-2*$^{b}$ (C57BL/6 and C57BL/10) haplotypes, and resistance is thought to be controlled by two loci in the *H-2* region (Chalmer et al., 1977; Osborn, 1982; Price et al., 1987; Quinnan and Manischewitz, 1987).

Numerous models of human cytomegalovirus have been produced by varying the strain, dose, and route of MCMV inoculation into laboratory mice of different ages and strains. These include models of subclinical infection (Osborn and Medearis, 1967; Osborn et al., 1968; Osborn and Shahidi, 1973), intrauterine infection (Medearis, 1964; Johnson, 1969; Basker et al., 1987), fetal and neonatal ear disease (Davis and Hawrisiak, 1977; Davis et al., 1979; Baskar et al., 1983), encephalitis (Lussier, 1973, 1975), glomerulonephritis (Lussier, 1975; Wehner and Smith, 1983), and interstitial pneumonitis (Jordan, 1978; Rose et al., 1982; Shanley et al., 1982).

Athymic (*nu/nu*) mice (Starr and Allison, 1977) and beige (*bg/bg*) mice (Shellam et al., 1981; Papadimitriou et al., 1982) are far more susceptible than their immunocompetent counterparts. The induction of natural killer cells and interferon early after infection are thought to be most important in non-specific defense against MCMV infection (Griffiths and Grundy, 1987). Cellular immunity is thought to be of pivotal importance in MCMV infection, particularly MCMV-specific cytotoxic T lymphocytes, nonspecific natural killer cells, and antibody-dependent killer cells (Quinnan et al., 1978, 1980; Quinnan and Manischewitz, 1979; Bukowski et al., 1984). $CD8^{+}$ $CD4^{-}$ T lymphocytes against early MCMV antigens are thought to be most important in specific defense (Reddehase et al., 1987, 1988; Mutter et al., 1988). Subclinical or latent infections have been activated by many regimens of immunosuppression, most notably antilymphocyte serum alone or in combination with cortisone or cyclophosphamide (Brody and Craighead, 1974; Gardner et al., 1974; Lussier, 1976; Howard et al., 1979; Shanley et al., 1979; Jordan et al., 1982).

### *Diagnosis*

The prevalence of MCMV in contemporary laboratory mice is generally thought to be negligible except in instances in which stocks may have been contaminated by contact with wild mice. Enzyme-linked immunosorbent assays (ELISAs) for MCMV have been developed and compared with the CF and IFA tests for detection of antibodies in mice experimentally infected with the virus (Anderson et al., 1983; Classen et al., 1987; Lussier et al., 1987b). The IFA and CF tests were found to be more sensitive for detecting acute infection, and the ELISAs were more sensitive for detecting persistent infection (Anderson et al., 1983; Lussier et al., 1987b). These methods may prove useful for monitoring laboratory or wild mice for MCMV infection in selected situations (Anderson et al., 1986; Classen et al, 1987; Lussier et al., 1987).

Virus isolation can be accomplished by using mouse embryo fibroblasts and other tissue culture systems (Osborn, 1982).

*Control*

Complete exclusion of wild mice from rodent facilities is essential. In experimental infections of mice, the virus is readily transmitted between cage mates but not from one cage to another. Therefore, with appropriate measures of containment (such as use of filtered cages, use of a hood while cages are changed, and handling the mice by sterile procedures), studies with this agent can be conducted in most facilities without the risk of contaminating other stocks (Osborn, 1982).

*Interference with Research*

Natural MCMV infection in laboratory mice has not been reported to interfere with research. However, acute MCMV infection in laboratory mice due to experimental inoculation of the virus is known to cause severe disturbances in immune responses.

Experimental MCMV infection results in depression of the following:

a. Antibody production (Osborn and Medearis, 1967; Osborn et al., 1968; Howard and Najarian, 1974; Tinghitella and Booss, 1979; Schilt, 1987).

b. Interferon induction (Osborn and Medearis, 1967; Kelsey et al., 1977).

c. Lymphocyte proliferation responses to mitogens (Howard et al., 1974; Selgrade et al., 1976; Booss and Wheelock, 1977a,b; Kelsey et al., 1977; Loh and Hudson, 1981, 1982; Allan et al., 1982) and in mixed lymphocyte cultures (Howard et al., 1974, 1977).

d. Allogeneic skin graft rejection (Howard et al., 1974, 1977; Lang et al., 1976; Dowling et al., 1977).

e. Reduced litter size and increased fetal abnormalities (Baskar et al., 1987).

Experimental MCMV infection can depress (Ho, 1980) or augment (Quinnan et al., 1982) cytotoxic lymphocyte responses.

Experimental MCMV infection increases susceptibility of mice to infection with *Pseudomonas aeruginosa*, *Klebsiella pneumoniae*, *Staphylococcus aureus*, or *Candida albicans* (Hamilton et al., 1976, 1977; Shanley and Pesanti, 1980; Leung and Hashimoto, 1986; Kournikakis and Babiuk, 1987) or Newcastle disease virus (Osborn and Medearis, 1967).

Experimental MCMV infection in mice can cause thrombocytopenia (Osborn and Shahidi, 1973).

Experimental MCMV infection has been reported to exacerbate the naturally occuring dystrophic cardiac calcification in BALB/c mice (Gang et al., 1986).

## Rat Cytomegalovirus

### *Significance*

Low

### *Perspective*

There are no known reports of natural cytomegalovirus (CMV) infections in laboratory rats. Acidophilic intranuclear inclusions thought to be due to CMV infection have been observed from time to time in the submaxillary salivary glands or kidneys of wild rats (Thompson, 1932; Kuttner and Wang, 1934; Syverton and Larson, 1947). More recently, three different CMV isolates have been obtained from wild rats: *Rattus norvegicus* in The Netherlands (Bruggemen et al., 1982) and England (Priscott and Tyrrell, 1982) and *Rattus rattus* in Panama (Rabson et al., 1969). These agents may have importance as potential contaminants of laboratory rats and as model infections for the study of CMV host-parasite relationships.

### *Agent*

Enveloped, double-stranded DNA virus, family Herpesviridae, subfamily Bethaherpesvirinae, CMV group. The rat CMV (RCMV) of Bruggeman et al. (1982) is the most extensively studied of the cytomegaloviruses isolated from *R. norvegicus*. Its morphologic and cultural characteristics are typical of the CMV group and comparable to those of mouse CMV (MCMV). However, RCMV appears to be distinctly different from MCMV based on results of DNA homology studies (Meijer et al., 1984).

### *Host*

RCMV strains have been reported to occur naturally only in wild rats, *R. norvegicus* (Bruggeman et al., 1982; Priscott and Tynell, 1982) and *R. rattus* (Rabson et al., 1969).

### *Epizootiology*

RCMV was originally isolated from the salivary glands of eight of ten wild rats (Bruggeman et al., 1982). After experimental infection of rats with RCMV by either subcutaneous or intraperitoneal inoculation, the virus appears at low titer in many organs, including brown fat (Bruggeman et al., 1987), during the first few weeks, and subsequently is found only in salivary glands (at high titer) where it persists for at least several months. The virus is shed in saliva and urine (Bruggeman et al., 1985). Although the salivary gland is the primary site of infection, persistent, latent infection is thought to occur in many organs (Bruning et al., 1986).

### *Clinical*

Natural infections of RCMV are subclinical (Bruggeman et al., 1982). Clinical illness does not occur even after the inoculation of rats with high doses of the virus (Bruggeman et al., 1985).

### *Pathology*

Experimental infections of RCMV were studied in LEW and BN rats by Bruggeman et al. (1983a). Four- to five-week-old rats were inoculated intraperitoneally with salivary gland suspensions containing the virus. Subsequently, rats were killed at intervals for attempted isolation of virus from salivary glands, spleens, and kidneys. Maximal virus titers were reached in salivary glands at 1 month post infection. Intranuclear inclusions typical of CMV infection were present in duct cells of the salivary glands, and clusters of virions typical of CMV were demonstrated in these cells by electron microscopy. Culture methods successfully detected virus in salivary glands of LEW rats for up to 12 months but in BN rats for only 5 months. Immunosuppression with cyclophosphamide or x-irradiation successfully reactivated the infection. Cocultivation of spleen cells from latently or chronically infected rats also was successful in recovering the virus. The intraperitoneal administration of interferon was shown to reduce the amount of virus recovered after experimental infection (Bruggeman et al., 1983b).

For purposes of differential diagnosis, it is imperative that morphologic peculiarities of the lacrimal glands in the rat be discussed here. Lyon et al. (1959) observed intranuclear inclusions and cytomegaly in the exorbital and intraorbital lacrimal glands of male rats from eight colonies and attributed them to CMV, although no virus was isolated. Meier (1960) observed cytomegalic inclusion body disease in the lacrimal glands of adult male and female SD (Sprague-Dawley®) rats from a cesarean-derived colony and claimed that passage of cell-free filtrates of these glands to newborn rats resulted in 20% of deaths due to systemic cytomegalic inclusion body disease. Meier's (1960) report, however, is probably best discounted altogether because it lacked both a meaningful morphologic description of the lesions and supporting evidence that a virus was involved.

The lesions described in the exorbital and intraorbital lacrimal glands of male rats by Lyon et al. (1959) are entirely compatible with the normal sexual dimorphism that occurs in these glands in the rat. The lacrimal glands of prepubertal rats are composed of small, closely packed acini of serous cells with small (5-7 µm), round to oval nuclei located in the basal position. At sexual maturity the lacrimal glands of male rats undergo dramatic changes. The acini and some of the nuclei enlarge, and the nuclei become more randomly distributed in the cytoplasm. Some of the acinar cells appear to be hypertrophic (cytomegalic) and contain markedly enlarged nuclei. The larger nuclei are often 20 µm or more in diameter; often irregular and lobulated in shape; and may contain inclusions or vacuoles of varying size, shape, and staining affinity. Under the light microscope these inclusions appear to be bounded by discrete basophilic membranes rather than halos, as are characteristically seen surrounding viral inclusions. The electron microscope, however, reveals that the discrete membrane is actually nuclear membrane; the inclusions, which contain varying amounts of cytoplasmic organelles, are formed by herniation of the nuclear membrane into the nucleus (Cordier and de Harven, 1960; Gaertner et al., 1988). In older animals patches of acini have uniformly small nuclei, foamy (vesicular-mucus) cytoplasm, and dilated acinar lumens, and thus resemble the Harderian gland. Similar but relatively very mild changes can be seen in the lacrimal glands of female rats (Walker, 1958; Baquiche, 1959; Cavallero, 1967; Klinge and Siveke, 1971; Paulini et al., 1972a, b; Paulini and Mohr, 1975; Gaertner et al., 1988).

### *Diagnosis*

An enzyme-linked immunosorbent assay has been found to be very sensitive for the detection of antibodies to RCMV after experimental infection (Bruggeman et al., 1983a), but is not generally available for routine use. In active infections, the virus can be isolated from tissues such as the salivary gland and the spleen by using the rat embryo fibroblast culture technique. Light and electron microscopy of salivary glands for inclusions and virions of CMV would also be of value. Latent infections can be activated by x-irradiation or cyclophosphamide-induced immunosuppression, followed by attempted virus isolation by using rat embryo fibroblasts (Bruggeman et al., 1983a).

### *Control*

Exclusion of wild rats from laboratory rodent facilities is apparently the only measure necessary to control RCMV infection.

*Interference with Research*

Natural infections of RCMV have not been reported in laboratory rats. Experimental RCMV infection has been reported to alter peritoneal macrophage functions (Hendrix et al., 1986) and transiently suppressed humoral response to sheep red blood cells during the weeks following infection (Bruggeman et al., 1985). Experimental infection with RCMV (strain of Priscott and Tyrrell, 1982) exacerbates the arthritis in type II collagen-induced arthritis in rats (Smith et al., 1986). RCMV infection can be transferred to recipient rats in organs transplanted from latently infected rats (Bruning et al., 1986).

## Mouse Thymic Virus

*Significance*

Uncertain, probably low.

*Perspective*

Rowe and Capps (1961) discovered this virus during studies in which specimens from mice suspected of containing mouse mammary tumor virus were being passaged in newborn mice. The only observed effect in the recipient mice was severe necrosis of the thymus, and the virus was named mouse thymic virus (MTV). Subsequent investigations of this agent have been severely hampered because no cell culture system has been found that will support its growth (Osborn, 1982).

*Agent*

MTV is considered a herpesvirus because of its ultrastructural features and its properties of heat and ether lability (Rowe and Capps, 1961; Parker et al., 1973). Intranuclear particles have a complete nucleoid and measure approximately 100 nm in diameter compared to cytoplasmic and extracellular particles, which are 135 nm in diameter. Large accumulations of intranuclear filaments measuring 10 nm in diameter also occur in the thymus of infected infant mice (Parker et al., 1973). Infectivity is destroyed by treatment with 20% ether for 2 hours at 2°C or by heating at 50°C for 30 minutes and is greatly reduced by storage at –60°C for short periods (Rowe and Capps, 1961).

MTV has been shown to be antigenically distinct from mouse

cytomegalovirus, another herpesvirus, by immunofluorescent antibody (IFA), complement fixation (CF) and neutralization tests (Cross et al., 1979).

MTV has not been grown successfully in cell cultures (Osborn, 1982).

### *Hosts*

Wild and laboratory mice (Rowe and Capps, 1961; Cross et al., 1979).

### *Epizootiology*

The prevalence of MTV in contemporary mouse stocks is unknown. However, the limited data available suggest that natural infections may be common in both wild and laboratory mice (Rowe and Capps, 1961; Cross, 1973; Lussier et al., 1988a). On the basis of virus isolations from saliva and the use of IFA and CF tests for serum antibody, Cross (1973) found 4 of 15 colonies of laboratory mice and 3 of 4 individual wild mice to be infected with MTV. In a more recent survey using an enzyme-linked immunosorbent assay (ELISA), Lussier et al. (1988a) reported finding 1 of 8 colonies of laboratory mice to be serologically positive for MTV. Wild mice frequently have dual infections of MTV and mouse cytomegalovirus (Rowe and Capps, 1961; Cross, 1973).

Information on the epizootiology of MTV in naturally infected mouse populations is very meager. The virus apparently occurs as a persistent, subclinical infection in the salivary glands with virus shedding in saliva (Cross et al., 1973; Osborn, 1982). MTV has been isolated on one occasion from mammary tissue of a lactating mouse, suggesting that it can be transmitted in milk (Morse, 1987).

Although of questionable applicability to the epizootiology of natural MTV infection, transmission of the virus following intraperitoneal inoculation has been studied (St.-Pierre et al., 1987). Under these conditions, low transmissibility of the virus occurred between cagemates, but not by the transplacental route. Thus, the weight of evidence presently suggests that horizontal transmission is most important, although vertical transmission cannot be ruled out.

### *Clinical*

Natural infections are subclinical (Rowe and Capps, 1961).

### *Pathology*

Although necrosis presumably occurs in the thymus, lymph nodes, and spleen of mice naturally infected with MTV as neonates (Cross, 1973; Wood et al., 1981), it usually goes unnoticed (Rowe and Capps, 1961).

Disease due to MTV infection is age-dependent, i.e., experimental inoculation of the virus causes morphologic lesions and depression of immunologic functions only in mice infected as neonates (before 72 hours of age). The characteristic lesion is lymphoid necrosis in the thymus, lymph nodes, and spleen, with the thymus being most severely affected (Cross, 1973; Wood et al., 1981). Following intraperitoneal inoculation of virus into 24 hour-old mice, virus is first detectable in the thymus on day 3, reaches peak titer on day 7, and disappears by day 14. Macroscopic necrosis of the thymus begins on day 7 and is most severe between days 10 and 14. Intranuclear inclusions are present in thymocytes on days 5 through 10. The weight of the thymus is reduced to only 25% of normal. Subsequently, the necrosis is superseded by a diffuse "granulomatous" response with giant cells. The thymus regains normal histology around day 21 and normal weight by day 42. Necrosis and repair follow similar patterns in the lymph nodes and spleen. After neonatal infection, persistent infection of the salivary glands occurs, but the mice do not produce serum antibody (Cross et al., 1979). In contrast, adult mice infected with the virus develop persistent infections of the salivary glands and produce serum antibody, without the occurrence of lymphoid necrosis (Cross, 1973, 1979; Wood et al., 1981).

The severe lymphoid necrosis seen in mice neonatally infected with MTV involves mainly helper T lymphocytes (Cohen et al., 1975; Mosier et al., 1977) and cytotoxic T lymphocytes (Cohen et al., 1975). There is reduced responsiveness to the T cell mitogens concanavalin A and phytohemagglutinin (Cohen et al., 1975), and reduced graft-versus-host response (Cross et al., 1976). Immunosuppression peaks at about 4 weeks and appears to return to normal by about 12 weeks after infection (Cohen et al., 1975). B lymphocyte functions appear to be unimpaired (Cohen et al., 1975; Morse et al., 1976), except that neonatally infected mice do not produce antibody to the virus (Cross et al., 1979).

### *Diagnosis*

Mice infected postnatally produce serum antibodies that can be detected by ELISA, IFA or CF tests, with the ELISA test being the most sensitive (Lussier et al., 1988 a,b). In cases where neonatal infection is suspected, evidence of MTV infection can be obtained by inoculating pathogen free neonatal mice with salivary gland homogenate, saliva, or other test material followed by histologic examination of their thymuses, lymph nodes, and spleens for lymphoid necrosis and intranuclear inclusions 10-14 days later (Cross, 1973; Wood et al., 1981). In vitro isolation of the virus is impossible as no cell culture system is known to support the growth of MTV (Osborn, 1982).

*Control*

Wild mice presumably serve as the main reservoir of infection and must be excluded from laboratory animal facilities (Lussier et al., 1988a). Periodic health surveillance testing of mouse stocks by ELISA is recommended (Lussier et al., 1988a,b). Elimination of the virus from infected mouse stocks might be possible through isolation of breeding pairs, with selection of progeny by ELISA testing (Lussier et al., 1988a,b) and passage of tissues in neonatal mice to test for development of lymphoid necrosis in thymus, lymph nodes, and spleen (Morse, 1987).

*Interference with Research*

The passage of tissues from mice subclinically infected with MTV in neonatal mice may be inadvertently complicated by the effects of this virus (Rose and Capps, 1961).

**Sialodacryoadenitis Virus**

*Significance*

High.

*Perspective*

*1961*: Innes and Stanton (1961) reported two epizootics in which weanling rats had swollen, thickened necks and red porphyrin pigment along the eyelid margins. Microscopically, there was severe inflammation and edema of the submaxillary salivary glands and Harderian glands (other lacrimal glands were not examined), and the disease was named sialodacryoadenitis. A viral etiology was suspected but virus isolation was not attempted.

*1963*: Hunt (1963) reported a disease in young rats from two shipments. Ten days after receipt, many of the rats had suborbital swelling and conjunctivitis, and a few had keratitis with corneal ulceration. The Harderian and intraorbital lacrimal glands were twice the normal size and were histologically characterized by loss of glandular tissue, hyperplasia and squamous metaplasia of the ductal epithelium, intense histiocytic inflammation, and acidophilic intranuclear inclusions in occasional epithelial cells. The disease was called dacryoadenitis.

*1969*: Jonas et al. (1969) reproduced the disease of salivary and lacrimal glands by intranasally inoculating gnotobiotic rats with an ultrafiltrate of the submaxillary gland from a rat with sialodacryoadenitis.

*1970*: Parker et al. (1970c) isolated and characterized a virus from the lungs of laboratory rats with mild interstitial pneumonia, carried out experimental infections in suckling and weanling F344 and WI (Wistar) rats, and named the virus rat coronavirus (RCV). [This virus is here considered a strain of sialodacryoadenitis virus (SDAV), the best studied of this group of closely related coronaviruses (Jacoby, 1986)].

*1972*: Bhatt et al. (1972) used primary rat kidney cells to isolate a virus from rats with sialodacryoadenitis, characterized the virus, identified it as a coronavirus, and named it SDAV.

*1977*: Weisbroth and Peress (1977) investigated an epizootic of SDAV infection in which lesions were limited to orbital tissues. They proposed the hypothesis that the variability in clinical and morphological expression of the disease due to SDAV was attributable to the occurrence of viral mutants with different tissue tropisms.

*1982*: Maru and Sato (1982) isolated and characterized a strain of SDAV from rats with sialoadenitis in Japan, and called it the causative agent of rat sialoadenitis (CARS). Unlike previous strains, it could be grown in 3T3 cells but not in primary rat kidney cells.

*1986*: Wojcinski and Percy (1986) demonstrated that SDAV produces significant albeit transient disease throughout the respiratory tract, and suggested that the respiratory disease due to SDAV had generally been overlooked except in the studies of RCV.

*1987*: Schoeb and Lindsey (1987) reported experimental evidence that SDAV can exacerbate murine respiratory mycoplasmosis in rats.

### *Agent*

SDAV is an RNA virus, family Coronaviridae, genus *Coronavirus*. It is antigenically related to many other coronaviruses, including mouse hepatitis virus (MHV) (Machii et al., 1988) and human coronavirus (strain OG38). SDAV, RCV, CARS, and other similar coronavirus isolates from rats are considered different strains of the same virus (Bhatt et al., 1977; Jacoby, 1986).

Virions of SDAV measure approximately 114 nm in diameter and have characteristic projections from the surface, giving a crown-like appearance. The virus is relatively unstable. Infectivity is quickly lost at room temperature, freezing to –20°C, heating to 56°C, and exposure to lipid solvents. It has been stored at –60°C for at least 7 years (Jacoby et al., 1979).

SDAV and RCV can be propagated in primary rat kidney and LBC cells (Parker et al., 1970c; Bhatt et al., 1972; Hirano et al., 1985, 1986). CARS grows in 3T3 cells (Maru and Sato, 1982).

### *Hosts*

Rats. Mice have been shown to be susceptible experimentally (Bhatt et al., 1977; Percy et al., 1986, 1988a), but natural infection in mice has not been reported. [A naturally occurring disease similar to SDAV in rats has been reported for mice (Wagner et al., 1969; Maronpot and Chavannes, 1977), but a causative agent was not identified.]

### *Epizootiology*

SDAV is one of the most common viruses in laboratory rats (Parker et al., 1970c). It is *highly contagious*, spreading rapidly within rooms of susceptible rats by contact and aerosol. It is not transmitted vertically. The virus is present in tissues of infected rats for only about 7 days, and there is no carrier state (Hanna et al., 1984; Wojcinski and Percy, 1986). Tissues affected by SDAV infection are mixed (submaxillary) and serous (parotid) salivary glands, lacrimal glands (Harderian, intraorbital, and exorbital), cervical lymph nodes, thymus, and the mucosa of the respiratory tract (Jacoby et al., 1979; Wojcinski and Percy, 1986).

LEW, WAG/Rij, and SHR rats are more susceptible than other strains (Tuchi et al., 1977; Weisbroth and Peress, 1977; Jacoby et al., 1979; Carthew and Slinger, 1981). Less susceptible rat strains include WI (Wistar), SD (Sprague-Dawley®), LE (Long Evans), and F344; they are approximately equal in susceptibility (Percy et al., 1984).

### *Clinical*

Natural infections usually take one of two forms:

a. *Enzootic infection in breeding colonies.* Adults are immune due to previous infection. Suckling rats have transient (1 week or less) conjunctivitis characterized by winking and blinking. Eyelids may adhere together due to exudate. Signs of this form of disease usually are mild and subtle, escaping detection by most observers. All clinical signs usually have disappeared by the time the investigator receives weanlings or older animals (Jacoby et al., 1979).

b. *Epizootic disease in fully susceptible weanlings or adults.* The incubation period is often less than 1 week. Sudden high prevalence of overt disease heralds an explosive outbreak. Signs can include any or all of the following: cervical edema, sneezing, photophobia, nasal and ocular discharge (serous to seropurulent, often porphyrin stained), corneal ulceration, and keratoconus. Characteristically, there is high morbidity and no mortality. Most clinical signs disappear in about a week, but the eyes may be more prominent than normal for 1 or 2 weeks due to inflammation of retro-orbital tissues (Jacoby et al., 1979).

The possibility has been raised that some outbreaks of SDAV infection may be completely asymptomatic (Eisenbrandt et al., 1982). This may be true, but one must remember that enzootic infections can be very mild and transient, and easily overlooked. Severe clinical disease characterized by cervical edema and eye lesions may be the exception rather than the rule.

### *Pathology*

SDAV has a tissue tropism for tubuloalveolar glands of the serous or mixed serous-mucous types, with the submaxillary and parotid salivary glands, exorbital lacrimal, Harderian, and intraorbital lacrimal glands being the major target organs. The cervical lymph nodes, thymus, and respiratory tract also are affected but usually by relatively mild changes (Jacoby et al., 1979; Wojcinski and Percy, 1986; Schoeb and Lindsey, 1987).

SDAV strains from different natural outbreaks also differ in organ tropism; i.e., they vary greatly in relative incidence and severity of disease produced in three organ systems: salivary glands, lacrimal glands, and the respiratory tract. Presumably, such differences in organ tropism explain, at least in part, the variations in pathological (and clinical) expression seen in the natural disease. There is no clear evidence that virus mutation has a role (Weisbroth and Peress, 1977), although this is still an interesting hypothesis. Differences in virulence of SDAV strains and host factors may be important (Nunoya et al., 1977; Tuchi et al., 1977; Utsumi et al., 1978; Jacoby et al., 1979).

The histopathologic changes in salivary and lacrimal glands are characteristic. Diffuse necrosis of alveolar and ductal epithelium occurs about 5 days post infection. Rapid infiltration of polymorphonuclear leukocytes into the necrotic debris and interstitium is accompanied by varying degrees of interstitial edema. Repair of ductal epithelium quickly ensues, becoming hyperplastic and squamous in appearance by 10 days post infection. Intranuclear inclusions are occasionally observed in the ductal epithelium. Continued glandular repair and lymphohistiocytic inflammation follow, with complete restoration of normal glandular architecture by about 30 days post infection (Jonas et al., 1969; Jacoby et al, 1975; Doi et al., 1980).

Eye lesions can include interstitial keratitis, corneal ulceration, keratoconus, synechia, hypopyon, hyphema, and conjunctivitis. Sequelae of the infection can include megaloglobus with lenticular and retinal degeneration (Innes and Stanton, 1961; Hunt, 1963; Jonas et al., 1969; Jacoby et al., 1975, 1979; Lai et al., 1976; Weisbroth and Peress, 1977).

Thymic lesions are limited to focal necrosis of the cortex and medulla with some widening of interlobular septae. Focal necrosis and lymphoid hyperplasia occur in the cervical lymph nodes. Mild interstitial pneumonia has been seen in experimental cases (Jacoby et al., 1975; Bhatt and Jacoby, 1977; Wojcinski and Percy, 1986; Schoeb and Lindsey, 1987).

It has been suggested that SDAV can act as a copathogen in murine respiratory mycoplasmosis due to *Mycoplasma pulmonis* (Jacoby et al., 1975; Bhatt and Jacoby, 1977; Wojcinski and Percy, 1986). Schoeb and Lindsey (1987) have shown experimentally that SDAV infection can exacerbate *Mycoplasma pulmonis* infection in rats.

### *Diagnosis*

Serologic tests are invaluable because subclinical infection is very common. The complement fixation (CF) test was the standard procedure for many years. The enzyme-linked immunosorbent assay (Peters and Collins, 1981, 1983) and indirect immunofluorescence test (Smith, 1983) are more sensitive than the CF test and are now standard in most laboratories. It must be emphasized, however, that a positive result from any or all of these tests is merely indicative of anti-coronavirus antibodies, not prior infection by a specific coronavirus (e.g., SDAV, RCV, CARS, or MHV). Experimental SDAV infections in mice have been shown to result in positive CF tests for SDAV and MHV (Bhatt et al., 1977).

In routine health monitoring it is recommended that histologic sections be taken of both Harderian glands and the submaxillary and parotid salivary glands of each animal. A presumptive diagnosis of SDAV infection often can be based on the characteristic histologic changes in these glands. Lesions may be bilateral or unilateral and are frequently found in animals with negative serologic tests for coronavirus antibody (i.e., lesions appear before seroconversion).

SDAV virus can be isolated by culture methods using primary rat kidney, 3T3 or LBC cells, or by intracerebral inoculation of neonatal mice (Bhatt et al., 1972; Kojima et al., 1980, 1983; Maru and Sato, 1982; Hirano et al., 1985, 1986). The virus can be demonstrated in affected tissues by immunofluorescence for about 7 days postinoculation (Jacoby et al., 1975).

### *Control*

The key to effective control in infected colonies is recognition that SDAV spreads rapidly through rat populations, infected rats shed virus for only about 7 days, and latent infections do not occur. Thus, infections in breeding colonies can be eliminated by quarantining the room, suspending breeding completely, and destroying all newborn pups for 6 to 8 weeks. The same result is achieved in nonbreeding populations through a 6- to 8-week quarantine period during which no new animals are introduced. Recovered rats are considered free of virus. However, there is some question as to the possibility of later reinfection with the same strain or a different strain of SDAV (Jacoby et al., 1979).

Since SDAV is not transmitted vertically, cesarean derivation is a very effective method of control; however, the disease runs its course so rapidly that this technique is usually impractical.

SDAV resists environmental conditions poorly, so fomites probably do not play an important role in transmission (Jacoby et al., 1979).

### *Interference with Research*

SDAV infection can seriously complicate studies involving the eyes, salivary glands, lacrimal glands, or the respiratory tract of rats (Jacoby, 1986). It causes depletion of epidermal growth factor in submaxillary salivary glands that could affect carcinogenesis studies (Percy et al., 1988b). It reduces interleukin-1 production by alveolar macrophages (Boschert et al., 1988) and exacerbates *Mycoplasma pulmonis* infection (Schoeb and Lindsey, 1987). Additional effects of infection that have been reported include reduced food consumption and weight loss (Nunoya et al., 1977; Utsumi et al., 1978, 1980), and reduced breeding performance and slowing of growth rate in young rats (Utsumi et al., 1978, 1980).

## Mouse Hepatitis Virus

### *Significance*

Very high.

### *Perspective*

*1949:* Cheever et al. (1949) at Harvard reported discovery of the JHM strain of mouse hepatitis virus (MHV), and Bailey et al. (1949) associated it with naturally occurring encephalomyelitis in mice.

*1951:* Gledhill and Andrewes (1951) in England discovered a viral agent (later designated MHV-1) that caused fatal hepatitis when passaged in young mice. Subsequently, Gledhill and associates (Gledhill and Dick, 1955; Gledhill and Niven, 1955; Gledhill et al., 1955) showed that the fatal hepatitis was actually due to combined MHV-1 and *Eperythrozoon coccoides* infections, and that several mouse strains differed in susceptibility to MHV-1 infection.

*1960:* Bang and Warwick (1960) showed that the inherited capacity of the mouse macrophage to restrict virus growth was important in the resistance of certain strains of mice to MHV.

*1962:* Kraft (1962a) described a new viral agent that caused diarrhea in suckling mice and named it the lethal intestinal virus of infant mice (LIVIM).

*1963:* Rowe et al. (1963) used a variety of methods to survey seven mouse colonies (including one germfree colony) for MHV and found that five had the infection. They also compared the effectiveness of Trexler-type plastic isolators, filter-covered cages, and open cages in controlling the spread of MHV within their experimental mouse room. Two of the most important conclusions from their work were that MHV was recognized as "a highly contagious, prevalent, enteric infection of mice," and that "precise animal experimentation with these viruses cannot be done without strict isolation facilities and known virus-free mice."

*1963:* East et al. (1963) reported that neonatal thymectomy of mice led to a wasting syndrome resulting from increased susceptibility to MHV.

*1974:* Sebesteny and Hill (1974) reported that MHV was responsible for the wasting syndrome in athymic (*nu/nu*) mice.

*1976:* Broderson et al. (1976b) reported that LIVIM was actually MHV, a concept later confirmed by Carthew (1977).

*1979:* Peters et al. (1979) described a highly sensitive serologic test for MHV, the enzyme-linked immunosorbent assay (ELISA), bringing to an end the long era of reliance on a very insensitive test, complement fixation (CF). The practical result was that MHV soon became recognized as being ubiquitous in contemporary mouse stocks.

*1984:* Barthold and Smith (1984) presented evidence supporting two basic patterns of natural MHV pathogenesis depending on the tropism of virus strains: respiratory and enteric.

### *Agent*

The term mouse hepatitis virus (MHV) is used to designate a large group of single-stranded RNA viruses belonging to the family Coronaviridae, genus *Coronavirus*. Like other coronaviruses, they are surrounded by an envelope with a corona of surface projections called peplomers. The virions are pleomorphic and measure 80-160 nm in diameter. Each peplomer is about 20 nm long by 7 nm wide at the tip (Robb and Bond, 1979; Matthews, 1982; Sturman and Holmes, 1983; Holmes et at., 1986a).

Approximately 25 different strains or isolates of MHV have been described. Of that number, six have been studied most extensively and are generally considered the prototype strains: MHV-1, MHV-2, MHV-3, JHM (MHV-4), A59, and S. The other strains and new isolates of MHV are often compared to the prototype strains by cross-neutralization tests, but antigenic relatedness, as determined by that method, correlates poorly with pathogenicity and has limited usefulness for epizootiologic studies. Other coronaviruses that are antigenically related to MHV include sialodacryoadenitis virus, human coronavirus OC43, hemagglutinating encephalomyelitis virus of pigs, and neonatal calf diarrhea coronavirus (Robb and Bond, 1979; Sturman and Holmes, 1983; Barthold, 1986a,b).

MHV is relatively resistant to repeated freezing and thawing, heating (56°C for 30 minutes), and acid pH but is sensitive to lipid solvents, drying, and disinfectants. It can be stored for 30 days at 4°C and indefinitely at –70°C (Hirano et al., 1978; Robb and Bond, 1979).

MHV is commonly grown in cell cultures, but some strains grow better in certain cell lines than others. Cell lines that have been found to be most useful are NCTC 1469, 17Cl-1, DBT, BALB/c-3T3, and CMT-93 (Barthold et al., 1985).

### *Hosts*

Mice (*Mus musculus*) are considered the natural hosts. Suckling rats have been found to be modestly susceptible to experimental intranasal infection; the virus replicated briefly in the nasal mucosa and there was seroconversion but no clinical signs (Taguchi et al., 1979b). When given the virus intranasally, deer mice (*Peromyscus maniculatus*) developed positive antibody titers but failed to develop clinical illness or transmit the virus to sentinel laboratory mice (Silverman et al., 1982).

### *Epizootiology*

MHV is *extremely contagious*. Infection of the majority of mice housed under conventional conditions in multipurpose facilities is the norm. It is one of the most ubiquitous infections of laboratory mice worldwide, with reported prevalence rates frequently exceeding 80% (Parker, 1980; Lindsey, 1986).

The epizootiology of natural MHV infections has not been studied well because sensitive detection methods were not available until very recently. Numerous factors such as virus strain and mouse strain are known to influence the pathogenesis of MHV infection and may be important determinants of its epizootiology. However, current evidence indicates that in immunocompetent mice the infection runs its course within 2-3 weeks, and there is no carrier state (Barthold, 1986a,b). During active infection virus is shed in the feces and by aerosol. Direct contact, fomites, and airborne particles are all probably very important in transmission (Rowe et al., 1963; Robb and Bond, 1979; Barthold, 1986b). Transplacental transmission is of doubtful importance in natural infections (Piccinino et al., 1966), although it has been achieved by the intravenous inoculation of MHV into pregnant dams (Katami et al., 1978).

MHV has been a frequent contaminant of transplantable tumors (Braunsteiner and Friend, 1954; Nelson, 1959; Manaker et al., 1961; Collins and Parker, 1972; Fox et al., 1977a) and cell lines (Sabesin, 1972; Stohlman and Weiner, 1978; Yoshikura and Taguchi, 1979; Holmes, 1986a).

*Clinical*

MHV infections in immunocompetent mice are usually subclinical. However, inasmuch as numerous factors related to the virus (e.g., virulence and organotropism) and the host (e.g., age, genotype, pathogen status, and experimental modifications) affect disease expression due to MHV, a range of clinical diseases can be anticipated (Barthold, 1986a,b). Most infections follow one of the following clinical patterns:

a. *Enzootic (subclinical) infection.* This has been the most common pattern in the United States because of the high prevalence of MHV in breeding populations. Adults are immune due to prior infection. Newborn mice are protected by maternally derived passive immunity that wanes by weaning age. Infection is perpetuated among partially protected weanlings with little or no clinical disease (unless they are compromised immunologically such as by experimental procedures) (Manaker et al., 1961; Hierholzer et al., 1979; Ishida and Fujiwara, 1982; Barthold, 1986a,b).

b. *Epizootic (clinically apparent) infection.* This is the pattern usually seen in infant mice of naive breeding populations housed in open cages. The infection spreads rapidly through the entire population. In infections due to the more virulent enterotropic strains, diarrhea with high (up to 100%) mortality can be seen in infant mice, whereas only moderate losses of infant mice are usually incurred due to the nonenterotropic strains. Infections in naive adults are usually subclinical (Rowe et al., 1963; Barthold et al., 1982; Barthold, 1986a,b).

c. *Wasting syndrome in athymic (nu/nu) mice.* Athymic mice develop severe generalized disease characterized clinically by progressive emaciation (wasting) leading ultimately to debility and death (Sebesteny and Hill, 1974; Hirano et al., 1975b; Fujiwara et al., 1977; Ward et al., 1977). Jaundice may be observed in some cases. Diarrhea may be a leading sign in cases with enterotropic MHV infection (Barthold et al., 1985).

*Pathology*

Much of the vast literature on MHV infection is not helpful in understanding the pathogenesis of natural MHV infections. In many published studies, inordinately high doses of the virus were inoculated by unnatural routes, mice of unknown (or unstated) pathogen status were used, and few target organs were examined for lesions (Barthold and Smith, 1984). Nevertheless, much has been learned about MHV infection. Strains of MHV differ greatly in virulence and tissue tropism (Taguchi et al., 1983; Barthold and Smith, 1984; Boyle et al., 1987), mouse strains differ greatly in susceptibility to MHV (Knobler et al., 1981; Smith et al., 1984; Barthold, 1986a,b), and these factors interact with host age, and route and dose of virus inoculation to determine the outcome of infection (Barthold, 1986a; Holmes et al., 1986b; Barthold, 1987). Because disease expression depends on interaction of host genotype with virus strain, it is not possible to strictly categorize mouse strains as susceptible or resistant (Barthold, 1986b).

The presence (or absence) of virus receptors on host cells appears to be very important in pathogenesis. SJL/J mice appear to be completely resistant to infection with MHV strain A59 because they lack a specific receptor that is present on plasma membranes of target cells from genetically susceptible mice (Boyle et al., 1987). Such receptors also may explain tissue tropisms of the virus. Barthold and Associates (Barthold et al., 1982, 1985; Barthold and Smith, 1984; Barthold, 1986a,b) have shown that there are two major disease patterns depending on the tropism of virus strains:

a. *Respiratory pattern.* MHV infection consistently involves the nasal passages and lungs with dissemination to other organs by the blood vascular system; intestinal involvement, if present, is minimal. After experimental infection, the virus appears sequentially in nasal mucosa; then lungs; and then other organs including lymph nodes, thymus, spleen, bone marrow, brain, liver, and intestine. The majority of MHV strains are thought to follow this pattern, but the evidence is best for MHV-1, MHV-2, MHV-3, A59, S, JHM, Tettnang, and wt-1 (Barthold and Smith, 1984; Barthold, 1986a,b).

b. *Enteric pattern.* MHV infection is primarily restricted to the nasal passages and bowel, with variable spread to other abdominal organs such as the liver and abdominal lymph nodes but usually not to the lungs, although a few strains are known to spread to other sites such as brain. MHV strains that follow this pattern include LIVIM, MHV-S/CDC, MHV-D, DVIM, MHV-Y, and wt-2 (Barthold and Smith, 1984; Barthold, 1986a,b).

The respiratory and enteric patterns of disease are considered basic, relative patterns of pathogenesis because some overlap between the two patterns is known to occur in infections caused by some strains of MHV. Variations in these patterns also can occur because of other factors such as host age, genotype, and immune status and concurrent infections (Barthold and Smith, 1983, 1984; Barthold, 1986a,b).

In immunocompetent mice, not immunosuppressed by an experimental regimen or by another infection, the lesions of MHV infection are present for only a brief period (7-10 days) following infection. Also, they are usually nonspecific and subtle, particularly those that follow the respiratory pattern. For example, the following lesions have been observed in 3-week-old mice following the intranasal inoculation of MHV-S, a strain with respiratory tropism: mild olfactory mucosal necrosis, neuronal necrosis of olfactory bulbs and tracts, lymphoplasmacytic infiltrates and vacuolation in the brain, multifocal interstitial pneumonia with mild perivascular lymphoid infiltrates, and multifocal necrotizing hepatitis (Taguchi et al., 1979a; Barthold and Smith, 1983). Lesions caused by the enterotropic strains of MHV are mainly confined to the intestinal tract and are most severe in neonatal mice because of their relatively slow kinetics of mucosal epithelium turnover (or replacement). Varying degrees of epithelial lysis and blunting of villi occur in the small intestine. Numerous multinucleate syncytial giant cells (balloon cells) may occur on the villi as well as in the crypts. Ulcerations of the mucosa may be seen in the more severe cases. A similar lytic process with the presence of syncytial giant cells occurs in the cecum and ascending colon. Severe typhlocolitis has been observed in some outbreaks. On occasion cases may be seen with multifocal necrotizing hepatitis and/or encephalitis (Biggers et al., 1964; Ishida et al., 1978; Hierholzer et al., 1979; Ishida and Fujiwara, 1979; Sugiyama and Amano, 1981; Barthold et al., 1982; Perlman et al., 1987, 1988).

The pathogenesis of MHV infection in athymic (*nu/nu*) and neonatally thymectomized mice also appears to follow the basic respiratory and enteric patterns. However, in these T-cell-deficient mice the infection and resulting disease tend to become progressively more generalized, severe, and chronic, with involvement of many organs, including brain, liver, lungs, bone marrow, lymphoreticular organs, vascular endothelium, and intestine. In the liver areas of multifocal necrosis appear with a zone of acute inflammatory cells and variable numbers of multinucleate giant cells at their periphery, followed by partial replacement of hepatocytes and continuing necrosis, leading to chronic active hepatitis if the animal survives long enough. Grossly, the liver appears shrunken, with the darker pits and grooves representing areas of hepatocyte loss and the lighter ridges representing areas of relatively normal hepatocytes. Small proliferative lesions with few to several syncytial cells may be seen on endothelial surfaces of many organs, particularly lungs and brain. Syncytial giant cells can occur in lymph nodes, on mesothelial surfaces, and at other sites. Splenomegaly may occur because of compensatory myelopoiesis, and large numbers of myelopoietic cells may appear in the liver (Hirano et al., 1975b; Fujiwara et al., 1977; Tamura et al., 1977; Ward et al., 1977; Ishida et al., 1978; Furuta et al., 1979; Barthold, 1986a). One outbreak has been reported in which athymic (*nu/nu*) mice were found to be infected with an enterotropic strain of MHV and had chronic hyperplastic typhlocolitis as the predominant lesion (Barthold et al., 1985).

The mechanisms of host resistance to MHV infection are poorly understood. There is strong evidence that mice are fully susceptible to the virus as neonates, but some strains acquire resistance at 2-3 weeks of age as lymphoreticular function matures, with the result that older mice have a spectrum of relative susceptibility ranging from susceptible to highly resistant (Shif and Bang, 1970; Hirano et al., 1975a; Taguchi et al., 1977, 1979c). Humoral immunity is considered relatively unimportant. Cell-mediated immunity is clearly important because of the high susceptibility of athymic (*nu/nu*) mice. Also, there is evidence that macrophages (Bang and Warwick, 1960; Weiser and Bang, 1977), interferon (Robb and Bond, 1979; Garlinghouse et al., 1984; Garlinghouse and Smith, 1985), and natural killer cells (Bukowski et al., 1983; Pereira et al., 1984) have important roles. Infection of mice with one strain of virus confers strong resistance to that strain, but not necessarily to other strains (Barthold and Beck, 1987).

*Diagnosis*

The enzyme-linked immunosorbent assay (ELISA) is the test of choice for routine serologic monitoring because it is far more sensitive than the CF or serum neutralization tests (Peters et al., 1979; Peters and Collins, 1983). An immunofluorescent antibody (IFA) test also is available and is about equal to the ELISA in sensitivity (Smith, 1983). The heterozygotes of nude mice or sentinel mice should be used in testing nude mouse stocks; nude mice do not develop CF antibody in response to MHV and only weak and variable ELISA or serum neutralization antibody responses (Barthold, 1986a).

A presumptive necropsy diagnosis of active enterotropic MHV infection in either clinical or subclinical infections is relatively easy to make based on typical lesions in the small and/or large intestine. The blunting of intestinal villi due to the loss of villous epithelium plus the presence of large, multinucleate syncytial giant cells in the mucosal epithelium of the small intestine, cecum, and/or ascending colon are virtually diagnostic. Lesions of MHV infection in other organs are usually nonspecific and often very subtle. An immunofluorescence method has been developed for identifying MHV antigen in formalin-fixed, paraffin-embedded tissue, but it is not practical for routine diagnostic purposes (Brownstein and Barthold, 1982).

MHV can often be isolated by cell culture methods by using NCTC 1469, 17C1-1, DBT, BALB/c-3T3, or CMT-93 cells; but all strains do not grow equally well in all cell lines (Barthold et al., 1985). It also is essential that tissues with a high titer of virus be used for attempted virus isolations. Frequently, the best approach is to expose pathogen-free athymic (*nu/nu*) mice to animals with suspected infection and use the livers from the nude mice with clinical disease for virus isolation (Barthold, 1986b). Cross-neutralization testing may be used for determining the antigenic relatedness of wild-type isolates to prototype strains (Barthold and Smith, 1984).

Transplantable tumors and other biologic materials from mice may be screened for MHV by isolating the virus in cell cultures and/or by the mouse antibody production (MAP) test (Rowe et al., 1959a, 1962).

*Control*

MHV is both highly contagious and highly prevalent in breeding populations of mice. Therefore, the strictest adherence to systematic measures of pathogen exclusion is required to prevent entrance of this agent into research facilities. MHV-free mice must be identified by regular health monitoring of supplier subpopulations, transported to the user facility in filter-protected cartons to prevent infection en route, quarantined in a barrier room at the receiving institution until tested and shown to be free of infection, and subsequently maintained by strict barrier protocol with regular health surveillance testing to check the effectiveness of the barrier. In addition, all biologic materials from mice such as transplantable tumors coming into the institution must be screened and shown to be free of infectious agents before experimental use in animals (Collins and Parker, 1972).

Once MHV infection has been diagnosed in a facility, the affected population should be either promptly eliminated or quarantined in an area or facility completely away from pathogen-free mice as MHV is highly contagious. Cesarean derivation followed by barrier maintenance has traditionally been recommended for rederivation of breeding stocks. However, recent evidence suggests that MHV infections in immunocompetent mice may have an acute course, with complete elimination of the virus in about 2 weeks (Weir et al., 1987; Barthold, 1986b). Thus, a practical alternative to cesarean derivation is the isolation of individual breeding pairs of mice from MHV-infected populations in separate containment devices such as filter-top cage systems (Sedlacek et al., 1981), with subsequent selection of seronegative progeny as breeders (Weir et al., 1987).

### *Interference with Research*

An extremely large number of effects of MHV on mice and their biologic responses to experimental treatments have been observed. Some occurred as a result of natural infections or conditions simulating natural infections, while others were observed under somewhat artificial experimental circumstances (e.g., large doses of virus inoculated by unnatural routes such as intraperitoneally). Both types of examples are included in the following extensive (albeit incomplete) lists.

In athymic (*nu/nu*) mice, MHV infection:

a. Can cause *severe* destructive lesions in many organs, including intestine, liver, brain, lungs, spleen, lymph nodes, and bone marrow (Sebesteny and Hill, 1974; Fujiwara et al., 1977; Ward et al., 1977; Ishida et al., 1978).

b. Causes spontaneous differentiation of lymphocytes bearing T-cell markers (Scheid et al., 1975; Tamura et al., 1978b).

c. Alters IgM and IgG responses to sheep erythrocytes (Tamura et al., 1978b; Tamura and Fujiwara, 1979).

d. Enhances phagocytic activity of macrophages (Tamura et al., 1980).

e. Is made more severe by experimental insults, such as injection of silica dust, that interfere with macrophage function (Tamura et al., 1979).

f. Causes rejection of xenograft tumors (Kyriazis et al., 1979; Akimaru et al., 1981).

g. Impairs liver regeneration after partial hepatectomy (Carthew, 1981).

h. Causes hepatosplenic myelopoiesis (Ishida et al., 1978).

In immunocompetent mice, MHV infection:

a. Causes immunosuppression or immunostimulation during acute infection and chronic immunodepression in persistent infection (Virelizier et al., 1976).

b. Inhibits lymphocyte proliferative responses in mixed lymphocyte cultures and mitogen-stimulated cells (Krzystyniak and Dupuy, 1983).

c. Inhibits immunoglobulin secretion by Peyer's patch B cells (Casebolt et al., 1987).

d. Depresses phagocytic activity (Gledhill et al., 1965; Williams and DiLuzzio, 1980).

e. Increases the number and tumoricidal activity of peritoneal macrophages in infected mice (Boorman et al., 1982).

f. Increases hepatic uptake of injected iron (Tiensiwakul and Husain, 1979).

g. Increases susceptibility to other indigenous mouse pathogens (and vice versa), including *Eperythrozoon coccoides* (Niven et al., 1952; Gledhill et al., 1965; Lavelle and Bang, 1973), K virus (Tisdale, 1963), leukoviruses (Nelson, 1952a,b; Braunsteiner and Friend, 1954; Gledhill, 1961; Manaker et al., 1961), and *Schistosoma mansoni* (Warren et al., 1969).

h. Activates natural killer cells and production of local and circulating interferon (Mallucci, 1964; Tardieu et al., 1980; Schindler et al., 1982).

i. Diminishes the production of interferon in response to infection with Sendai virus (Virelizier et al., 1976).

j. Alters the course of concurrent viral infections due to pneumonia virus of mice or Sendai virus (Carrano et al., 1984).

k. Alters the course of experimental ascites myeloma (Nelson, 1959; Fox et al., 1977a).

l. Alters hepatic enzyme activity (Ruebner and Hirano, 1965; Cacciatore and Antoniello, 1971; Budillon et al., 1972, 1973; Paradisi et al., 1972; Carter et al., 1977).

m. Slows liver regeneration after partial hepatectomy (Carthew, 1981) and increases proliferative activity of liver and bowel during the recovery phase of infection (Carthew, 1981; Barthold et al., 1982).

n. Induces production of serum $\alpha$-fetoprotein (Piazza et al., 1965).

o. Induces macrophage procoagulant activity (Levy et al., 1981).

p. Causes anemia, leukopenia, and thrombocytopenia (Piazza et al., 1965; Hunstein et al., 1969; Namiki et al., 1977).

q. Delays the increase in plasma lactic dehydrogenase activity following infection with lactic dehydrogenase virus (Dillberger et al., 1987).

r. Subclinical infections (of MHV) are transformed into severe disease with mortality by thymectomy (East et al., 1963; Dupuy et al., 1975; Sheets et al., 1978), cortisone (Starr and Pollard, 1958; Gallily et al., 1964; Vella and Starr, 1965; Taylor et al., 1981), cyclophosphamide (Willenborg et al., 1973), whole body irradiation (Vella and Starr, 1965; Dupuy et al., 1975), anti-lymphocyte serum (Riet et al., 1973; Dupuy et al., 1975; Levy-Leblond and Dupuy, 1977), reticuloendothelial blockade by iron salts (Warren et al., 1968), chemotherapeutic agents (Braunsteiner and Friend, 1954), and halothane anesthesia (Moudgil, 1973).

s. Resistance (to MHV) in mice is increased by giving glucan, a macrophage stimulant (Williams and DiLuzzio, 1980); concanavalin A, a mitogen (Weiser and Bang, 1977); triolein (Lavelle and Starr, 1969); *Corynebacterium parvum* (Schindler et al., 1981); and silica (Schindler et al., 1984).

MHV is notorious as a contaminant of transplantable tumors (Braunsteiner and Friend, 1954; Nelson, 1959; Manaker et al., 1961; Collins and Parker, 1972; Fox et al., 1977a) and cell lines (Sabesin, 1972; Stohlman and Weiner, 1978; Yoshikura and Taguchi, 1979), including hybridomas (Holmes, 1986a).

## Mouse Rotavirus

### *Significance*

Low.

### *Perspective*

There are three main phases in the work concerned with mouse rotavirus (MRV) and the disease it causes:

*1947-1956:* Discovery of MRV infection and other early work of Cheever, Papenheimer, and colleagues at Harvard (Cheever and Mueller, 1947, 1948; Papenheimer and Enders, 1947; Papenheimer and Cheever, 1948; Cheever, 1956). The disease was called epidemic diarrheal disease of suckling mice. The infectious nature of the disease, its clinical manifestations, and influence of parity of dams on survival of young were emphasized.

*1957-1967:* Work of Kraft and associates (Kraft, 1957, 1958, 1961, 1962a, 1966; Adams and Kraft, 1963, 1967; Biggers et al., 1964; Kraft et al., 1964). The disease name was changed to epizootic diarrhea of infant mice (EDIM), and the causative agent was shown to be a virus. The clinical syndrome was described and contrasted with a second diarrheal syndrome caused by lethal intestinal virus of infant mice (LIVIM). Filter-top cages were introduced for control of the two diarrheal syndromes.

*1968-1988:* Period of improving diagnostic methodology for distinguishing MRV and mouse hepatitis virus (MHV) infections, and recognizing the relatively low importance of MRV as a natural infection of mice. LIVIM was shown to be MHV (Broderson et al., 1976; Carthew, 1977a). No natural epizootic of clinical disease due to MRV was reported in mice during this period.

### *Agent*

MRV is a double-stranded RNA virus, family Reoviridae, genus *Rotavirus*, group A. Although MRV shares a common antigen(s) with the group A rotaviruses, it is serotypically distinct from them. Also, serotypic and genomic differences have been found among isolates of MRV (Greenberg et al., 1986). Spherical virus particles 65-80 nm in diameter occur in the cytoplasm of the intestinal epithelium, and tubular structures about 60 nm in diameter occur in both the cytoplasm and the nucleus. It is unstable at –24, 4, and 37°C. It is not resistant to environmental conditions (Banfield et al., 1968; Woode et al., 1976; Flewett and Woode, 1978; Much and Zajac, 1978; Wolf et al., 1981; Kraft, 1982; Greenberg et al., 1983).

MRV has been grown successfully in trypsinized primary monkey kidney cells and in the continuous rhesus monkey kidney cell line MA 104 (Tajima et al., 1984; Greenberg et al., 1986).

### *Hosts*

Mice (Carthew, 1977b; Flewett and Woode, 1978; Kraft, 1982). Other rotaviruses are recognized as important causes of neonatal diarrhea in children, rabbits, piglets, calves, lambs, foals, and many other young animals.

### *Epizootiology*

MRV is generally held to be a widely prevalent, important pathogen of mice, but this has not been documented for contemporary mouse stocks. Carthew (1977b) reported a small survey in England in which complement-fixing antibodies to rotavirus were found in 47% of mouse colonies and 16% of rat colonies.

Transmission is by airborne infection in which contaminated dust and bedding from adjacent cages probably play key roles (Kraft, 1957), hence the reason that filter-top cages are useful. Mice are most susceptible to infection from birth to about 17 days of age. Infected neonates shed high concentrations of virus in the feces from about 2 days to 8-10 days post infection. Transient viremia and viruria can occur. Mice infected after about 17 days of age shed lower concentrations of virus in the feces for 2-4 days. It is not known whether there is persistent infection or whether very low concentrations of virus are shed in the feces beyond these time points. There is no evidence of transplacental transmission (Malherbe, 1978; Kraft, 1982; Little and Shadduck, 1982; Eydelloth et al., 1984; Eiden et al., 1986a; Starkey et al., 1986; Riepenhoff-Talty et al., 1987; Osborne et al., 1988).

### *Clinical*

Diarrhea during the first two weeks of life is considered the only consistent sign of disease. Watery, yellow stools usually begin around 48 hours post infection and persist for about one week. Varying amounts of stool accumulate around the anus and base of the tail, and soil the coats of neonates and dams. Affected neonates may appear lethargic and have distended abdomens. Usually there is no mortality. Mice infected with MRV as adults show no clinical signs (Kraft, 1982; Little and Shadduck, 1982).

Some clinical manifestations, particularly the mortality sometimes attributed to MRV in the earlier literature, do not fit with current knowledge. For example, Cheever and Mueller (1948) observed high infant mortality. Survival of young increased with increasing parity of the dams: approximately one-third of infants survived in first litters, one-half in second and third litters, and three-quarters in fourth and fifth litters, presumably because of increasing maternal antibody in the milk. This high mortality was more likely due to some other intercurrent infection(s), possibly mouse hepatitis virus (Kraft, 1982). The observation that increasing age and parity of dams in infected colonies was associated with protection of young can not be fully explained although it has now been shown that some degree of protection against infection (not disease) is afforded infected neonates suckled by dams with pre-existing antibody to MRV (Runner and Palm, 1953; Little and Shadduck, 1982).

### *Pathology*

Susceptibility to infection and disease (diarrhea) due to MRV is age dependent, and occurs from birth to about 17 days of age with the peak period of susceptibility being from four days to 14 days of age (Wolf et al., 1981; Eydelloth et al., 1984). During this time enterocytes in the small intestine are particularly susceptible to infection and support maximal cytoplasmic replication of the virus, possibly due in part to the high pinocytotic activity of enterocytes (Clark, 1959; Wolf et al., 1981) or availability of viral receptors on enterocytes (Reipenhoff-Talty et al., 1982).

The occurrence of diarrhea and histopathologic changes in the small intestine parallel virus concentrations in the epithelium. In animals older than about 18 days of age, small numbers of enterocytes become infected, there is little replication of virus and diarrhea does not occur (Little and Shadduck, 1982; Eydelloth et al., 1984; Starkey et al., 1986; Osborne et al., 1988).

Infection progresses from proximal to distal parts of the intestine, involving sequentially the duodenum, jejunum, ileum, and colon. Virus infects primarily enterocytes in the apical one-fourth to one-third of intestinal villi, causing degeneration and sloughing of these cells into the lumen. Thus, the major pathologic change is mild villous atrophy. Since the crypt epithelium is spared, regeneration occurs rapidly. Grossly, the intestines usually contain watery fluid and gas bubbles during the period of clinical diarrhea (Moon, 1978; Little and Shadduck, 1982).

Although the precise mechanisms are unknown, both passively and actively acquired humoral immunity are thought to be important in host defense. Infant mice that nurse rotavirus seropositive dams have partial resistance to experimental MRV infection for three to four days after birth, presumably due to specific IgG and/or IgA in colostrum (Little and Shadduck, 1982; Sheridan et al., 1983). Also, diarrhea and shedding of virus in the feces occur 2 or 3 days longer in infant mice nursing seronegative dams (Little and Shadduck, 1982). In neonates nursed on seronegative dams anti-rotavirus IgA appears in the intestine by seven days post infection and specific IgG appears around 14 days post infection (Sheridan et al., 1983). Neonatal athymic (*nu*/*nu*) mice experimentally infected with MRV experience a self-limiting infection identical to that seen in age-matched immunocompetent mice (Eiden et al., 1986a). In contrast, severe combined immunodeficient (*scid*/*scid*) mice have higher percentages of enterocytes infected, achieve greater concentrations of virus in intestinal epithelium, shed higher concentrations of virus for longer periods of time in the feces, and remain persistently infected (Riepenhoff-Talty et al., 1987a,b). Vacuolation (lipid droplets) in the epithelium of the small intestine has been emphasized as a response to MRV (Adams and Kraft, 1967). In MRV infection numerous cytoplasmic vacuoles of varying size and distribution occur in the mucosal epithelium, near the tips of villi (Starkey et al., 1986; Osborne et al., 1988), a change that should not be confused with the orderly distension of the cytoplasm by very large vacuoles seen in the intestinal epithelium of entire villi in normal neonatal animals (Moon, 1972), including mice (T. R. Schoeb and J. R. Lindsey, Department of Comparative Medicine, University of Alabama at Birmingham, unpublished). Papenheimer and Enders (1947) described intranuclear inclusions in the intestinal epithelium of infected mice that are compatible with inclusions now recognized as being due to mouse adenovirus-2 (Van der Veen and Mes, 1974; Luethans and Wagner, 1983; Hamelin et al., 1988).

*Diagnosis*

Detection of anti-rotaviral antibodies can be accomplished by complement fixation (CF) (Blackwell, 1966; Wilsnack et al., 1969; Carthew, 1977b), radioimmunoassay (Wolf et al., 1981), immunofluorescent antibody (IFA) test (Smith et al., 1983), enzyme-linked immunosorbent assay (ELISA) (Ghose et al., 1978; Sheridan et al., 1983; Smith et al., 1983), and numerous other methods (Kraft, 1982; Ferner et al., 1987). A homologous enzyme immunoassay inhibition method utilizing MRV-derived reagents has been considered the most efficient (Ferner et al., 1987) The ELISA and IFA are available commercially.

Definitive diagnosis of diarrheal disease due to MRV can be made by demonstration of lesions compatible with MRV infection in the small intestine, demonstration of MRV antigen in the intestine or feces, and isolation of the virus by using trypsinized primary monkey kidney cells (Tajima et al., 1984; Greenberg et al., 1986). Radioimmunoassay (Cukor et al., 1978; Wolf et al., 1981), immunofluorescence (Wilsnack et al., 1969), electron microscopy (Wolf et al., 1981), and polyacrylamide gel electrophoresis of the viral genome (Smith et al., 1983) have been used to demonstrate rotaviruses in the intestinal tract. A commercially available ELISA (Rotazyme II, Abbott Laboratories, North Chicago, Ill.) for this purpose has been found to give a high proportion of false positives in testing fecal specimens from mice, but the problem could be eliminated by pretreatment of test beads with 0.1% bovine serum albumin (Jure et al., 1987).

*Control*

Cesarean derivation followed by barrier maintenance has traditionally been recommended for rederivation of breeding stocks, but it is not known whether this approach is necessary to eliminate MRV. It probably would be necessary for *scid/scid* mice that are known to become persistently infected and to shed the virus in feces for many months, perhaps for life (Riepenhoff-Talty et al., 1987a,b). For immunocompetent and athymic (*nu/nu*) mice, it may be that virus is shed for only a few weeks after the acute infection. If so, this would permit the isolation and quarantine of individual breeding pairs with subsequent selection of MRV seronegative progeny for breeding, as has been achieved with certain other agents (Lipman et al., 1987; Weir et al., 1987).

Use of filter-top cage systems can be beneficial in controlling transmission of infection between subpopulations in the same room. To be most effective these systems require that rooms be closed to the entry of outside animals, that filter covers be removed from one cage at a time (and only while the cage is inside a transfer cabinet within the room), and that measures be taken to avoid cross-contamination between cages during handling of mice (Kraft, 1958; Jennings and Rumpf, 1965; Schneider and Collins, 1966; Poiley, 1967).

Vaccination may be useful in the control of MRV in some instances. Neonatal mice born to dams that have been vaccinated with purified empty capsids of simian rotavirus SA-11 have been found to be protected from diarrheal disease when challenged with MRV (Sheridan et al., 1984).

### *Interference with Research*

Infection can alter results of studies with infant mice. Protein-calorie deprivation of nursing dams has been found to result in increased severity of diarrhea, increased mortality, and reduced weight gains of their infant pups infected with MRV (Noble et al., 1983; Offor et al., 1985). Folic acid deficiency also has been reported to increase the severity of diarrheal disease due to MRV (Morrey et al., 1984). Infant mice with MRV infection have increased mortality when challenged with enterotoxigenic *Escherichia coli* (Newsome and Coney, 1985). MRV infection alters intestinal absorption (Ijaz et al., 1987) and intestinal enzyme profiles (Collins et al., 1988).

## Rat Rotavirus-Like Agent

### *Significance*

Uncertain.

### *Perspective*

Rat rotavirus-like agent (RVLA) was recently discovered as the cause of a spontaneous outbreak of diarrhea in suckling rats in Baltimore, Maryland (Vonderfecht et al., 1984). A similar, if not identical, virus was subsequently found to be a prevalent infection associated with diarrhea in human adults and children in that city (Eiden et al., 1985).

### *Agent*

RVLA is a double-stranded RNA virus, family Reoviridae, genus *Rotavirus*, group B (tentative classification). Virions are spherical, 65-80 nm in diameter, and composed of capsomeres with cubic symmetry. It is antigenically and genetically related to group B rotaviruses from pigs and calves with diarrhea (Eiden et al., 1986b) and Chinese group B rotavirus from diarrheic human patients (Hung et al., 1984). RVLA resists treatment with ether or acidification to pH 5 but is inactivated by pH 3 or heating at 56°C for 30 minutes. It has not been grown in cell cultures (Vonderfecht et al., 1984, 1985).

*Hosts*

Rats and man (Vonderfecht et al., 1984; Eiden et al., 1985).

*Epizootiology*

Unknown. During the diarrheal phase of the infection, the feces contain a high titer of virus, and fecal-oral transmission is undoubtedly most important. Presumably, transmission between rat cages involves airborne infection as in mouse rotavirus infection (Kraft, 1982). Personnel may be the major source of infection for rat colonies (Eiden et al., 1985; Vonderfecht et al., 1985).

*Clinical*

The disease syndrome in rats has been called infectious diarrhea of infant rats (IDIR). Diarrhea occurs in suckling rats 1-11 days old. The feces of affected rats consist of poorly formed pellets, liquid, and gas. Diarrhea persists for 5-6 days, during which there is erythema, cracking, and bleeding of the perianal skin. Growth retardation and drying and flaking of the perianal skin are apparent for several more days. There is no mortality (Vonderfecht et al., 1984).

*Pathology*

At necropsy affected suckling rats always have stomachs filled with milk. The contents of the proximal small intestine are watery and tan to green in color. The distal small intestine and colon contain fluid, poorly formed pellets, gas, and mucinous material (Vonderfecht et al., 1984).

In histologic sections lesions are restricted to the small intestine and consist of villous epithelial necrosis, formation of epithelial syncytial cells, and villous atrophy. Epithelial necrosis involves the luminal one-third of the villi. Syncytial cells are found on the villi but never in the crypts. The cytoplasm of the syncytial cells often contain an abundance of 1- to 2-μm eosinophilic inclusions. By electron microscopy, the cytoplasm of epithelial syncytial cells contains large numbers of 80-nm viral particles associated with reticular and amorphous aggregates of electron-dense material (Vonderfecht et al., 1984).

*Diagnosis*

The specialized methods for definitive diagnosis of RVLA are not available in most rodent diagnostic laboratories. The preferred methods presently are the indirect enzyme immunoassays (Vonderfecht et al., 1984) and the enzyme immunoassay inhibition test (Vonderfecht et al., 1985) for detection of the virus in intestinal and fecal specimens. Although the enzyme immunoassay inhibition test has been found to be excellent for this purpose, its usefulness may be somewhat limited in diagnosing RVLA infection as fecal shedding of the virus occurs for only a few days after infection and the timing of sample collection is of critical importance (Vonderfecht et al., 1988). Light and electron microscopic methods provide important supporting data for diagnosis (Vonderfecht et al., 1984).

### *Control*

Uncertain. Infected personnel may be an important source of infection.

### *Interference with Research*

RVLA could interfere with studies involving the intestinal tract, but no examples have been reported. Presumably, infected rats can serve as a source of infection for personnel.

## Reovirus-3

### *Significance*

Natural infections due to this virus have little significance for most studies with mice and rats but can interfere with studies involving transplantable tumors and in vitro test systems that use cells from these animals. The chief importance of reovirus-3 is that experimental infections with this agent, particularly in mice, provide a large number of models of human disease and test systems for studying the molecular biology of the virus.

### *Perspective*

The literature on reovirus-3 infections in rodents is so dominated by studies of mice experimentally infected with the virus that experimental and natural infections are best considered separately.

### *Experimental Infections and Models*

*1953:* Stanley et al. (1953) carried out animal inoculations using a virus isolated from the feces of a child in Australia. Suckling mice inoculated with the virus developed hepatitis, encephalitis, diarrhea, oily coats, alopecia, and jaundice; and the agent was called the hepato-encephalomyelitis virus or HEV. It was later identified as reovirus-3 (Stanley, 1961).

*1954-1986:* During this period further studies of experimental infections in mice were conducted by Stanley and colleagues (Stanley et al., 1954, 1964). Subsequently, experimental infections of reovirus-3 were proposed as models of many diseases in humans, including acute and chronic hepatitis, chronic biliary obstruction, pancreatitis, and lymphoma (reviewed by Stanley, 1974). Also, experimental infection models using mice were used extensively in studies relating the molecular biology of reovirus-1 and -3 to viral pathogenesis (reviewed by Sharpe and Fields, 1985).

### *Natural Infections and Disease*

*1960:* Bennette (1960) and Nelson and Tarnowski (1960) reported that a viral contaminant was oncolytic for their transplantable ascites tumors in mice; the causative agent was later identified as reovirus-3 (Hartley et al., 1961; Bennette et al., 1967). Nelson and Tarnowski (1960) also observed that some of the uninoculated suckling mice in their colony had "oily coats and yellow foci in the liver," and concluded that this was probably a natural occurrence of the disease produced earlier (Stanley et al., 1953) by the inoculation of reovirus-3 into suckling mice.

*1961:* Hartley et al. (1961) isolated reovirus-3 from two populations of laboratory mice and five of seven mouse leukemia cell lines.

*1963:* In Australia, Cook (1963) described two epizootics in suckling mice characterized by runting, diarrhea, oily coats, alopecia, focal hepatic necrosis, and jaundice. Reovirus-3 was isolated and considered the causative agent, but additional diagnostic procedures were not done.

*1964:* Nelson (1964) was unable to reproduce the experimental disease syndrome described by Stanley et al. (1953) by inoculating the reovirus-3 isolate of Nelson and Tarnowski (1960) into infant mice. Later, Bennette et al. (1967) reported similar failures using their isolate of the virus (Bennette, 1960).

*1972:* Collins and Parker (1972) reported reovirus-3 to be a contaminant in 2% of 465 murine leukemia cell lines and transplantable tumors.

Thus, the literature contains only two instances that seem to implicate reovirus-3 as the cause of spontaneous disease in mice (i.e., mice not inoculated with the virus), those reported by Cook (1963) and Nelson and Tarnowski (1960). Also, there are only two reported instances in which reovirus-3 was found to interfere with research involving transplantable tumors in mice (Bennette, 1960; Nelson and Tarnowski, 1960).

### *Agent*

The reoviruses are double-stranded RNA viruses, family Reoviridae, genus *Reovirus*. Other genera of the Reoviridae are *Orbivirus* and *Rotavirus*. The three genera are morphologically similar but differ in structure, antigenicity (i.e., are not immunologically related), stability, and preferred hosts. The reoviruses have a wide host range and are considered ubiquitous in nature. The orbiviruses multiply in insects and include blue tongue virus of ruminants and Colorado tick virus of people. The rotaviruses cause mainly infantile diarrheas of humans and animals (Davis et al., 1980).

The genus *Reovirus* contains mammalian and avian serotypes. The mammalian reoviruses are divided into serotypes 1, 2, and 3, which are distinguished by the neutralization and hemagglutination tests (Rosen, 1960). The major or type-specific antigen is the sigma 1 outer capsid protein. Serologic types 1, 2, and 3 share a common group antigen and cross-react in the complement fixation (CF) test. Types 1 and 2 agglutinate human erythrocytes, and type 3 agglutinates bovine erythrocytes. There are five serotypes of avian reoviruses; they are not serologically related to the mammalian reoviruses (Jackson and Muldoon, 1973; Ramig and Fields, 1977; Matthews, 1982; Sharpe and Fields, 1985).

Reovirus virions are spherical particles 75-80 nm in diameter, consisting of an outer and an inner capsid, or core, measuring about 52 nm in diameter. There is no lipoprotein envelope. Reoviruses are highly resistant to lipid solvents, acid pH, heating (56°C for two hours or 60°C for 30 minutes), and many disinfectants (Stanley et al., 1953; Fenner et al., 1974; Buxton and Fraser, 1977a).

Mammalian reoviruses have been grown in a wide range of cells but most commonly in L cells and primary monkey kidney cells (Kraft, 1982).

### *Hosts*

Mice, rats, hamsters, and guinea pigs (Carthew and Verstraete, 1978; Parker, 1980; Suzuki et al., 1982). Reovirus-2 has been isolated from wild mice (Hartley et al., 1961). Mammalian reoviruses have also been found in many other species because they have a broad host range (Buxton and Fraser, 1977a; Davis et al., 1980).

### *Epizootiology*

Based on recent serologic surveys using either the CF or hemagglutination inhibition (HAI) test, one or more of the reoviruses may be quite prevalent in contemporary rodents. The combined data from Canada, England, Japan, and the United States give the following ranges in percentages of colonies found infected: mice, 8-100%; rats, 6-44%; hamsters, 30-33%; and guinea pigs, 33-77% (Descoteaux et al., 1977; Carthew and Verstraete, 1978; Parker, 1980; Suzuki et al., 1982; Lindsey, 1986). Prevalence values based on the HAI test may have overstated the true prevalences of reovirus-3 infection because of false positive results (Kraft and Meyer, 1986; Van Der Logt, 1986).

Natural infections caused by reoviruses in rodents are assumed to involve mainly the respiratory and gastrointestinal tracts as they do in people. Therefore, transmission probably involves the aerosol as well as the fecal-oral route. Infected fomites may have an important role because reoviruses resist environmental conditions moderately well (Davis et al., 1980).

*Clinical*

Natural infections of mice and rats due to reoviruses are almost always subclinical.

The following clinical manifestations were observed in the colony studied by Cook (1963). For more than 9 years litters 10-14 days old frequently showed stunting, diarrheic yellow stools, oily coats, abdominal alopecia, and jaundice. Signs usually were confined to first litters of parents mated at 7-8 weeks of age. At least 1 and up to 5 per litter were stunted (i.e., weights of 3 grams instead of the expected 10 grams). Jaundice persisted in some mice to 5 or 6 weeks of age.

*Pathology*

The mammalian reoviruses are not considered important pathogens because they are commonly isolated from the feces or respiratory tracts of healthy humans and animals. However, on occasion they have been associated with minor respiratory and gastrointestinal illnesses (Davis et al., 1980).

In the natural outbreak studied by Cook (1963), stunted mice had enlarged black protruding gall bladders, yellow necrotic areas in the livers, and yellow kidneys. Unfortunately, no efforts were made to detect other infectious agents, and no histopathologic studies were done.

Nelson (1964) and Nelson and Tarnowski (1960) described a few gross lesions associated with the transplantation of reovirus-3-contaminated ascites tumors. On the seventh day after intraperitoneal inoculation of infant or weanling mice with uninfected tumors, copious amounts of ascitic fluid and large numbers of tumor cells were present. In contrast, after inoculation of reovirus-3-contaminated tumors the ascitic fluid was slightly turbid and contained many inflammatory cells but reduced numbers of tumor cells. Fibrinous exudate covered the liver, and chalky foci of necrosis were present in peritoneal fat deposits. A few animals had multifocal hepatic necrosis and jaundice.

Numerous morphologic lesions have been observed in mice inoculated experimentally with reovirus-3, including emaciation, stunting, encephalitis, pneumonia, hepatitis, cholangitis, pancreatitis, adrenalitis, myocarditis, ascites, and many others (Stanley et al., 1953, 1954, 1964; Walters et al., 1963, 1973; Jenson et al., 1965; Papadimitriou, 1966, 1968; Papadimitriou and Walters, 1967; Stanley and Joske, 1975a,b; Papadimitriou and Robertson, 1976; Ondera et al., 1978; Bangaru et al., 1980).

A large research effort during the past decade has focused on relating the molecular components of reovirus, particularly types 1 and 3, to pathogenesis in mice. Among the major findings has been the fact that each of the three outer capsid proteins has a distinct role in pathogenesis. The sigma 1 protein is the determinant of cell and tissue tropism, and both humoral and cellular immune responses to the reoviruses. Protein mu 1C determines viral sensitivity to intestinal proteases. Sigma 3 protein is an inhibitor of host cell RNA and protein synthesis and participates in mutations related to lytic versus persistent infections by the virus. The mechanisms of protective immunity are not well understood; however, it is known that athymic (*nu/nu*) mice resist reovirus infections as well as immunocompetent mice (Sharpe and Fields, 1984, 1985).

### *Diagnosis*

The CF and HAI tests for antibodies to reovirus-3 have been the standards for routine health monitoring for many years, but the more sensitive enzyme-linked immunosorbent assay (ELISA) is now used by most laboratories (London et al., 1983; Parker, 1983). The CF test is not reovirus type specific, as is probably true of most ELISAs currently in use. Also, the HAI test is prone to give false positive results (Kraft and Meyer, 1986; Van Der Logt, 1986).

Virus isolations can be performed with L cells or embryonic kidney cells (Kraft, 1982). Transplantable tumors and cell lines can be screened for reoviruses by using tissue culture methods or the mouse antibody production test (Rowe et al., 1962).

### *Control*

Cesarean derivation and barrier maintenance have proven effective. However, the common occurrence of reoviruses in man suggests that personnel may be a source of contamination for reovirus-free rodent stocks.

### *Interference with Research*

There are relatively few published examples in which natural infections of reovirus in mice and rats were found to interfere with research, i.e., only one alleged clinical outbreak in mice that was incompletely studied and of totally unknown pathogen status (Cook, 1963), and two instances of interference with transplantable ascites tumor studies in mice (Bennette, 1960; Nelson and Tarnowski, 1960). More recently, reovirus-3 has been reported to be an occasional contaminant of transplantable tumors and cell lines (Collins and Parker, 1972).

Experimental infections of reovirus-3 have been reported to result in the following altered biological responses:

a. Reduced pulmonary clearance of *Staphylococcus aureus* (Klein et al., 1969).
b. Suppression of pulmonary carcinogenesis due to urethan (Theiss et al., 1978).
c. Enhancement of tumor-specific immunity (Kollmorgen et al., 1976; Sansing et al., 1977).

## Adenoviruses

### *Significance*

Low.

### *Perspective*

Two distinct strains of so-called "mouse" adenovirus have been recognized in mice. The FL strain (MAd-1) )was first isolated by Hartley and Rowe (1960) in the United States during attempts to establish the Friend leukemia virus in tissue culture. The K87 strain (MAd-2) was first isolated in Japan by Hashimoto et al. (1966) while searching for cytopathic viruses in the feces of healthy mice. Neither agent appears to be an important pathogen in contemporary rodents.

### *Agent*

These agents are DNA viruses, family Adenoviridae, genus *Mastadenovirus*. Adenovirus virions measure 70-90 nm in diameter and have icosahedral symmetry. There is no envelope surrounding the nucleocapsid. More than 80 different adenovirus species have been isolated from mammalian hosts. Adenoviruses generally have strong host specificity (Wigand et al., 1977; Matthews, 1982; Otten and Tennant, 1982).

Determination of the species (formerly, type designation) of adenoviruses traditionally has been based on immunological distinctiveness as determined by quantitative neutralization with animal antisera (Wigand and Adrian, 1986). Conflicting reports have been published on the antigenic relationship between the FL and K87 strains (Van der Veen and Mes 1974; Wigand et al., 1977; Smith et al., 1986; Wigand and Adrian, 1986; Lussier et al., 1987a). Nevertheless, there is general agreement that the two agents represent distinct species; the FL strain is designated mouse adenovirus-1 (MAd-1) and the K87 strain as mouse adenovirus-2 (MAd-2), as originally proposed by Van der Veen and Mes (1974). More recently, restriction endonuclease cleavage studies of DNA from the two strains have confirmed their distinctiveness and separation into two species (Hamelin and Lussier, 1988; Hamelin et al., 1988).

Adenoviruses are resistant to ether and acid pH. Stability is retained for over 2 months at 4°C, 2 weeks at room temperature, and 1 week at 37°C, but the viruses are inactivated by 50°C for 15 minutes (Buxton and Fraser, 1977b).

*Hosts*

Mice and rats. Inclusion of the rat as a host is based on serologic (Jacoby et al., 1979; Parker, 1980; Suzuki et al., 1982) and morphologic (Ward and Young, 1976) evidence, but rats have been reported to be refractory to experimental infection with either MAd-1 or MAd-2 (Smith and Barthold, 1987).

*Epizootiology*

The prevalence of these viruses in contemporary mouse and rat stocks is not well understood. Recent data obtained by using the time-honored complement fixation (CF) test for antibody to the MAd-1 (alone) suggest that the prevalence of this agent in mice is quite low. Using this test, Parker (1980) found all of 21 mouse colonies to be negative in the United States, and Suzuki et al. (1982) reported that all of 196 mouse colonies in Japan were negative. For rats, Parker (1980) reported 36% of 25 colonies in the United States to be positive, and Suzuki et al. (1982) found 8% of colonies in Japan to be positive. More recently, Smith et al. (1986), using an immunofluorescent antibody (IFA) test for both MAd-1 and MAd-2, reported serological evidence of MAd-2 in mice from 1 of 6 commercial sources, MAd-1 in rats from 2 of 6 sources, and MAd-2 in rats from 3 of 6 sources surveyed in the United States.

Few surveys have been done using a serological test known to be reliable for detecting antibodies to MAd-2. However, that agent may be more prevalent than presently suspected as intestinal inclusions compatible with MAd-2 infection have been observed infrequently in mice in The Netherlands (Cohen and de Groot, 1976) and the United States (Takeuchi and Hashimoto, 1976; Luethans and Wagner, 1983), and in rats in the United States (Ward and Young, 1976).

MAd-1 is said to be shed in the urine. Viruria has been reported to persist for periods ranging from 2 weeks to as long as 2 years post infection (Van der Veen and Mes, 1973).

MAd-2 infects the intestinal tract and is shed for only about 3 weeks post infection in immunocompetent mice (Hashimoto et al., 1970). Athymic (*nu/nu*) mice shed the virus for about 6 weeks post infection and thereafter intermittently for at least 6 months (Umehara et al., 1984). Thus, fecal-oral transmission is most important.

*Clinical*

Neither MAd-1 nor MAd-2 is known to cause clinical disease in naturally infected immunocompetent rodents. MAd-1 (Winters and Brown, 1980) and MAd-2 (Cohen and deGroot, 1976) have been associated with wasting in athymic (*nu/nu*) mice.

*Pathology*

All reports of pathology caused by MAd-1 have been the result of experimental infections. Intraperitoneal, intracranial, or intranasal inoculation can produce a systemic fatal disease in suckling mice born to mothers without antibody (Hartley and Rowe, 1960; Heck et al., 1972; Wigand, 1980). In 28-day-old mice inoculated intraperitoneally, most animals showed no clinical disease, although some became ill and 10 of 250 animals died (Van der Veen and Mes, 1973). MAd-1 has tropisms for adrenal gland, myocardium, endocardium, heart valves, brown fat, kidney, salivary gland, and brain. Thus, experimental infections of mice with this virus have been proposed as models of human diseases such as Addison's disease (Margolis et al., 1974) and nonrheumatic endocarditis (Blailock et al., 1967, 1968). Intranuclear inclusions are frequently observed in infected tissues (Heck et al., 1972; Hoenig et al., 1974; Margolis et al., 1974).

The proclivity of MAd-1 to produce systemic infection contrasts sharply with the strict intestinal tropism of MAd-2. Inoculation of MAd-2 into mice, including neonates and athymic (*nu/nu*) mice, by any route results in subclinical infection during which virus replication occurs exclusively in the intestine (Sugiyama et al., 1967; Umehara et al., 1984). Viral antigen appears in the feces of immunocompetent mice about three days post infection and peaks between seven and 14 days post infection. At that time large numbers of amphophilic, intranuclear inclusions can be found in the mucosal epithelium of both the small and large intestine, but particularly in the small intestine, involving both crypt and villous cells. Little inflammatory response occurs. Ultrastructurally, the inclusions contain densely packed crystalline arrays of angular-shaped, homogeneous virions, each measuring about 85 nm (Takeuchi and Hashimoto, 1976). Host resistance has been attributed to locally produced neutralizing antibody of the IgA class (Hashimoto and Umehara, 1977). Cyclophosphamide administration delays the onset of resistance (Hashimoto et al., 1973).

### *Diagnosis*

The CF test for detection of antibodies to only MAd-1 was the standard test used in health surveillance testing until very recently. With the recognition of two distinct adenovirus species in mice and rats, it is now standard practice to test sera against antigens of both MAd-1 and MAd-2 (Smith et al., 1986; Lussier et al., 1987a). The prefered methods are IFA (Smith et al., 1986; Lussier et al., 1987a) and enzyme-linked immunosorbent assay. The IFA has been shown to give antibody titers to MAd that are approximately 10-fold higher than those determined by CF test (Lussier et al., 1987a).

No histologic lesions have been reported for natural infections of MAd-1 in mice and rats. Presumptive diagnosis of MAd-2 infection can be made by finding the characteristic intranuclear inclusions in histologic sections of intestinal epithelium (Cohen and de Groot, 1976; Ward and Young, 1976; Luethans and Wagner, 1983). A fluorescent antibody method has been used for the detection of MAd-2 antigen in the intestine (Takeuchi and Hashimoto, 1976).

Definitive diagnosis of mouse adenovirus infections requires virus isolation. MAd-1 can be grown in primary mouse kidney cells, L 929 murine fibroblasts, and CMT-93 murine rectal carcinoma cells (Wigand et al., 1977; Otten and Tennant, 1982; Smith et al., 1986). MAd-2 grows in mouse kidney and CMT-93 cells (Hashimoto et al., 1966; Smith et al., 1986).

### *Control*

Definitive information is lacking. Casarean derivation and barrier maintenance apparently have been very effective in eliminating these agents from infected stocks in the past.

### *Interference with Research*

MAd-1 has been reported to produce extensive persistent lesions in the kidneys of adult mice and to render them more susceptible to experimental *Escherichia coli*-induced pyelonephritis (Ginder, 1964). MAd (strain not given) infection has been reported to accelerate experimental scrapie in mice (Ehresmann and Hogan, 1986).

## ***Bacillus piliformis***

### *Significance*

Unknown. Outbreaks of disease caused by this agent have occurred occasionally, but the actual prevalence of the infection in contemporary mice and rats remains unknown.

*Perspective*

Clinical disease caused by *B. piliformis*, commonly called Tyzzer's disease, was first recognized by Tyzzer (1917) at Harvard in a colony of *Mus bactrianus*. Since then several outbreaks of the disease in laboratory mice and rats have been reported, and a few occurrences of the disease have been seen in other species. Unfortunately, little progress has been made in understanding the natural history and prevalence of the infection (Ganaway et al., 1971; Weisbroth, 1979; Ganaway, 1982).

*Agent*

*B. piliformis* is an unclassified bacterium. It occurs in vegetative and spore forms. The vegetative form is a Gram negative, motile, pleomorphic, slender rod measuring 0.5 × 8-10 μm. Also, it is silver positive, weakly periodic acid-Schiff positive, and forms subterminal spores (Ganaway, 1980).

The vegetative form is an obligate intracellular parasite. It loses infectivity in host tissues quickly after the host's death and is very unstable to environmental conditions. The spores survive at room temperature for a year or longer (Allen et al., 1965; Craigie, 1966a) and at 60°C for 30 minutes (Ganaway, 1980). Spores are inactivated by 70°C for 30 minutes, 80°C for 15 minutes, and treatment with 0.3% sodium hypochlorite or 2% peracetic acid (with 0.025% sodium alkylarylsulfonate as the wetting agent) for 5 minutes. Solutions of formaldehyde, iodophor, benzalkonium chloride, ethanol, or phenolic disinfectant have little or no sporicidal effect (Ganaway, 1980).

*B. piliformis* is generally considered not cultivable in cell-free media, although there have been reports to the contrary (Kanazawa and Imai, 1959; Simon, 1977). It can be cultivated in the yolk sac of embryonating hen's eggs (Craigie, 1966a; Ganaway et al., 1971; Fries, 1977b) and in primary cultures of hepatocytes (Kawamura et al., 1983; Thunert, 1984).

A number of methods have been found useful for the laboratory maintenance of *B. piliformis*, including the following:

a. infected tissues such as liver from a diseased animal can be harvested shortly after the animal's death and frozen at –70°C;

b. the organism can be passaged in the yolk sac of 6- to 9-day-old embryonated hen's eggs and harvested at about the time of embryo death, and the yolk sac suspensions can be frozen at –70°C;

c. suspensions of infected tissue can be passaged in immunocompetent mice given a concurrent dose of 100-200 mg/kg of cortisone acetate; and

d. suspensions of infected tissue can be passaged in immunodeficient CBA/N-*xid* or C3.CBA/N-*xid* homozygous female or hemizygous male mice, with or without concurrent administration of cortisone (Waggie et al., 1981).

### *Hosts*

Mice, rats, gerbils, hamsters, guinea pigs, rabbits, cats, dogs, nonhuman primates, horses, and others (Ganaway et al., 1971; Weisbroth, 1979).

### *Epizootiology*

Tyzzer's disease has been reported in Europe, North America, and Asia (Ganaway et al., 1971), suggesting that *B. piliformis* has a worldwide distribution. Most of the outbreaks in laboratory mice and rats have occurred in conventional colonies, but a few have been seen in cesarean-derived, barrier-maintained colonies (Mullink, 1968; Hunter, 1971; Tsuchitani et al., 1983; Thunert et al., 1985; Gibson et al., 1987).

Surveys based on serologic tests suggest that subclinical infection is common even in cesarean-derived, barrier-maintained rodents. Fujiwara (1980) reported that 5% of 80 mouse colonies and 47% of 83 rat colonies in Japan were seropositive by the complement fixation (CF) test for *B. piliformis*. Using an indirect immunofluorescent antibody (IFA) test for serum antibody, Fries (1980) found seven of eight mouse colonies and all of six rat colonies in Europe, representing both conventional and specific-pathogen-free colonies, to be serologically positive. Both of these investigators have confirmed the presence of *B. piliformis* in representative seropositive mouse and rat colonies by use of cortisone administration to provoke the expression of Tyzzer's disease or by other methods (Fujiwara, 1967; Fries, 1977a, 1979; Fries and Svendsen, 1978; Fujiwara et al., 1981).

The spores are passed in the feces and retain infectivity at room temperature for 1 year or more (Allen et al., 1965; Craigie, 1966a). Natural infection is thought to be by ingestion of spore-contaminated food or bedding. Thus, a high concentration of spores in the animal environment, due to poor sanitation practices and crowding of animals, provides an ideal setting for the occurrence of clinical disease (Ganaway et al., 1971).

Very little is known about the epizootiology and natural history of *B. piliformis* in nature. However, the occurrence of Tyzzer's disease in wild animals (e.g., muskrats in Iowa and Wisconsin and cottontail rabbits in Maryland) and domestic animals (e.g., foals in at least seven states in the United States, as well as in Canada and Europe) from numerous geographic locations strongly suggests that the organism is widely distributed in nature (Ganaway et al., 1976; Turk et al., 1981). Thus, it is possible that laboratory animal diets could contain spores of *B. piliformis* when made from ingredients such as grains and alfalfa hay that have been contaminated by the feces of infected rodents or other animals (Ganaway et al., 1976). If so, inadequate sterilization of spore-contaminated diet or bedding may be a major cause of *B. piliformis* infection in cesarean-derived, barrier-maintained rodents.

*Clinical*

Based on the results of serologic surveys, subclinical infection is probably far more common than clinical disease (Fujiwara, 1967, 1980; Fries and Svendsen, 1978; Fries, 1979, 1980; Fujiwara et al., 1979, 1981).

Numerous environmental and host factors have been recognized as important contributors to the expression of disease caused by *B. piliformis*, including poor sanitation, overcrowding, transportation stress, food deprivation, dietary modifications, and altered host immune status (Tuffery, 1956; Takagaki et al., 1966; Fujiwara et al., 1973; Weisbroth, 1979; Ganaway, 1982).

Clinical disease occurs most frequently in sucklings and weanlings, but animals of any age can be affected. Unexpected deaths, watery diarrhea, pasting of feces around the perineum, ruffled fur, and inactivity are the most common signs. Morbidity and mortality can vary from low to high (Tyzzer, 1917; Gard, 1944; Rights et al., 1947; Mullink, 1968; Jonas et al., 1970; Stedham and Bucci, 1970; Tsuchitani et al., 1983; Thunert et al., 1985; Gibson et al., 1987).

*Pathology*

There are three main phases in the evolution of Tyzzer's disease: the establishment of primary infection in the ileum and cecum, the ascension of organisms by the portal vein to the liver, and bacteremic spread to other tissues, most notably the myocardium. The organism preferentially replicates in intestinal epithelium, intestinal smooth muscle, hepatocytes, and myocardium; but the degree of replication (and lesions) in the three major organs involved varies considerably from case to case and between species. Intestinal lesions are usually more severe in rats (and in gerbils, hamsters, and rabbits) than in mice. Myocardial lesions occur inconsistently in all species except for, possibly, the gerbil, which is considered the most susceptible of the common laboratory animal species (Allen et al., 1965; Takagaki and Fujiwara, 1968; Ganaway, 1971; Fujiwara et al., 1973; Weisbroth, 1979; Tsuchitani et al., 1983; Waggie et al., 1984).

Gross lesions range from none to severe involvement of the intestine, liver, and/or heart. In mice the most consistent finding is multiple pale to yellow foci in the liver. Infrequently, the ileum and cecum may appear thickened, edematous, and hyperemic; and the myocardium may contain circumscribed pale gray areas. Lesions in rats are similar, except that the ileum often appears dilated, atonic, and edematous (megaloileitis). The mesenteric lymph nodes usually are enlarged (Yamada et al., 1969; Jonas et al., 1970; Weisbroth, 1979; Ganaway et al., 1982; Tsuchitani et al., 1983).

Microscopically, intestinal lesions are found in the ileum, cecum, and sometimes the proximal colon. There is mild to severe loss of the mucosal epithelium, with blunting of villi in the ileum, thinning of the surface epithelium, and even severe ulceration and hemorrhage. In the more advanced stages there is hyperplasia of the crypt epithelium. In areas of severe epithelial loss there is transmural acute to subacute inflammation. In the liver there are multiple discrete foci of coagulative necrosis that are rapidly converted to microabscesses but that may contain varying numbers of macrophages and lymphocytes in the more advanced stages. If the myocardium is affected, there is focal to diffuse myocardial necrosis with intense acute to subacute inflammation. In each of the affected tissues, the characteristic large, filamentous bacilli are best demonstrated in the cytoplasm of viable cells along the margin of the necrotic tissues. Silver stains (e.g., the Warthin-Starry and methenamine silver methods) are preferred (Jonas et al., 1970; Stedham and Bucci, 1970; Ganaway et al., 1971; Weisbroth, 1979; Tsuchitani et al., 1983).

B-cell deficient CBA/N-*xid* and C3.CBA/N-*xid* homozygous female and hemizygous male mice are highly susceptible, whereas T-cell deficient athymic (*nu*/*nu*) male and female mice are as resistant as immunocompetent mice. Thus, resistance to *B. piliformis* infection in the mouse appears to be mainly dependent on B-cell function (Waggie et al., 1981). The passive transfer of immune serum to mice protects against experimental infection (Fujiwara et al., 1969). Athymic rats are reported to be highly susceptible (Thunert et al., 1985).

### *Diagnosis*

The diagnosis of Tyzzer's disease is made by necropsy and is based on the finding of characteristic gross and microscopic lesions and the demonstration of the characteristic organisms in silver-stained histologic sections (Allen et al., 1965; Jonas et al., 1970; Stedham and Bucci, 1970; Weisbroth, 1979).

IFA (Fries, 1977a, 1980), CF (Fujiwara, 1967, 1980) and enzyme-linked immunosorbent assay (Toriumi et al., 1986) tests have been used for the diagnosis of subclinical infections, but none of these tests is currently available commercially in the United States. Alternatively, weanling animals can be immunosuppressed by the administration of cortisone acetate (100-200 mg/kg) to provoke active disease, and killed 7 days later for demonstration of characteristic lesions and organisms (Kaneko et al., 1960; Fujiwara et al., 1963, 1973; Takagaki et al., 1966). Tissues suspected of containing *B. piliformis* can be passaged in gerbils or in homozygous female or hemizygous male *xid* mice (CBA/N or C3.CBA/N), which are killed 5 to 7 days later for the demonstration of lesions and organisms (Waggie et al., 1981, 1984).

### *Control*

The use of cesarean-derivation and barrier-maintenance procedures appears to have minimized the occurrence of clinical disease, but the true prevalence of subclinical *B. piliformis* infection in contemporary rodent colonies in the United States is unknown. If subclinical infections are found to be widespread, major revisions in current control methods might be required.

A number of practical approaches have been recommended for reducing losses due to Tyzzer's disease in conventional colonies. Good sanitation practices, avoidance of crowding, autoclaving of food and bedding, and the use of 0.3% sodium hypochlorite for disinfecting room surfaces are recommended for reducing spore contamination in the animal environment (Ganaway et al., 1971; Ganaway, 1980). The oral administration of tetracycline can be helpful in controlling losses during outbreaks (Hunter, 1971; Yokoiyama and Fujiwara, 1971).

### *Interference with Research*

Tyzzer's disease has been reported to cause high mortality in breeding colonies of mice (Gard, 1944) and in mice used in long-term carcinogenesis studies (Hunter, 1971). However, it appears that both the provocation of overt disease from subclinical disease and the exacerbation of clinical disease by immunosuppressive treatments have been particularly troublesome.

The administration of cortisone or adrenocorticotropic hormone to animals with subclinical infection has provoked severe clinical disease (Kaneko et al., 1960; Fujiwara et al., 1963, 1973; Takagaki et al., 1966; Yamada et al., 1969).

Whole body x-irradiation has provoked severe clinical disease with high mortality (Tuffery, 1956; Takagaki et al., 1966; Taffs, 1974).

Transplantation of ascites tumors has provoked Tyzzer's disease in recipient mice (Craigie, 1966b).

Tyzzer's disease has been reported to alter the pharmacokinetics of warfarin and trimethoprim (Fries and Ladefoged, 1979), and the activity of hepatic transaminases (Naiki et al., 1965) in mice.

A high-protein diet has exacerbated Tyzzer's disease in mice (Maejima et al., 1965).

Experimental Tyzzer's disease in weanling mice was exacerbated by treatment of the mice with carbon tetrachloride (Takenaka and Fujiwara, 1975).

## *Salmonella enteritidis*

### *Significance*

Uncertain because the prevalence of subclinical infection is unknown.

### *Perspective*

*Salmonella enteritidis* serotypes enteritidis and typhimurium ranked among the most important causes of epizootic and enzootic disease in laboratory mice and rats during the first half of the twentieth century (Edwards et al., 1948; Habermann and Williams, 1958; Weisbroth, 1979). More recently, clinical disease caused by these serotypes has virtually disappeared, while subclinical infections caused by weakly pathogenic *S. enteritidis* of many other serotypes have been recognized as relatively common (Werner, 1957; Wetmore and Hoag, 1960; Margard and Litchfield, 1963; Brennan et al., 1965; Morello et al., 1965; Franklin and Richter, 1968; Kirchner et al., 1982; Steffen and Wagner, 1983).

### *Agent*

Salmonellosis in rodents is caused by a bacterium, family Enterobacteriaceae, tribe Salmonellae, *Salmonella enteritidis* (with more than 1,500 serotypes, see below). Members of the genus *Salmonella* are Gram-negative, non-spore-forming, usually motile, facultatively anaerobic, straight rods, measuring 0.7-1.5 × 2.0-5.0 µm. They reduce nitrites, produce gas from glucose, usually produce hydrogen sulfide on triple sugar iron agar, and usually utilize citrate as a sole source of carbon. They are indole and urease negative (LeMinor, 1984; Farmer et al., 1985).

According to the classification system of the Centers for Disease Control (Ewing, 1972; Farmer et al., 1985), all salmonellae belong to three species: *Salmonella choleraesuis*, *Salmonella typhi*, and *Salmonella enteritidis*. *S. choleraesuis* and *S. typhi* are distinct serotypes. All other serotypes, of which there are over 1,500, are defined as serotypes of *S. enteritidis*. Thus, organisms previously designated *S. enteritidis* are technically "*S. enteritidis* serotype enteritidis"; *S. typhimurium* is "*S. enteritidis* serotype typhimurium;" and so on. However, this system proved to be confusing and cumbersome, and is commonly simplified in laboratory reports so that "*S. enteritidis* serotype typhimurium" is reported as "*Salmonella* serotype typhimurium". In scientific articles the designations are often simplified further by artificially treating *Salmonella* serotypes as if they are species. Thus, "*S. enteritidis* serotype typhimurium" becomes simply "*S. typhimurium*" (Farmer et al., 1985). In the following paragraphs *S. enteritidis* refers exclusively to genus and species, and serotypes are always so designated.

*S. enteritidis* serotypes typhimurium and enteritidis were the serotypes most commonly isolated from laboratory mice and rats during the first half of the twentieth century (Edwards et al., 1948). Serotypes most commonly isolated from these hosts in recent years have included agona, amsterdam, anatum, binza, blockley, bredeney, california, cerro, infantis, kentucky, livingstone, montevideo, oranienburg, poona, senftenberg, tennessee, and others (Werner, 1957; Brennan et al., 1965; Morello et al., 1965; Weisbroth, 1979; Simmons and Simpson, 1980; Simpson and Simmons, 1981; Ganaway, 1982; Kirchner et al., 1982; Lentsch et al., 1983).

### *Hosts*

Mice, rats, humans, and many others (Edwards et al., 1948; LeMinor, 1984).

### *Epizootiology*

The prevalence of *S. enteritidis* in contemporary stocks of mice and rats is not well known, but there is evidence that subclinical infections due to weakly virulent strains of *S. enteritidis* may be common in the United States. Kirchner et al. (1982) isolated *S. enteritidis* serotypes agona, anatum, or oranienburg from the feces of mice at 11 of 22 breeding and research facilities. These isolates were found to be only mildly pathogenic when inoculated into mice. Steffen and Wagner (1983) reported the occurrence of subclinical *S. enteritidis* serotype amsterdam infection in rats of a large commercial breeding facility. However, Casebolt and Schoeb (1988) recently have reported an outbreak in mice of severe disease with high mortality due to *S. enteritidis* serotype enteritidis.

*Salmonella* infections are acquired primarily by ingestion. Contaminated food, water, and bedding are usually considered the major sources of infection for barrier-maintained rodent stocks. The inadvertent use of contaminated animal products in the preparation of rodent diets traditionally has been very troublesome (Hoag et al., 1964). Stott et al. (1975) found 19% of animal diets in the United Kingdom to be contaminated with *Salmonella* spp., the source being contaminated meat and bone meal. Although the pasteurization procedures currently used for rodent diets in the United States are thought to be highly effective, they may not eliminate all salmonellas. Where sources other than municipal water supplies are used for rodent facilities, rigorous measures must be taken to assure *Salmonella*-free water by filtration or other methods (Steffen and Wagner, 1983). Only sterilized bedding should be used in order to avoid the use of bedding contaminated by wild rodents or other hosts.

Infected hosts shed large numbers of salmonellas in the feces during early phases of their infections but may subsequently become chronic carriers, shedding organisms continuously or intermittently for many months. Thus, infected rodent and other hosts, including personnel, may be sources of infection for rodents. Such risks are especially great in multipurpose research facilities that house animals of varying pathogen status, including wild or random source animals (Fox and Beaucage, 1979).

### *Clinical*

The majority of *S. enteritidis* infections in mice and rats are subclinical. Clinical infections are rare in contemporary rodent stocks (Margard et al., 1963; Morello et al., 1965; Weisbroth, 1979). According to Weisbroth (1979), no natural outbreak of clinical disease caused by *S. enteritidis* has been reported for laboratory rats in the United States since 1939.

Lentsch et al. (1983) have reported an outbreak caused by serotype oranienburg in a breeding colony of mice that had reduced weaning rate as the leading clinical sign. Two outbreaks in which enteritis and deaths of mice up to 3 weeks of age were allegedly due to either serotype montevideo (Simmons and Simpson, 1980) or serotype livingstone (Simpson and Simmons, 1981) must be questioned because diagnostic procedures were not done to rule out other causes or contributing agents such as mouse hepatitis virus infection.

Following ingestion of an infectious dose of the organism, clinical signs may appear after an incubation period of 2-6 days. The signs are nonspecific and may include ruffled fur, hunched posture, reduced activity, weight loss, conjunctivitis, diarrhea, and variable mortality. Diarrhea is inconstant, usually occurring in no more than 20% of animals. Following the acute phase of the infection, 5% or more may become asymptomatic chronic carriers, shedding the organisms in the feces for many months. Enzootically infected breeding colonies may have alternating periods of inapparent infection and overt clinical disease with mortality. Litter sizes and birth weights may be reduced (Ratcliffe, 1949; Habermann and Williams, 1958; Rabstein, 1958; Margard et al., 1963; Jenkin et al., 1964; Morello et al., 1965; Lentsch et al., 1983).

### *Pathology*

Many factors are known to affect the expression of disease caused by *S. enteritidis* infection, including virulence and dose of the organism, host age and genotype, intestinal microflora, nutritional state, immune status, and intercurrent infections. Weanling mice are more susceptible than adults (Tannock and Smith, 1971). The normal intestinal microflora has an inhibitory effect on the establishment of infection by the oral route. Whereas more than $10^6$ organisms are required to establish infection in 50% of mice with a normal flora, less than 10 organisms are required in axenic mice or mice pretreated with oral antibiotics (Bohnhoff and Miller, 1962; Collins and Carter, 1978). Susceptibility to infection is increased by food and water deprivation (Miller and Bohnhoff, 1962; Maenza et al., 1970; Collins, 1972; Tannock and Smith, 1972), nutritional iron deficiency in rats (Newberne et al., 1968; Baggs and Miller, 1974), nutritional iron overload in mice (Jones et al., 1977), pretreatment with sodium bicarbonate by gavage (Collins, 1972), and administration of morphine sulfate to slow gastrointestinal motility (Miller and Bohnhoff, 1962).

Inbred strains of mice have a wide range of susceptibility to *S. enteritidis*. Based on the results of subcutaneous, intravenous, or intraperitoneal inoculations of virulent *S. enteritidis* serotype typhimurium, O'Brien et al. (1980) separated mouse strains into two groups. Relatively resistant strains were those having an $LD_{50}$ (the dose required to cause the deaths of 50% of the animals) of greater than $1 \times 10^3$ organisms, including C3H/HeN, C3H/St, C3H/Bi, CBA/Ca, BRVR, A/J, A/HeN, SWR/J, and DBA/2. Relatively susceptible strains were those having an $LD_{50}$ of less than $2 \times 101$ organisms, including BSVS, DBA/1, BALB/c, C57BL/6, C3H/HeJ, and CBA/N. Three distinct genetic loci that affect susceptibility to virulent strains of serotype typhimurium have been identified as follows:

a. *Ity (immunity to S. typhimurium) locus on chromosome 1.* This locus is thought to influence control of initial (less than 10 days post infection) replication of the organism in the spleen and liver, possibly through modulation of uptake and/or killing by macrophages. There are two alleles, $Ity^r$ (resistant) in A/J, BRVR, C3H/HeJ, and DBA/2 and $Ity^s$ (susceptible) in BSVS and C57BL/6 (O'Brien et al., 1980; Briles et al., 1981).

b. *Lps (lipopolysaccharide response) locus on chromosome 4.* This locus has to do with response to lipopolysaccharide and also appears to influence control of the initial (less than 10 days post infection) replication of serotype typhimurium in the spleen and liver. The allele designated $Lps^n$ (endotoxin sensitive) confers normal responsiveness and is found in most mouse strains. $Lps^d$ (endotoxin insensitive) is a mutant gene that results in the inability of the host's macrophages and B cells to be stimulated by bacterial endotoxin. It occurs in strains C3H/HeJ and C57BL/10/ScCr. This gene explains the relative susceptibility of C3H/HeJ, although that strain is $Ity^r$ (O'Brien et al., 1980; Briles, 1981).

c. *xid (X-linked immune deficiency) locus.* The mutant allele *xid* confers a B lymphocyte functional defect on CBA/N mice, making them susceptible. It controls antibody production and is thought to influence control of late (more than 10 days post infection) replication of salmonellae (O'Brien et al., 1980).

The pathogenesis of natural salmonellosis has been simulated by experimental studies in which *S. enteritidis* was inoculated intragastrically into mice (Collins, 1972; Carter and Collins, 1974). Following the inoculation of virulent organisms, more than 99% of the original dose is inactivated or voided from the gastrointestinal tract within 48 hours. The cecum and large intestine are exposed to large numbers of organisms for longer time periods than the small intestine, but the mucosa and Peyer's patches in the distal ileum are the primary sites of invasion. Organisms reach the mesenteric lymph nodes that drain this region in 24 hours, and the liver and spleen in 48 hours. Bacteremia occurs by 72 hours. Acute inflammation begins in the ileum and cecum by 24 hours, but the gut becomes heavily infected and develops severe lesions only as a result of the generalized septicemia. The cervical lymph nodes may be infected in some animals by 36 hours following ingestion or intragastric inoculation of organisms (Carter et al., 1975).

Gross lesions are extremely variable, depending on the stage of disease. Animals that die of acute infection may have only hyperemia and congestion of visceral organs, as seen in any septicemia. Animals that survive a week or longer often appear emaciated, have hyperemia and thickening of the ileal and cecal walls, an empty or fluid-filled large intestine, multiple white or yellow foci in the liver, splenomegaly, enlarged mesenteric lymph nodes, and scanty fibrinous exudate in the peritoneal cavity. Chronic carriers usually do not have gross lesions (Buchbinder et al., 1935; Ratcliffe, 1949; Habermann and Williams, 1958; Maenza et al., 1970; Casebolt and Schoeb, 1988).

The predominant microscopic lesions of salmonellosis are ileocecitis, mesenteric lymphadenitis, and multifocal inflammation in the liver and spleen, each varying in character depending on the stage of disease. There is multifocal to diffuse destruction of villous epithelium in the ileum, with blunting of villi and hyperplasia of crypt epithelium and purulent to pyogranulomatous inflammation in the lamina propria. Similar changes occur in the cecum. The cecum is more severely affected in rats. Ulcerative cecitis with severe pyogranulomatous inflammation in the lamina propria and purulent to chronic inflammation leading to atrophy and cyst formation in the paracecal lymph nodes are characteristic of salmonellosis in rats. Multifocal purulent, pyogranulomatous, or granulomatous inflammation occurs in the mesenteric lymph nodes, liver, and spleen. So-called cell fragment thrombi commonly occur in those organs in which necrotic foci break into venous channels. Peritonitis is commonly seen due to extension of the infection through the capsule of the liver, lymph nodes, or spleen. Cholangitis and cholecystitis are seen infrequently. Pyogranulomatous inflammation occasionally occurs in other organs such as the lungs (Buchbinder et al., 1935; Ratcliffe, 1949; Bakken and Vogelsang, 1950; Habermann and Williams, 1958; Bohme et al., 1959; Miller and Bohnhoff,

1962; Abrams et al., 1963; Maenza et al., 1970; Carter et al., 1975; Weisbroth, 1979; Casebolt and Schoeb, 1988).

The mechanisms of immunity to *S. enteritidis* have been studied extensively in mice (as the best animal models of typhoid fever in humans). According to Eisenstein and Sultzer (1983), many important conclusions can be made from this vast literature. There is a wide spectrum (10,000-fold range) of genetically determined susceptibility among different mouse strains to *S. enteritidis* infection. The genetic diversity (at the *Ity*, *Lps*, *xid*, and probably other loci) among mouse strains accounts for many of the discrepancies in results on protective immunity. In resistant stocks, such as Crl:ICR (CD®-1), humoral immunity alone is protective; but in strains that are highly susceptible, such as C3H/HeJ, antibody alone gives poor protection and cellular immunity is required. Living organisms are required for cellular immunity. Humoral immunity appears to be dependent on O antigens and can be produced by the inoculation of killed organisms. Monoclonal antibodies to O antigens have been found to be protective for C3H/HeN but not C3H/HeJ mice (Colwell et al., 1984).

*Diagnosis*

The diagnosis of *S. enteritidis* infection is dependent upon cultural isolation and identification of the organism. Typing of isolates is done by serology. Organs with suspicious lesions should be cultured, but it is usually best to culture liver, spleen, intestine, feces, and blood. Histopathology should be done to demonstrate the characteristic microscopic lesions of salmonellosis and to help rule out those diseases that can have similar gross lesions (e.g., mousepox, Tyzzer's disease, and streptobacillosis in mice) or exacerbate disease caused by *S. enteritidis*.

The detection of carrier animals is a special problem because few (less than 5%) animals in a population may be infected, and cultural isolation is necessary because there is no satisfactory serologic method for testing suspected carriers. The preferred procedure is to culture recently voided fecal pellets from individual mice or cages of mice in selenite F enrichment broth, followed by the inoculation of selective agar plates (brilliant green, salmonella shigella, or bismuth sulfite), and to test selected colonies on triple sugar iron agar (Margard and Litchfield, 1963; Margard et al., 1963). Sampling is a major problem in the detection of carriers. Assuming a carrier rate of 5% and random sampling of a population, 58 mice must be cultured to achieve 95% confidence of detecting one carrier mouse (Ganaway, 1982).

*Control*

Rodent populations infected with *S. enteritidis* are a zoonotic risk to personnel, a source of infection for other animals in the facility, and unsuitable for research purposes. There are only two effective methods of eliminating the infection. The usual method is to destroy the entire population and replace them with animals from a pathogen-free source. In the case of extremely valuable stocks, cesarean derivations can be attempted. This requires the maintenance of all breeders in an isolation system (e.g., a Trexler-type plastic film isolator) to prevent the spread of the infection, housing of individual cesarean-derived litters and their foster dams in separate isolators, and repeated fecal cultures (see above) to assure that any litter to be used for restocking purposes is free of *S. enteritidis*.

Prevention of *S. enteritidis* infection is accomplished through barrier maintenance of rodent stocks. Particular attention must be given to the avoidance of *Salmonella*-contaminated food and water, and the exclusion of infected animals and wild rodents from the facility (Ganaway, 1982). Regular monitoring of all rodent populations must be done to assure that all rodents are free of *S. enteritidis*. Studies involving experimental infection of animals with *S. enteritidis* must be done by using appropriate containment systems (Habermann and Williams, 1958; Steffen and Wagner, 1983).

### *Interference with Research*

Rodents infected with *S. enteritidis* can serve as a source of infection for other laboratory animals and humans. In addition, the infection can alter a number of biologic responses.

a. *S. enteritidis*-infected mice can have nonspecific resistance to challenge with other intracellular parasites such as *Listeria monocytogenes* (Blanden et al., 1966; Zinkernagel, 1976).

b. Prior immunization of mice with viable *S. enteritidis* results in the suppression of growth of transplantable tumors (Ashley et al., 1976).

c. Concurrent infections of *S. enteritidis* and *Plasmodium berghei* in mice result in higher mortality than infection by either agent alone (Kaye et al., 1965).

d. Concurrent infections of *S. enteritidis* and *Schistosoma japonicum* in mice result in higher mortality than infection by either agent alone (Tuazon et al., 1986).

e. *S. enteritidis* infection results in reduced blood glucose and hepatic enzyme levels (Moore et al., 1977).

f. Mice orally infected with *S. enteritidis* have reduced intestinal enzyme activities (Madge, 1973).

g. Susceptibility to *S. enteritidis* infection is increased by:

- lack of a gastrointestinal microflora (Bohnhoff and Miller, 1962; Margard and Peters, 1964; Ruitenberg et al., 1971; Collins and Carter, 1978);

- pretreatment with oral antibiotics (Bohnhoff et al., 1954; Bohnhoff and Miller, 1962; Watson, 1970; Collins and Carter, 1978);
- food and/or water deprivation (Miller and Bohnhoff, 1962; Maenza et al., 1970; Collins, 1972; Tannock and Smith, 1972).
- pretreatment with sodium bicarbonate by gavage (Collins, 1972);
- slowing of gastrointestinal motility by morphine sulfate (Miller and Bohnhoff, 1962); or
- iron deficiency in rats (Newberne et al., 1968; Baggs and Miller, 1974) and iron overload in mice (Jones et al., 1977).
- cecetomy of mice (Voravuthikunchai and Lee, 1987).

### *Citrobacter freundii (Biotype 4280)*

#### *Significance*

Low.

#### *Perspective*

*1965:* Brennan et al. (1965c) associated *Citrobacter freundii* with an outbreak of diarrhea in laboratory mice.

*1974:* Ediger et al. (1974) reported an epizootic characterized by colitis, colonic mucosal hyperplasia, and rectal prolapse. *C. freundii* was isolated and given orally to pathogen-free mice, resulting in reproduction of the clinical and histopathologic features of the natural disease.

*1976:* Barthold et al. (1976) named the disease transmissible murine colonic hyperplasia and identified a biochemical variant (4280) of *C. freundii* as the etiologic agent. Bieniek and Tober-Meyer (1976) characterized the disease and also incriminated a biotype of *C. freundii* as the causative agent.

*1977:* Barthold and Jonas (1977) demonstrated that infection with *C. freundii* (Biotype 4280) enhances the responsiveness of mice to the colon carcinogen 1,2-dimethylhydrazine.

#### *Agent*

The agent is a bacterium, family Enterobacteriaceae, *C. freundii* (Biotype 4280). They are straight, Gram-negative, facultatively anaerobic rods, measuring 1.0 µm wide × 2.0 to 6.0 µm long, which occur singly and in pairs, and grow on ordinary medium. They may be a normal inhabitant of the gastrointestinal tract in humans and other species. *C. freundii* (Biotype 4280) is usually considered an opportunistic pathogen (Sakazaki, 1984).

Only one biotype (4280), defined on the basis of in vitro biochemical reactions, is recognized as being pathogenic in mice. This biotype is positive for ornithine decarboxylase, ferments rhamnose, produces hydrogen sulfide, and reduces nitrite. This is in contrast to the nonpathogenic biotype which is negative for these reactions (Barthold et al., 1976).

*Hosts*

Mice. The organism does not colonize the intestines of rats or hamsters (Barthold et al., 1977).

*Epizootiology*

The natural history of this infection is poorly understood. Transmission has been shown to occur between cage contacts (Brennan et al., 1965c), presumably via fecal contamination and ingestion. It has been stated that the organism persisted in one colony for at least 3 years (Ediger et al., 1974). It is rarely found in cesarean-derived, barrier-maintained mouse populations.

*Clinical*

Signs are nonspecific. They include ruffled fur; listlessness; weight loss; stunting; pasty feces about the anus, base of the tail, and the perineum; and rectal prolapse (Brennan et al., 1965c; Ediger et al., 1974; Bieniek and Tober-Meyer, 1976; Barthold et al., 1977).

Suckling mice are more susceptible than adults. Mortality may reach 60% and rectal prolapse 15%. Mortality is significantly higher in C3H/HeJ than in DBA/2J, NIHS (Swiss), or C57BL/6J mice (Barthold et al., 1977).

*Pathology*

*C. freundii* (Biotype 4280) produces a transient infection in mice lasting only about 4 weeks. Even if the infection is eliminated as early as 2 days post infection by administration of neomycin sulfate and tetracycline hydrochloride, mucosal hyperplasia still occurs. Presence of the infection in the intestine for 10 days results in maximum hyperplasia (Barthold, 1980).

Following experimental infection, the organism attaches to the surface of the colonic mucosa within 4 to 10 days, hyperplasia is most severe at 16 days, and the mucosa reverts to normal by 45 days. Colonic hyperplasia possibly serves as a defense mechanism for replacement of infected epithelial cells (Johnson and Barthold, 1979).

The descending colon is most commonly affected, but the entire colon and cecum may be involved. Grossly, the affected bowel is thickened and rigid in appearance. Microscopically, there is increased crypt height (to 3 times normal), increased mitotic activity, decreased numbers of goblet cells, and increased basophilia of the epithelium. Crypt abscesses are common, and mucosal erosions and ulcers can occur. Occurrence of necrotizing and inflammatory lesions tend to parallel mortality. Variable numbers of neutrophils or mononuclear leukocytes may be present in the lamina propria, but there is often a paucity of inflammatory cells. During regression of mucosal hyperplasia, goblet cell hyperplasia with mucinous distension of crypts and streaming of mucin into the gut lumen can occur (Brynjolfsson and Lombard, 1969; Bieniek and Tober-Meyer, 1976; Barthold et al., 1978).

#### *Diagnosis*

Diagnosis is made by demonstration of characteristic lesions in the large intestine and isolation of *C. freundii* (Biotype 4280). However, the organism may not be recovered from all cases because lesions persist beyond the period of infection. Both the pathogenic and the nonpathogenic biotypes may be isolated from a given animal (Barthold et al., 1976).

#### *Control*

Definitive data are lacking. Elimination of the organism from an infected colony probably requires depopulation and restocking with cesarean-derived mice. Neomycin and tetracycline in drinking water reduce losses during outbreaks but probably do not completely eliminate the infection.

#### *Interference with Research*

Cytokinetics of the mucosal epithelium in the large intestine is profoundly altered in infected mice. Susceptibility to the carcinogen 1,2-dimethylhydrazine is increased, and the latent period for neoplasia induction is reduced (Barthold and Jonas, 1977).

### ***Pseudomonas aeruginosa***

#### *Significance*

Low, except in immunosuppressed hosts.

#### *Perspective*

*Pseudomonas aeruginosa*, and to a lesser extent other species of *Pseudomonas* and coliform bacteria, are normal inhabitants of the nasopharynx and lower digestive tract; however, they are occasionally associated with disease, primarily as opportunistic pathogens in immunosuppressed hosts (Weisbroth, 1979). *P. aeruginosa* has been particularly troublesome in mice following whole body irradiation (Hammond et al., 1954; Vincent et al., 1955; Wensinck et al., 1957; Flynn, 1963a,c; Hammond, 1963; Hightower et al., 1966) or administration of cyclophosphamide (Pierson et al., 1976; Hazlett et al., 1977; Rosen and Berk, 1977; Urano and Maejima, 1978; Harada et al., 1979). In addition, there are a few reported instances in which clinical inner ear disease in mice has been attributed to natural *P. aeruginosa* infection (Ediger et al., 1971; Kohn and MacKenzie, 1980).

*Agent*

*P. aeruginosa* is a bacterium, class Schizomycetes, order Eubacteriales, family Pseudomonadaceae. The organisms are Gram-negative, straight or slightly curved rods measuring 0.5-1.0 μm in diameter × 1.5-5.0 μm in length. They are motile and catalase and oxidase positive. Most strains produce a bluish green phenazine pigment (pyocyanin), as well as fluorescein, a greenish yellow pteridine that fluoresces. The organisms grow readily on media used in the routine isolation of bacteria (Palleroni, 1984; Gilardi, 1985).

Different strains of *P. aeruginosa* vary widely in virulence for mice (Pennington and Williams, 1979), and flagella appear to have a role in virulence (Montie et al., 1982). *P. aeruginosa* elaborates three potent exotoxins that are more pathogenic than endotoxin. Exotoxin A is thought to be the major toxin involved in virulence. In addition, the organism produces a variety of other toxins and enzymes that can contribute to its pathogenesis (Palleroni, 1984; Gilardi, 1985).

*Hosts*

Laboratory and wild mice and rats, humans, and numerous other species (Palleroni, 1984).

*Epizootiology*

The organism is ubiquitous, occurring widely in soil, water, sewage, and air. It frequently is present in small numbers in the normal intestinal flora of people, and also occurs normally on the human skin (Gilardi, 1985). It is widely distributed in conventional stocks of rodents. In one 10-year survey in Japan it was found in 20-50% of the rodent colonies (Nakagawa et al., 1984). In the same survey *P. aeruginosa* was isolated from nasal passages, oropharynx, large intestine, and skin in many healthy rodent colonies.

*P. aeruginosa* can be transmitted by fomites (such as food, bedding, and water), human carriers, and contact with infected rodents (either wild rodents or other laboratory animals). There is frequent shedding of the organism in infected, clinically normal rodents, but the normal flora of the nasopharynx and the gastrointestinal tract are effective in controlling the population in vivo. Disease occurs when this normal flora is altered or host defenses are impaired (Vincent et al., 1955; Hoag et al., 1965; Hightower et al., 1966).

### *Clinical*

Under usual circumstances the organism is part of the normal flora in the digestive tract and clinical signs are not present. After immunosuppression fulminating septicemia can occur, resulting in death with few clinical signs (Flynn, 1963c). There are a few reports of "circling" or "rolling" in mice associated with otitis media and interna due to *P. aeruginosa* (Ediger et al., 1971; Olson and Ediger, 1972; Kohn and MacKenzie, 1980).

### *Pathology*

In immunosuppressed animals the organism invades from the normal sites of localization into deeper tissues, resulting in bacteremia and high mortality (Hammond et al., 1954; Vincent et al., 1955; Hightower et al., 1966). There is disagreement on whether the major site of entry is via the intestine and portal circulation (Urano and Maejima, 1978) or through the nasal mucosa (Brownstein, 1978). Gross and histopathologic lesions are nonspecific (Flynn, 1963b).

There are two reported instances of inner ear disease in mice attributed to *P. aeruginosa* and characterized clinically by either circling (Ediger et al., 1971) or rolling (Kohn and MacKenzie, 1980). In both instances, affected animals had suppurative otitis media with extension into the inner ears and to the adjacent meninges or brain. *P. aeruginosa* was consistently isolated from the middle ears and associated lesions (Olson and Ediger, 1972; Kohn and MacKenzie, 1980). A similar disease has been produced experimentally by inoculating *P. aeruginosa* intravenously into mice (Gorrill, 1956; Ediger et al., 1971).

B-lymphocyte-deficient mice are more susceptible to *P. aeruginosa* infection than B-lymphocyte-immunocompetent mice and have been used as a model for studying the protective efficacy of monoclonal antibodies against the organism (Zweerink et al., 1988). Other models of increased susceptibility of mice to the organism have included whole body irradiation (Flynn, 1963a,b,c; Hammond, 1963; Hightower et al., 1966), administration of cyclosphosphamide (Buhles and Shifrine, 1977; Urano and Maejima, 1978), local burns (Stieritz and Holder, 1975; Cryz et al., 1984), and administration of ferric ions (Forsberg and Bullen, 1972).

### *Diagnosis*

Diagnosis is dependent on isolation and identification of the organism and exclusion of other possible causes of disease. In animals previously immunosuppressed, septicemia due to *P. aeruginosa* (or other opportunists) should be demonstrated by culture (Flynn, 1963b).

### *Control*

Control of *P. aeruginosa* infection is not necessary for most studies using mice and rats, but it can be of great importance to the success of studies in which these animals are immunosuppressed by whole body irradiation or the administration of chemotherapeutic agents such as cyclophosphamide (Flynn, 1963b; Urano and Maejima, 1978).

*P. aeruginosa* can be completely eliminated from mice and rats by cesarean derivation followed by maintenance under gnotobiotic conditions (Trentin et al., 1966). However, for most studies employing immunosuppressive regimens, the complications caused by this organism can be avoided through more practical measures.

When mice and rats are maintained by standard husbandry practices, the nasopharynx and lower digestive tract frequently become colonized by *P. aeruginosa*. Maintenance of this colonized state depends on the repeated ingestion of large numbers of *P. aeruginosa* in the drinking water. Water provided by either water bottles or automatic watering systems can serve as an excellent medium for growth of the organism. The colonized state can be virtually eliminated by preventing the repeated ingestion of organisms through rigorous sanitation measures coupled with acidification and/or hyperchlorination of the water. However, hyperchlorination/acidification of water will not eliminate an established infection. Cages, water bottles, sipper tubes, and bedding should be autoclaved. The water can be treated with sodium hypochlorite to provide 10-12 μg/ml (ppm) chlorine or acidified to pH 2.5 to 2.8 with hydrochloric acid to prevent growth of *P. aeruginosa*. Water bottles must be changed and automatic water lines flushed frequently to assure these effective levels of chlorination or acidification (Wensinck et al., 1957; Beck, 1963; Flynn, 1963c; McPherson, 1963; Woodward, 1963; Hoag et al., 1965; Hightower et al., 1966; McDougall et al., 1967; Weisbroth, 1979). Hyperchlorination of drinking water to prevent infection with *P. aeruginosa* has been reported to depress macrophage function in mice (Fidler, 1977). Acidification and chlorination of drinking water does not adversely affect reproduction in mice (Les, 1968).

A number of vaccines against *P. aeruginosa* have been shown to have some protective effect in mice and rats (Lusis and Soltys, 1971; Pavlovskis et al., 1981; Joo et al., 1982; Leiberman et al., 1986) but appear to be of doubtful value for use in rodents.

*Interference with Research*

Indigenous infections of *P. aeruginosa* in laboratory mice and rats are generally of little importance except when immunosuppressive regimens are carried out:

a. Mice and rats naturally or experimentally infected with *P. aeruginosa* typically show the early death syndrome (i.e., on average they die several days earlier than comparable animals not infected with this organism) when exposed to lethal doses of whole body irradiation (Hammond et al., 1954, 1955; Vincent et al., 1955; Wensinck et al., 1957; Flynn, 1963a,b,c; Hammond, 1963; Hightower et al., 1966). Similar early deaths in mice exposed to lethal irradiation have occasionally been attributed to other enteric bacteria including *Enterobacter cloacae*, *Escherichia coli*, *Klebsiella pneumonia*, and *Proteus vulgaris* (Matsumoto, 1980, 1982). In general, axenic rodents can tolerate more radiation than animals with a normal flora, i.e., they survive higher median lethal doses and have increased survival times (McLaughlin et al., 1964).

b. Mice and rats infected naturally or experimentally with *P. aeruginosa* can have high mortality due to *P. aeruginosa* bacteremia following administration of cyclophosphamide (Pierson et al., 1976; Hazlett et al., 1977; Rosen and Berk, 1977; Urano and Maejima, 1978; Harada et al., 1979), cortisone (Millican, 1963), or other chemical immunosuppressants (Schook et al., 1977).

c. Mice with streptozotocin-induced diabetes mellitus have been reported to have increased susceptibility to *P. aeruginosa* infection (Kitahara et al., 1981).

d. Mice previously infected with murine cytomegalovirus have been reported to be more susceptible to experimental *P. aeruginosa* infection (Hamilton and Overall, 1978).

e. Mice given *P. aeruginosa* intraperitoneally have depressed contact sensitivity to oxazolone (Campa et al., 1975, 1976, 1977).

f. Mice given *P. aeruginosa* by gavage have reduced survival when exposed to cold stress of –20°C for 2.5 hours (Halkett et al., 1968).

g. Indwelling jugular catheters in rats may become infected with *P. aeruginosa* and be causally associated with septic pulmonary emboli (Wyand and Jonas, 1967).

## COMMON ENDOPARASITES

Traditionally, publications concerned with endoparasites of laboratory mice and rats have tended to be encyclopedic in coverage and monolithic in treatment of reports from older versus recent literature. That approach is no longer acceptable inasmuch as earlier reports often reflected the diverse parasite flora of wild mice and rats, which persisted for many years after these species were adapted for laboratory use. The majority of parasites that were commonplace in rodent colonies only a few decades ago have now been either eliminated or greatly reduced in prevalence through the application of cesarean derivation and barrier maintenance methodologies. Occasional exceptions may be encountered in conventional colonies that have never been rederived by cesarean section and in cesarean-derived stocks that have been contaminated by wild rodents. Thus, those parasites of the digestive tract that are regularly encountered in contemporary stocks of laboratory mice and rats in the United States are listed in Table 11. Among parasites of this group only two, *Spironucleus muris* and *Giardia muris,* are considered important pathogens and have been reported to interfere significantly with research. The other pathogen in the group, *Hymenolepis nana,* is only considered a mild pathogen. The remainder (*Syphacia obvelata, Syphacia muris, Aspicularis tetraptera, Entamoeba muris,* and *Tritrichomonas muris*) are nonpathogenic under usual circumstances. These eight parasites are reviewed below.

## *Spironucleus muris*

### *Significance*

*Spironucleus muris* is a common intestinal parasite in laboratory rodents, including those maintained by barrier methods, and there is increasing evidence that it alters immune responses (see below).

### *Agent*

*S. muris* (formerly *Hexamita muris*) is a flagellated protozoan, subphylum Mastigophora, class Zoomastigophorea, order Diplomonadida, family Hexamitidae, subfamily Hexamitinae. The trophozoite is elongated, torpedo-shaped, bilaterally symmetrical, and measures 3-4 × 10-15 μm. It has six actively beating anterior flagella and two slow-moving flagella at the posterior tip. The cysts measure 4 × 7 μm (Kunstyr, 1977; Brugerolle et al., 1980).

### *Life Cycle*

The life cycle is direct. The trophozoites reproduce by longitudinal fission and form highly resistant cysts. The minimal infectious dose for a mouse is one cyst (Kunstyr, 1977; Stachan and Kunstyr, 1983).

*Hosts*

Mice, rats, and hamsters (Wagner et al., 1974; Kunstyr et al., 1977a; Kunstyr and Friedhoff, 1980).

*Epizootiology*

Young mice, 2-6 weeks old, are most susceptible. The trophozoites usually inhabit the crypts of Lieberkuhn in the small intestine, but in young animals the lumen can also contain large numbers. In older mice and rats very few trophozoites may be present, and they can be found only in the glands of the gastric pylorus (J. R. Lindsey, Department of Comparative Medicine, University of Alabama at Birmingham, unpublished).

Transmission is by ingestion of the cysts. The cysts are shed in the feces, in greatest numbers by young or immunocompromised hosts, e.g., athymic (*nu/nu*) or lethally irradiated mice (Kunstyr et al., 1977b). The cysts are inactivated by some disinfectants and high temperature (45°C for 30 minutes) but are highly resistant to most other environmental conditions. They retain infectivity after –20°C for 6 months, pH 2.2 for 1 day, room temperature for 14 days, and 0.1% glutaraldehyde for 1 hour (Kunstyr and Ammerpohl, 1978).

*Clinical*

The infection is usually subclinical in immunocompetent hosts. Severe chronic enteritis with weight loss has been associated with *S. muris* infection in athymic (*nu/nu*) and lethally irradiated mice (Meshorer, 1969; Kunstyr et al., 1977b).

Young mice infected with *S. muris* have been reported to have diarrhea, dehydration, rough hair coats, weight loss, listlessness, hunched posture, abdominal distension, and sporadic mortality (Sebesteny, 1969; Lussier and Loew, 1970; Boorman et al., 1973a; Csiza and Abelseth, 1973; Wagner et al., 1974; von Mattheisen et al., 1976; Flatt et al., 1978; Van Kruiningen et al., 1978; Eisenbrandt and Russell, 1979). However, none of these studies excluded other possible causes such as mouse hepatitis virus infection. It is doubtful whether *S. muris* alone causes clinical disease in otherwise healthy hosts (Kunstyr and Friedhoff, 1980).

*Pathology*

Immunocompetent mice are susceptible to experimental infection until about 8 or 10 weeks of age, and rats are susceptible until 12 weeks of age. Athymic (*nu/nu*) mice are fully susceptible at any age. After ingestion of cysts by the host, trophozoite (and cyst) numbers in the intestines of

TABLE 11 Common Endoparasites of Mice and Rats

| Site and Parasite (Common name, if any) | Type of Parasite | Stage Most Useful in Diagnosis (Size) | Ecological Niche in Host | Histologic Features | Other Diagnostic Methods |
|---|---|---|---|---|---|
| Small Intestine | | | | | |
| *Spironucleus muris* | Flagellated protozoan | Trophozoite (2-3 μm wide wide × 7-9 μm long) | Intervillous spaces and crypts of small intestine, glands of gastric pylorus | Charcteristic granular appearance of trophozoites in crypts of small intestine and glands of pylorus; stain with periodic acid-Schiff and silver methods | Demonstrate characteristic trophozoites in saline mounts of small intestine contents or cysts (4.0 × 7.4 μm) in wet mounts of feces: phase-contrast preferred |
| *Giardia muris* | Flagellated protozoan | Trophozoite (5-10 μm wide × 7-13 μm long) | Along and between villi of small intesine | Size, shape, and location of trophozoites; stain with periodic acid-Schiff and silver methods | Same as for *S. muris* |
| *Hymenolepis nana* (dwarf tapeworm) | Tapeworm | Adults (25-40 μm long × 0.75 μm wide) | Small intestine attached to mucosa [Note: larval stage (cercocystis) can be seen in mucosa of small intestine] | Adults have scolices with armed rostellum, segments, no body cavity or digestive tract, calcareous corpuscles present; cercocystis in intestinal villi | Demonstrate eggs (37-41 × 50-53 μm) by fecal flotation |

| | | | | | |
|---|---|---|---|---|---|
| Large Intestine | | | | | |
| *Syphacia obvelata* (mouse pinworm) | Nematode | Adults (female, 3.4-5.8 µm long; male, 1.1-1.5 µm long), egg | Cecum and colon | Nematodes have a digestive tract and a single layer of muscle cells; genus and species identification based on morphology of intact adults | Demonstrate eggs (36 × 134 µm, flat on one side) by cellophane tape preparation of periannal area |
| *Syphacia muris* rat pinworm) | Nematode | Adults (female, 2.8-4.0 mm long; male, 1.2-2.3 mm long), egg | Cecum and colon | Same as *S. obvelata* | Same as for *S. obvelata;* eggs are 29 × 75 µm, football shaped to slightly flat on one side |
| *Aspicularis tetraptera* (mouse pinworm) | Nematode | Adults (female, 2.6-4.7 µm long; male, 2.0-2.6 µm long), egg | Large intestine, *except* cecum | Same as *S. obvelata* | Demonstrate eggs (41 × 90 µm, ellipsoidal shape) by fecal flotation |
| *Entamoeba muris* | Amoeba | Trophozoite (8-30 µm diam.) | Fecal/mucosal interface, cecum, and colon | Trophozoites have distinct magenta nucleus and vacuolated violet cytoplasm; cell membrane indistinct (hematoxylin and eosin stain) | Demonstrate characteristic trophozoites in saline mounts of cecal or colon contents, cysts (9-20 µm diameter) in feces |
| *Tritrichomonas muris* | Flagellated protozoan | Trophozoite (10-15 µm × 16-26 µm) | In fecal stream of cecum and colon | Trophozoites have indistinct nucleus and no cytoplasmic vacuolation; outer membrane is distinct and may appear wrinkled (hematoxylin and eosin stain) | Demonstrate trophozoites with characteristic wobbly movement in saline mount of cecal or colon contents, fresh feces |

immunocompetent rodents peak at 1-2 weeks and decline to low numbers by 4-5 weeks (BALB/c mice), 7-9 weeks (CBA, SJL, and C3H/He mice), or 13 weeks (A and B.B10 mice). By comparison, the numbers in athymic (*nu/nu*) mice persist indefinitely at high levels (Kunstyr et al., 1977a,b; Kunstyr and Friedhoff, 1980; Brett and Cox, 1982a).

In severe infections, such as those in athymic (*nu/nu*) mice, the small intestine may appear reddened and contain watery fluid and gas. Wet mounts of the contents of the small intestine are useful for demonstrating the motile trophozoites; the cysts can be demonstrated in the contents of the cecum and colon. In hematoxylin and eosin-stained sections of the small intestine, the best indicator of *S. muris* infection is distension of the crypts of Lieberkuhn by masses of granular-appearing trophozoites. They are seen less frequently in the intervillous spaces and gut lumen. The trophozoites can cause shortening of microvilli on the crypt epithelium and increased turnover of enterocytes. There usually is little or no inflammatory response in immunocompetent animals, but heavily parasitized animals that are immunodeficient can have moderate to severe enteritis (Kunstyr et al., 1977a,b; Brugerolle et al., 1980; Kunstyr and Friedhoff, 1980).

### *Diagnosis*

Definitive diagnosis of disease caused by *S. muris* requires exclusion of other possible causes of digestive tract disease, e.g., enterotrophic strains of mouse hepatitis virus. In many laboratories the diagnosis is made by using wet mounts to demonstrate the characteristic trophozoites in contents of the small intestine or cysts in contents of the large intestine or feces (Kunstyr, 1977). For routine health surveillance that includes histopathology, the examination of multiple histologic sections of small intestine and gastric pylorus is probably superior to other methods because very few parasites may be present and they may be localized in distribution. The trophozoites can be stained by silver or periodic acid-Schiff methods (Flatt et al., 1978).

### *Control*

Cesarean derivation and barrier maintenance are the recommended procedures. Treatment of spironucleosis in mice with 0.04-0.1% dimetridazole in drinking water for 14 days can ameliorate clinical signs but does not completely eliminate the infection (Herweg and Kunstyr, 1979).

### *Interference with Research*

There is considerable evidence that *S. muris* infection interferes with research, including the following:

a. *S. muris* can increase the severity and mortality of wasting syndrome (presumably due to mouse hepatitis virus) in athymic (*nu/nu*) mice (Boorman et al., 1973a,b).

b. Susceptibility to *S. muris* infection and disease is greatly enhanced by whole body irradiation (Meshorer, 1969; Meyers, 1973; Kunstyr et al., 1977b; Gruber and Osborne, 1979).

c. *S. muris* infection increases mortality in cadmium-treated mice (Exon et al., 1975).

d. *S. muris* infection alters macrophage function (Keast and Chesterman, 1972; Ruitenberg and Kruyt, 1975).

e. *S. muris* infection reduces spleen plaque-forming cell responses to sheep erythrocytes (Brett, 1983) and lymphocyte responsiveness to mitogens such as phytohemagglutinin, concanavalin A, and pokeweed mitogen (Kunstyr and Friedhoff, 1980).

f. *S. muris* infection alters immune responsiveness to tetanus toxoid and type 3 pneumococcal polysaccharide in mice (Ruitenberg and Kruyt, 1975) but not in rats (Mullink et al., 1980).

g. Concurrent infections of *Babesia microti*, *Plasmodium yoelii*, or *Plasmodium berghei* with *S. muris* decreases the numbers of *S. muris* trophozoites and cysts (Brett and Cox, 1982b).

## *Giardia muris*

### *Significance*

*Giardia muris* causes a common, subclinical infection of laboratory rodents that has been shown in recent years to alter a number of immune responses in mice (Belosevic et al., 1985).

### *Agent*

*G. muris* is a flagellated protozoan, subphylum Mastigophora, class Zoomastigophorea, order Diplomonadida, family Hexamitidae, subfamily Giardinae. The trophozoite is 7-13 μm long × 5-10 μm wide, pear-shaped, and bilaterally symmetrical. The anterior end is broadly rounded, while the posterior end is drawn out. There are two dark-staining median bodies that are small and round and located just posterior to the nucleus. The trophozoites are easily recognized in wet preparations of intestinal contents because of their characteristic cupped shape and rolling and tumbling motion. The cysts are ellipsoidal, 15 × 17 μm, have thick walls and 4 nuclei, and are found in the large intestine and feces (Hsu, 1979, 1982; Brugerolle et al., 1980).

### *Life Cycle*

The life cycle is direct. The trophozoites reproduce by longitudinal fission and form cysts that are passed in the feces. Transmission is by ingestion of cysts. The minimal infectious dose for a mouse is approximately 10 cysts (Hsu, 1979, 1982; Stachan and Kunstyr, 1983).

### *Hosts*

Mice, rats, hamsters, humans, and many other species (Kunstyr and Friedhoff, 1980).

### *Epizootiology*

The trophozoites colonize the proximal one-fourth of the small intestine in which they are found mainly adhering to columnar cells near the bases of villi and free in the adjacent mucus layer. The number of trophozoites in the small intestine correlates directly with the number of cysts in the large intestine and feces (Owen et al., 1979; Brett and Cox, 1982a; Belosevic and Faubert, 1983; Belosevic et al., 1984).

The cysts are resistant to most environmental conditions but are inactivated by treatment with a 2.5% phenol solution and by temperatures above 50°C (Hsu, 1979).

### *Clinical*

*G. muris* infections in mice and rats are usually subclinical but can cause reduced weight gain, rough hair coats, and enlarged abdomens (Sebesteny, 1969; Roberts-Thomson et al., 1976b; Owen et al., 1979). Infection has been associated with morbidity and mortality in athymic (*nu*/*nu*) and thymectomized mice (Boorman et al., 1973a), and in mice immunocompromised by x-irradiation or protein-deficient diets (Owen et al., 1979). However, these studies did not exclude concurrent infection(s) by other enteric pathogens.

### *Pathology*

Pathogenesis of *G. muris* infection has been studied most extensively in mice. The acute phase of the infection involves the proliferation of trophozoites in the small intestine and the peak period of cyst release during week 2 of infection. The elimination phase is the period during which the cysts released in the feces are reduced to undetectable levels. The DBA/2, B10.A, C57BL/6, BALB/c, and SJL/J strains eliminate the infection in 5 weeks and are said to be resistant, whereas the C3H/He, A/J, and Crl:ICR

(CD®-1) mice require 10 weeks and are considered susceptible (Brett and Cox, 1982a; Belosevic et al., 1984). Genetic analyses have shown that resistance during the acute phase of the infection may be controlled by several genes not linked to the *H-2* locus (Belosevic et al., 1984), while resistance during the elimination phase is inherited as a dominant trait (Roberts-Thomson et al., 1980; Belosevic et al., 1984).

Protective immunity is thought to be dependent upon both antibody- and cell-mediated mechanisms (Brett and Cox, 1982a; Stevens, 1982). Both IgA and IgG antibodies against *G. muris* have been demonstrated in milk of immune mice (Andrews et al., 1980), and such milk conveys passive protection (Stevens and Frank, 1978; Roberts-Thomson and Mitchell, 1979). Athymic (*nu/nu*) mice also are highly susceptible and have prolonged infections (Roberts-Thomson and Mitchell, 1978; Stevens et al., 1978).

The morphologic changes in the small intestine associated with uncomplicated *G. muris* infection are usually minimal. The villus to crypt ratio may be reduced and variable numbers of lymphocytes may be present (Roberts-Thomson et al., 1976b; Stevens and Roberts-Thomson, 1978; Brett and Cox, 1982a).

### *Diagnosis*

Definitive diagnosis of overt disease thought to be attributable to *G. muris* requires exclusion of other possible primary or contributing pathogens. Infection due to *G. muris* can be diagnosed histologically by identifying the characteristic "monkey-faced" trophozoites in sections of small intestine. The trophozoites also can be demonstrated in wet mounts of intestinal contents, and the cysts can be demonstrated in wet mounts of feces (Hsu, 1979, 1982).

### *Control*

The most practical approach is procurement of rodents from breeding populations shown by health surveillance testing to be free of *G. muris*, followed by barrier maintenance in the user facility. Cesarean derivation is required to eliminate the parasite from infected stocks. Metronidazole can be used for treatment of infected animals (Belosevic et al., 1985) but does not completely eradicate the infection.

### *Interference with Research*

*G. muris* infection can alter research results, and the course of experimental *G. muris* infections can be influenced by a variety of experimental procedures as follows:

a. *G. muris* infection causes a transient reduction in the immunoresponsiveness of mice to sheep erythrocytes during weeks 2 and 3 of infection (Brett, 1983; Belosevic et al., 1985).

b. *G. muris* infection alters intestinal fluid accumulation and mucosal immune responses caused by cholera toxin in mice (Ljungstrom et al., 1985).

c. Concurrent *G. muris* and *Trichinella spiralis* infection in mice results in suppression of the *G. muris* infection (Roberts-Thomson et al., 1976a).

d. Concurrent infections of *Babesia microti, Plasmodium yoelii,* or *Plasmodium berghei* with *G. muris* decreases the number of *G. muris* trophozoites and cysts (Brett and Cox, 1982b).

e. Susceptibility to *G. muris* infection is increased by x-irradiation or protein-deficient diets (Owen et al., 1979).

f. *G. muris* infection can increase the severity and mortality of wasting syndrome (presumably due to mouse hepatitis virus) in athymic (*nu/nu*) mice (Boorman et al., 1973a).

## *Hymenolepis nana* (Dwarf Tapeworm)

### *Significance*

*Hymenolepis nana* is a small tapeworm found infrequently in contemporary rodents. It is only mildly pathogenic but has importance as a zoonotic agent for humans.

### *Agent*

*H. nana* belongs to the order Cyclophyllidea, family Hymenolepididae. The adult is a slender, white worm, 25-40 mm long and less than 1 mm wide. It has a scolex with 4 suckers and an armed, retractable rostellum with a row of 20-27 hooks. Mature proglottids are trapezoidal in shape. The eggs are oval, thin shelled, and colorless and have prominent polar filaments. They contain an oncosphere with 3 pairs of hooklets enclosed in an inner envelope. They measure 30-56 × 44-62 μm and are unable to survive long outside the host. The spherical embryo measures 16-25 × 24-30 μm and possesses 3 pairs of hooks (Flynn, 1973b; Wescott, 1982).

### *Life Cycle*

The life cycle includes adult, egg (with embryo or oncosphere), and larval (cercocystis) stages. The life cycle can be direct. Eggs in the feces of a definitive host are directly infectious when ingested by another potential definitive host, or the eggs hatch within the intestine of the definitive host, resulting in autoinfection of the same host. In either case, the eggs hatch in the small intestine, the larvae penetrate and develop in the intestinal villi as cercocystis, and return to the lumen to become mature adults. By direct transmission the life cycle requires only 14-16 days. Alternatively, the cycle can be indirect. The egg is ingested by an arthropod intermediate host such as a flour beetle, the cercocystis develops in the intestine of the beetle, the intermediate host is eaten by the definitive host, and the adult develops in the lumen of the small intestine. The entire life cycle by indirect transmission requires 20-30 days (Flynn, 1973b; Wescott, 1982).

*Hosts*

Mice, rats, hamsters, other rodents, simian primates, and humans (Hsu, 1979; Kunstyr and Friedhoff, 1980; Wescott, 1982).

*Epizootiology*

Weanling and young adult rodents are most frequently infected. The duration of infection by the adult worms in the small intestine is usually only a few weeks (Flynn, 1973b; Wescott, 1982).

*Clinical*

Most infections are subclinical. However, severe infections have been reported to cause retarded growth and weight loss in mice and intestinal occlusion, impaction, and death in hamsters (Flynn, 1973b; Wescott, 1982).

*Pathology*

The presence of adult worms in the small intestine is usually associated with mild enteritis. The finding of typical cercocystis with an armed rostellum in the intestinal villi of a rodent is diagnostic of *H. nana*.

Larval stages occasionally reach the mesenteric lymph nodes, liver, or lung where they incite a granulomatous inflammatory response (Flynn, 1973b; Hsu, 1979; Wescott, 1982). This is reportedly a common occurrence in mice of the RFM strain (C. Zurcher, Institute for Experimental Gerontology TNO, Rijswijk, The Netherlands, unpublished).

*Diagnosis*

The most common method is demonstration and identification of the adult tapeworms in the small intestine. Eggs may be demonstrated in the feces. Also, histologic sections occasionally are successful in demonstrating the cercocystis in intestinal villi and mesenteric nodes (Flynn, 1973b; Hsu, 1979; Wescott, 1982).

### *Control*

The most practical method usually is to obtain rodents from stocks that have been demonstrated to be free of *H. nana*. Cesarean derivation and barrier maintenance are the most effective methods for eliminating the infection from infected rodent stocks (Flynn, 1973b; Wescott, 1982).

### *Interference with Research*

Infected rodents are deemed unsuitable for research use because of the potential for zoonotic infection and the fact that *H. nana* is pathogenic. *H. nana* infection can interfere with studies involving the intestinal tract (Flynn, 1973b; Wescott, 1982).

## ***Syphacia obvelata* (Mouse Pinworm) and *Syphacia muris* (Rat Pinworm)**

### *Significance*

*Syphacia obvelata* and *Syphacia muris* are among the more common endoparasites of contemporary rodents, including stocks that have been derived by cesarean section and maintained in barrier facilities (Flynn, 1973c).

### *Agents*

These rodent pinworms belong to class Nematoda, order Ascarida, suborder Oxyurina, genus *Syphacia*. They are roundworms, with three broad lips; a prominent esophagus with a well-developed single bulb at the posterior end; and long, pointed tails. Male worms possess three mamelons; a long, prominent spicule; a gubernaculum; and a ventrally bent tail. On the female, the vulva is located on the anterior quarter of the body, behind the excretory pore. Eggs are asymmetrical, more or less flattened on one side, thin shelled, and transparent (Flynn, 1973c; Wescott, 1982).

For most purposes there is no reason to differentiate infections due to *S. obvelata* and those due to *S. muris;* however, the two species can be distinguished by the following criteria (Wescott, 1982):

a. *Male worms.* The adult male *S. obvelata* is 1.1-1.6 mm long and 125 μm wide. The adult male *S. muris* is 1.2-1.3 μm long and 100 μm wide. The tail length of *S. muris* is about two times its body width, whereas the tail length of *S. obvelata* is about equal to its body width.

b. *Female worms.* The adult female *S. obvelata* is 3.4-5.8 μm long and 240-400 μm wide. The adult female *S. muris* is 2.8-4.0 mm long and 250 μm wide. The vulva of *S. muris* is further posterior in relation to the esophageal bulb than that of *S. obvelata*.

c. *Eggs*. *S. muris* eggs (75 × 20 μm) are slightly more than half the length of *S. obvelata* eggs (134 × 36 μm), although nearly the same width. *S. muris* eggs are slightly asymmetrical, being slightly flatter on one side than the other, but somewhat football shaped. *S. obvelata* eggs are decidedly asymmetrical or somewhat banana shaped.

### *Life Cycle*

The life cycle is direct and requires only 11-15 days for completion. Gravid females migrate from the large intestine to deposit their eggs in the perianal area. The eggs become infective in about 6 hours. Following ingestion by another host, the eggs hatch in the small intestine, and the larvae reach the cecum in 24 hours. The parasites spend 10-11 days in the cecum where they mature and mate. Gravid females again migrate to the perianal area, deposit their eggs, and die (Wescott, 1982).

### *Hosts*

Laboratory mice, rats, hamsters, gerbils, and wild rodents. *S. obvelata* has been reported to occur in people, but it has no known public health significance (Flynn, 1973c; Wightman et al., 1978; Ross et al., 1980; Wescott, 1982).

### *Epizootiology*

The adults occur primarily in the cecum and colon of infected hosts. Eggs are deposited in the perianal area of the host, from which they are efficiently disseminated into the cage and room environments. The eggs can survive for weeks under most animal room conditions. Transmission is by ingestion of embryonated eggs (Flynn, 1973c; Wescott, 1982).

### *Clinical*

Infections due to *Syphacia* spp. alone are subclinical. Poor condition, rough hair coats, reduced growth rate, and rectal prolapse have been attributed to natural *Syphacia* infections in mice (Hoag, 1961; Harwell and Boyd, 1968; Jacobson and Reed, 1974). Unfortunately, such reports have failed to exclude other possible causes, e.g., *Citrobacter freundii* (Biotype 4280) infection, which has been shown to cause rectal prolapse in mice (Barthold et al., 1977). Clinical signs have not been observed in rodents experimentally infected with *S. obvelata* or *S. muris* (Flynn, 1973c; Wescott, 1982).

### *Pathology*

The prevalence of pinworms in an infected rodent population is a function of age, sex, and host immune status. In enzootically infected colonies, weanling animals develop the greatest parasite loads, males are more heavily parasitized than females, and *Syphacia* numbers diminish with increasing age of the host (Wescott, 1982).

Athymic (*nu/nu*) mice were reported by Jacobson and Reed (1974) to have increased susceptibility to pinworm infection. When naturally infected athymic and immunocompetent mice were housed together in the same room for 130 days, the athymic mice obtained increasingly heavy worm burdens, while the immunocompetent mice maintained consistently low worm counts.

Pinworms of laboratory rodents are generally not considered pathogens. Heavy infections have been reported to cause rectal prolapse, constipation, intussusception, or fecal impaction but usually without use of diagnostic procedures appropriate to exclude other intercurrent diseases as primary or contributing causes (Flynn, 1973c; Wescott, 1982).

### *Diagnosis*

Diagnosis is based on the demonstration of eggs on the perianal region (cellophane tape technique) or the finding of adult worms in the cecum and colon at necropsy (Flynn, 1973c; Wescott, 1982).

### *Control*

The use of cesarean derivation and barrier maintenance methods are effective (Phillips, 1960), but subsequent reinfection of such stocks with *Syphacia* spp. has been a common occurrence (Flynn, 1973c).

Hygienic methods, such as frequent cage and room sanitization, can aid in controlling the *Syphacia* burden in an infected rodent population. Cage-to-cage transmission can be prevented by the use of filter-top cages (Wescott et al., 1976). Several anthelminthics are effective in eliminating a high percentage of the adult worms but are inefficient in clearing immature worms or eggs. Thus, treatment must be repetitive and is not generally recommended, except in special circumstances (Wagner, 1970; Flynn, 1973c; Hsu, 1979; Wescott, 1982).

### *Interference with Research*

Pinworm infections in rats have been reported to reduce the occurrence of adjuvant-induced arthritis (Pearson and Taylor, 1975).

### ***Aspicularis tetraptera*** **(mouse pinworm)**

*Significance*

*Aspicularis tetraptera* ranks second (after *Syphacia obvelata*) in prevalence in contemporary rodents, but like the other rodent pinworms, it is considered nonpathogenic (Flynn, 1973c; Wescott, 1982).

*Agent*

These rodent pinworms belong to class Nematoda, order Ascarida, suborder Oxyurina, genus *Aspicularis*. The males are 2.0-2.6 mm long and 120-190 µm wide; the females are 2.6-4.7 mm long and 215-275 µm wide. Both sexes have broad cervical alae and conical tails. The vulva in the female is located near the center of the body. The males lack spicules and mamelons. The eggs are ellipsoidal and measure 41 × 90 µm (Flynn, 1973c; Hsu, 1979; Wescott, 1982).

*Life Cycle*

The life cycle is direct and requires 23-25 days. The adults reside in the colon. Females lay their eggs in the colon (not in the perianal area as is true of *Syphacia* spp.), and the eggs subsequently leave the host on fecal pellets. The eggs become infective after 6-7 days at room temperature. Transmission occurs when the infective eggs are ingested by another host. The eggs hatch in the colon, where the larvae develop to maturity, and the cycle begins again (Flynn, 1973c; Wescott, 1982).

The life cycle of *A. tetraptera* differs from that of *Syphacia obvelata* and *Syphacia muris* in that it is 10-12 days longer, and the eggs of *A. tetraptera* require an additional 6 days for embryonation to the infective stage (Flynn, 1973c; Wescott, 1982).

*Hosts*

Mice, rats (rarely), and wild rodents (Flynn, 1973c; Wescott, 1982).

*Epizootiology*

Unlike *S. obvelata* and *S. muris*, which primarily inhabit the cecum (except for gravid females), *A. tetraptera* primarily inhabits the colon. *A. tetraptera* females lay eggs in the colon, not in the perianal area as is characteristic of *S. obvelata* and *S. muris*. Like the other pinworms, the eggs of *A. tetraptera* survive for weeks in animal room environments (Flynn, 1973c; Wescott, 1982).

*Clinical*

Same as for *S. obvelata* and *S. muris* (see above). Infections caused by *A. tetraptera* are subclinical.

*Pathology*

Same as for *S. obvelata* and *S. muris* (see above). *A. tetraptera* is not considered pathogenic.

*Diagnosis*

The more common methods are demonstration of the distinctive eggs by fecal flotation (the cellophane tape method is of no value) and demonstration and identification of the adult worms in the colon at necropsy (Flynn, 1973c; Wescott, 1982).

*Control*

Same as for *S. obvelata* and *S. muris* (see above).

*Interference with Research*

Same as for *S. obvelata* and *S. muris* (see above).

***Entamoeba muris***

*Significance*

*Entamoeba muris* is a commensal amoeba found in the large intestine of rodents. It lacks significance both in terms of public health and as a complication of research.

*Agent*

This organism is a protozoan, phylum Sarcomastigophora, subphylum Sarcodina, superclass Rhizopoda, order Amoebida, family Entamoebidae, genus *Entamoeba*. The trophozoites measure 8-30 μm in diameter and have 8 nuclei (Levine, 1961).

*Life Cycle*

The life cycle is direct. The trophozoites form cysts that are passed in the feces. Transmission is by ingestion of cysts. Excystment occurs in the intestinal tract, and the trophozoites inhabit the cecum and colon (Levine, 1961).

### *Hosts*

Mice, rats, hamsters, and other rodent species (Levine, 1961, 1974).

### *Epizootiology*

The trophozoites reside in the cecum and colon, where they are most commonly found at the interface between the fecal stream and the intestinal epithelium. The cysts are quite resistant to environmental conditions (Levine, 1961).

### *Clinical*

*E. muris* infections are always subclinical (Levine, 1961, 1974).

### *Pathology*

The organism is nonpathogenic (Levine, 1961, 1974).

### *Diagnosis*

The infection can be diagnosed by demonstrating the trophozoites in wet mounts of intestinal contents from the cecum or colon or the cysts in feces (Levine, 1961, 1974). In histologic sections of the cecum or large intestine prepared without disturbing the luminal contents, the trophozoites are readily identified at the margin of the fecal stream. In sections stained by hematoxylin and eosin, the trophozoites usually have a distinct magenta-stained nucleus and violet-stained cytoplasm that may or may not appear vacuolated. The outer cell membrane of the trophozoites is usually distinctly visible (J. R. Lindsey, Department of Comparative Medicine, University of Alabama at Birmingham, unpublished).

### *Control*

Infection with this amoeba is considered inconsequential, and control measures are not usually justified. The infection can be eliminated by cesarean derivation and barrier maintenance.

### *Interference with Research*

No examples have been reported.

### *Tritrichomonas muris*

#### *Significance*

*Tritrichomonas muris* is a commensal organism that occurs in the large intestine of rodents. It has no known significance as a complication of research. It is not known to infect people.

#### *Agent*

A flagellated protozoan, subphylum Mastigophora, class Zoomastigophorea, order Trichomonadida, genus *Tritrichomonas*. The trophozoite is pear-shaped and measures 10-14 × 16-26 μm. It has an anterior nucleus. More anteriorly there is a blepharoplast that gives rise to three anterior flagella and one posterior flagellum attached to the body by an undulating membrane. The trophozoite has a characteristic wobbly motility. Reproduction is by binary fission (Levine, 1974; Hsu, 1982). In the past, transmission has been thought to be by ingestion of the trophozoites, but there is a recent suggestion that *T. muris* forms cysts (Kunstyr and Friedhoff, 1980).

#### *Life Cycle*

In addition to the trophozoite stage, the organism may have a cyst stage (Kunstyr and Friedhoff, 1980). If so, the cyst stage is probably the one primarily involved in transmission.

#### *Hosts*

Mice, rats, hamsters, and rodents (Levine, 1974; Hsu, 1982).

#### *Epizootiology*

The trophozoites are found throughout the fecal mass in the cecum and colon (Levine, 1974; Hsu, 1982).

#### *Clinical*

*T. muris* infections are not known to cause clinical signs (Levine, 1974; Hsu, 1982).

#### *Pathology*

The organism is considered a commensal (Levine, 1974; Hsu, 1982).

*Diagnosis*

*T. muris* infection can be diagnosed by demonstrating the trophozoites in wet mounts of contents from the cecum or colon. Their wobbly or jerky movements are very characteristic (Levine, 1974; Hsu, 1982). In histologic sections of cecum or colon prepared without disturbing the luminal contents, the trophozoites are found dispersed throughout the fecal stream. In hematoxylin and eosin-stained sections, the nucleus stains poorly, the nuclear membrane is indistinct, and the cell wall often appears wrinkled or folded upon itself (J. R. Lindsey, Department of Comparative Medicine, University of Alabama at Birmingham, unpublished).

*Control*

The organism is a commensal, and control measures are not likely to be justified (Levine, 1974; Hsu, 1982).

*Interference with Research*

No examples have been reported.

**Other Endoparasites**

Numerous other endoparasites have been reported from wild mice and rats and are encountered occasionally in animals maintained by conventional methods. For information on those parasite species, more comprehensive works on this subject should be consulted (Levine and Ivens, 1965; Oldham, 1967; Griffiths, 1971; Owen, 1972; Flynn, 1973a; Levine, 1974; Hsu, 1979, 1982; Wescott, 1982).

# 8

# Skin and Joints

## Overview

Diseases affecting the skin and adnexal structures (e.g., mammary glands) account for many of the clinical abnormalities observed in mice and rats. As a group these diseases can be most perplexing to the clinician and pathologist concerned with rodents. Establishing definitive diagnoses frequently proves difficult or impossible, even in the most capable diagnostic laboratories, because of the complex interactions between some or all of the following: overt pathogens, opportunistic pathogens, host responses, genetic variations of hosts, environmental factors, social interactions, and other, often unknown factors.

A classification of these diseases and conditions is given in Table 12. There are 12 diseases attributed to infectious agents and 6 conditions due to other causes, such as social behavior or environmental factors. In addition to ectromelia virus, other causes of appendage amputations (*Mycoplasma arthritidis, Streptobacillus moniliformis, Corynebacterium kutscheri,* and "ringtail") are included because of clinical overlap with the pox diseases. Joint diseases, although rare in rodents, have been included here for clinical reasons.

By far the most frequently observed skin conditions are those categorized in Table 12 as "Dermatitis/Alopecias." It should be noted that this category is comprised of a heterogeneous group of conditions represented under both "Infectious Diseases" and "Noninfectious Conditions." The common ectoparasites (mites) and *Staphylococcus aureus,* a normal inhabitant of the

TABLE 12 Classification of Skin and Joint Diseases/Conditions

I. Infectious diseases
   A. Pox Diseases, Spontaneous Amputations in Some Cases
      1. Mousepox (ectromelia)
      2. Poxvirus disease(s) in rats
   B. Arthritis, Spontaneous Amputations Possible
      1. *Mycoplasma arthritidis*
      2. *Streptobacillus moniliformis*
      3. *Corynebacterium kutscheri*
   C. Dermatitis/Alopecias
      1. Common ectoparasites
      2. *Staphylococcus aureus*
      3. *Pasteurella pneumotropica*
      4. Dermatophytosis
      5. Mouse papule virus
      6. Self-mutilation associated with otitis media
   D. Neoplasms
      1. Mouse mammary tumor viruses

II. Noninfectious conditions
   A. Dermatitis/Alopecias
      1. Bite Wounds
         a. Adults (fighting)
         b. Weanlings (hunger ?)
      2. "Whisker trimming," "hair nibbling," and "barbering"
      3. Muzzle alopecia
      4. Hair growth arrest (?)
   B. Spontaneous Amputation Probable
      1. "Ringtail"

skin, are probably the leading causes of skin diseases in mice, while *S. aureus* alone probably holds that distinction in rats.

Although the diseases caused by poxviruses are extremely important because of high mortality, deleterious effects on research results, and their highly contagious nature, they are relatively infrequent in occurrence or are restricted in geographic distribution. Bacterial arthritis is extremely rare in rodent stocks.

## Ectromelia virus

### *Significance*

Low for most research uses of mice. High in those laboratories, such as immunogenetics and tumor biology laboratories, that exchange biologic materials from mice for research purposes.

*Perspective*

*1930:* Mousepox was first recognized by Marchal (1930) in England and called "infectious ectromelia". Since that time, mousepox has become the disease name and ectromelia virus has been accepted as the name of the virus.

Recorded major outbreaks of mousepox in the United States are as follows:

*1951-1953:* Yale University (Trentin and Briody, 1953; Briody, 1955)

*1954-1956:* Roswell Park Memorial Institute, Buffalo, New York (Shope, 1954; Briody, 1955; Fenner, 1981)

*1957-1958:* Epizootics in 10 laboratories (Briody, 1959)

*1960:* Yale University (Bhatt et al., 1981)

*1960-1974:* National Institutes of Health (NIH), Bethesda, Maryland (Whitney et al., 1981)

*1979-1980:* NIH and eight other institutions in five states: Utah, Maryland, Missouri, Illinois, and Minnesota (AALAS, 1981; Held, 1981; Whitney et al., 1981).

*1981:* An enzyme-linked immunosorbent assay (ELISA) for ectromelia virus infection was developed (Collins et al., 1981) and subsequently shown to be far more sensitive and specific than the hemagglutination inhibition (HAI) test that traditionally had been used for serologic diagnosis (Buller et al., 1983).

*Agent*

Ectromelia virus is a large DNA virus, family Poxviridae, genus *Orthopoxvirus.* Virions are shaped like ovals or bricks (175 × 290 nm), have a characteristic dumbbell-shaped nucleoid, and are morphologically indistinguishable from vaccinia virus (Fenner, 1982).

Many strains of ectromelia virus have been isolated. The Moscow and Hampstead strains have been studied most extensively. Moscow is the most virulent of the recognized strains. Strains are closely related antigenically. The virus is antigenically related to vaccinia (Fenner, 1982).

Ectromelia virus is cultivable in tissue cultures of several cell types, including HeLa, Vero, and mouse fibroblasts (L929), and on the chorioallantoic membrane of chick embryos (Fenner, 1982).

The virus is quite stable for extended periods under dry conditions at room temperature. It can be preserved for months at room temperature in glycerol and indefinitely at –70°C or by lyophilization (Fenner, 1982). The virus resists dry heat but is rapidly inactivated by moist heat. Heating of serum or other body fluids for 30 minutes at 60°C destroys infectivity (Bhatt and Jacoby, 1987c). Recommended disinfectants include sodium hypochlorite (100 µg/ml [ppm] available chlorine), vapor-phase formaldehyde (paraformaldehyde, 5-10 g/m3), and iodophores (150-300 µg/ml [ppm]) (Fenner, 1982; Allen et al., 1986; Bhatt and Jacoby, 1986).

### *Hosts*

Mice (*Mus musculus*). There is one unconfirmed report of the virus being recovered from wild rodents of three genera (*Microtus, Apodemus,* and *Clethrionomys*) in East Germany, but wild rodents are not known to serve as reservoir hosts. Some wild mouse species, including *Mus caroli*, *Mus cookii*, and *Mus cervicolor popaeus*, are highly susceptible to experimental infection. Limited replication of the virus and seroconversion occur in members of the genus *Rattus* after experimental infection (Burnet and Lush, 1936; Fenner, 1981, 1982; Buller et al., 1986).

### *Epizootiology*

Ectromelia virus infections have been reported in many countries. The infection is thought to be enzootic in some institutional mouse colonies in Europe. Periodic epizootics have occurred in the United States since 1950. Some have been traced to imported mice or mouse specimens (Fenner, 1981; Osterhaus et al., 1981).

Ectromelia virus infection has not been reported in commercial barrier colonies in the United States. The infection is most commonly seen in those research laboratories that exchange live mice, mouse tissues, mouse sera, and transplantable mouse tumors (e.g., immunogenetics and experimental oncology laboratories) (Fenner, 1981).

Natural transmission usually is dependent on direct contact and fomites (Wallace and Buller, 1986; Bhatt et al., 1988). Skin abrasions are thought to provide the main route of entry. Aerosol transmission and infection via the respiratory route also is thought to be possible but of relatively little importance (Briody, 1966; Bhatt and Jacoby, 1986; Bhatt et al., 1988). Infected animals begin shedding virus about 10 days after infection when characteristic skin lesions appear (Fenner, 1982).

Persistent infection ("the carrier state") was previously thought to be important in the epizootiology of mousepox. Recovered mice have been reported to shed virus in the feces or from skin lesions for up to 116 days (Gledhill, 1962). However, more recent data indicate that significant numbers of virus particles are shed from infected mice for only about 3 weeks even though the virus can persist for months in the spleen of an occasional mouse (Fenner, 1948c; Bhatt and Jacoby, 1987b). Thus, long-term persistent shedding of virus probably is not as important in the epizootiology of the infection as previously thought (Wallace and Buller, 1985). Cage-to-cage transmission is low unless favored by husbandry practices, e.g., mixing mice from different cages or handling mice from different cages without changing gloves (Wallace and Buller, 1986; Bhatt and Jacoby, 1987b).

### *Clinical*

*Inapparent infection.* This form of infection occurs mainly in the highly resistant strains, such as C57BL/6 or C57BL/10. Resistance of these strains to clinical disease (not to infection) has been reported to be due to a single dominant *H-2* linked gene (Schell, 1960a,b; Wallace et al., 1985; O'Neill and Brenan, 1987).

*Clinical disease.* Highly variable, ranging from less than 1% to nearly 100%, depending on many factors such as strain of mouse, strain of virus, length of time infection has been present in the colony, and husbandry practices (Briody et al., 1956; Briody, 1966). The spectrum includes:

a. *Minimal enzootic disease.* The disease can smolder for long periods in small subpopulations (e.g., 2-4% of cages or total mice within a room) with little spread of infection, few if any clinical signs, and negligible mortality (Werner et al., 1981).

b. *Explosive epizootic disease.* May result in sudden morbidity and mortality affecting 80-90% of a colony. This form of the disease most often has been seen in the more susceptible strains, including A, CBA, C3H, DBA/2, and BALB/c, as a result of the first introduction of the infection into a colony (Briody et al., 1956; Briody, 1966; AALAS, 1981; Bhatt and Jacoby, 1986; Wallace and Buller, 1986).

Clinical manifestations can include any or all of the following: variable (<1% to >80%) mortality; ruffled hair coat; hunched posture; facial edema; conjunctivitis; swelling of the feet; cutaneous papules, erosions, or encrustations mainly on face, ears, feet, or tail; or necrotic amputation (ectromelia) of limbs or tails (Werner et al., 1981; Fenner, 1982).

### *Pathology*

All mice are probably equal in susceptibility to infection, but clinical disease and mortality are virus- and mouse strain-dependent (Bhatt and Jacoby, 1986, 1987a). In general, mice of the A, CBA, C3H, DBA/2, and BALB/c strains are highly susceptible, the AKR and SJL strains are moderately susceptible, and the C57BL/6 and C57BL/10 strains are highly resistant to disease (Briody et al., 1956; Briody, 1966; AALAS, 1981; Wallace and Buller, 1985, 1986; Wallace et al., 1985; Bhatt and Jacoby, 1986, 1987a; Buller et al., 1987a).

The incubation period is 7 to 10 days. Virus ordinarily enters via the skin. There is local replication and extension to regional lymph nodes via lymphatics, where replication also occurs, resulting in a mild "primary viremia" as virus escapes into the blood via efferent lymphatics. Virus is taken up by splenic and hepatic macrophages, and extensive multiplication occurs in these target organs (sometimes with death due to diffuse splenic and hepatic necrosis), resulting in a massive "secondary viremia." Virus from the secondary viremia localizes in a wide variety of tissues, especially the skin (basal cells), and in the conjunctiva and lymphoid tissues. A primary lesion (frequently on the head) may appear at the site of skin inoculation about 4-7 days post infection. Foot swelling and secondary (generalized) rash (pocks) may appear 7-10 days post infection. Skin lesions heal rapidly (within 2 weeks), leaving scars on survivors (Fenner, 1948a,b, 1949).

In acute mousepox there is severe necrosis of the liver, spleen, lymph nodes, Peyer's patches, and thymus. Jejunal hemorrhage often results from mucosal erosions. Inclusions may be present in the cytoplasm of hepatocytes and other infected cells. Characteristic large eosinophilic cytoplasmic inclusions may be present in skin lesions. Necrotic amputation of limbs (ectromelia) and tails can be seen in mice that survive the acute disease (Roberts, 1962a,b, 1963; Allen et al., 1981).

### *Diagnosis*

Inapparent infections and low prevalence of enzootic disease may create major problems in establishing a diagnosis of mousepox. In the former, there may be no reason to suspect the infection. In the latter, extensive testing may be necessary to identify the low percentage of infected mice in a large population (Wallace et al., 1981; Werner et al., 1981).

Diagnosis of acute disease is based on the presence of typical lesions, with confirmation by: (a) demonstration of characteristic large virus particles in affected tissues by using transmission electron microscopy, or (b) serologic testing of survivors of acute disease (Allen et al., 1981; Bhatt and Jacoby, 1986). Differential diagnosis of the hepatic and splenic lesions should consider infections due to *Salmonella enteritidis* and *Streptobacillus moniliformis*. Differential diagnosis of skin lesions should exclude fight wounds, bite lesions of the type in mice described by Les (1972), and loss of limbs due to bacterial infections such as *Streptobacillus moniliformis* or *Mycoplasma arthritidis* (Freundt, 1959).

Serologic testing is of special value because of the feasibility of testing large numbers of animals rapidly in the event of a suspected outbreak. The enzyme-linked immunosorbent assay (ELISA) is particularly useful for this purpose in unvaccinated mice because it is sensitive and specific. The ELISA has been reported to give false-positive results in NZW and NZB mice. The hemagglutination inhibition (HAI) test is relatively insensitive but has the advantage that it does not give positive reactions in testing sera from mice that have been vaccinated with the IHD-T strain (Collins et al., 1981; Buller et al., 1983).

The indirect immunofluorescence assay (IFA) for many years was considered the most sensitive and specific procedure for serologic testing, but the impracticality of maintaining live antigen in the laboratory limited its usefulness for research purposes (Christensen et al., 1966). Recently, the ELISA was found to be 10-fold more sensitive than the IFA (Buller et al., 1983).

Biologic materials, such as cells and blood, can be screened for mousepox (and other agents) by injecting the tissue into known pathogen-free mice followed by serologic testing. Alternatively, virus isolation may be attempted using BS-C-1 and other cell lines (Bhatt and Jacoby, 1986). Failure of skin lesion development at the site of vaccination with vaccinia virus by scarification of tail skin is considered suggestive of prior infection with mousepox (Fenner, 1982).

### *Control*

Institutions that must receive mice, mouse tissues, or tumors from sources other than commercial barrier facilities should have a disease surveillance program for quarantine and testing of incoming mice and mouse tissues for infectious agents, including ectromelia virus. This approach constitutes the only practical way by which laboratories with a high risk of introducing ectromelia virus can effectively avoid the periodic disastrous consequences of mousepox outbreaks (Small and New, 1981).

In the past, accepted practice for eradicating mousepox required disposal of mouse colonies and all infected biologic materials (e.g., tumors and sera), plus rigorous decontamination of rooms and equipment (AALAS, 1981). Cesarean derivation of infected mouse stocks was not considered an acceptable alternative since it may not eliminate the virus; intrauterine infection is known to occur in mice infected during pregnancy (Fenner, 1982). More recently, it has been suggested that quarantine and cessation of breeding may be successful in eliminating ectromelia virus (Bhatt and Jacoby, 1987b).

Vaccination with a live virus vaccine, the IHD-T strain of vaccinia adapted to growth in embryonated eggs, may be useful in eliminating the infection from small, closed colonies where all offspring can be vaccinated at around 6 weeks of age (Tuffery, 1958; Trentin and Ferrigno, 1959; Flynn, 1963a). Vaccination can protect mice from fatal mousepox, but does not prevent infection or virus transmission (Wallace and Buller, 1986; Bhatt and Jacoby, 1987d). Vaccination with the IHD-T strain causes seroconversion and resultant false positive ELISA and IFA test results, but not to the HAI test because the vaccine does not stimulate production of HAI antibody (Collins et at., 1981; Buller et al., 1983). Immunodeficient mice are highly susceptible to infection with the IHD-T strain and must be protected when vaccinating.

### *Interference with Research*

Mousepox is one of the most feared diseases of mice because of (a) the potential for explosive outbreaks in which mortality can approach 100%, (b) known major effects on research results, and (c) known serious problems of detection once latent infection becomes established in a mouse population (AALAS, 1981).

Manipulations that have been reported to promote mousepox epizootics include: experimental infection with tubercle bacilli, x-irradiation, administration of various toxic chemicals, shipment, tissue transplantation, castration, and tumors (Briody, 1959). In addition:

a. Mousepox infection can alter phagocytic response (Blanden and Mims, 1973). Conversely, procedures that decrease phagocytosis may increase susceptibility to mousepox, e.g., large doses of endotoxin or splenectomy (Schell, 1960b).

b. Intraperitoneal injection of Freund's adjuvant enhances the severity of experimental mousepox (McNeill and Killen, 1971).

c. C57BL/6 mice infected experimentally with LP-BM5 murine leukemia virus had increased susceptibility to ectromelia virus, possibly due to inability to generate an ectromelia virus-specific cytotoxic T cell response (Buller et al., 1987c).

d. Ectromelia virus can replicate in vitro in lymphoma and hybridoma cell lines from mice. Potentially, passage of such contaminated cell lines in mice can introduce the virus into mouse colonies (Buller et al., 1987b; Wallace and Buller, 1986).

## Poxvirus(es) in Rats

### *Significance*

Unknown.

### *Perspective*

Two large outbreaks of a highly fatal poxvirus disease occurred in laboratory rats in the USSR during 1973 and 1974 (Marennikova and Shelukhina, 1976; Marennikova et al., 1978b). A poxvirus disease with symptoms resembling mousepox was reported in Romania in 1976 (Iftimovici et al.,

1976). More recently, rat tissues received from the USSR, but originating in Czechoslovakia, were found to contain poxvirus. The animals from which the tissues were obtained had a clinically inapparent poxvirus infection (Kraft et al., 1982). Whether these reports concerned the same or different viruses is unknown.

*Agent*

Poxvirus (or perhaps more than one virus). Possibly a virus of wild rodents, Turkmenia rodent poxvirus, that is related to cowpox virus but that is distinctly different from mousepox virus (Marennikova et al., 1978a). The strain isolated from rats in the USSR was designated 012-Moscow 73 (Krikun, 1977; Marennikova et al., 1978b; Kraft et al., 1982).

*Hosts*

Laboratory rats and wild rodents, Felidae (zoo animals fed infected rats), and humans (Marennikova and Shelukhina, 1976; Marennikova et al., 1978b). Laboratory mice are highly susceptible to experimental infection (Majboroda and Lobanova, 1980; Majboroda et al., 1980).

Of 40 personnel exposed to infected rats, four became ill. Symptoms included headache, fatigue, cough, rhinitis, tickling in the throat, and digestive upset. Two of the four had a rash on the head, shoulders, knees, and back of the hands (Marennikova et al., 1978b).

*Epizootiology*

Infections in rats have been reported only in animals from the USSR and Eastern Europe. Wild rodents might serve as reservoir hosts in the USSR. Outbreaks of disease in the USSR were explosive, possibly associated with the entry of wild rodents into animal facilities.

*Clinical*

Infection can be inapparent (Kraft et al., 1982) or occur as an epizootic with 50% mortality (Marennikova and Shelukhina, 1976; Marennikova et al., 1978b). Disease in rats during epizootics occurred in three forms: pulmonary, dermal, and mixed pulmonary and dermal.

a. *Pulmonary form.* Rats became anorexic, extremely dyspneic, and moribund, with death occurring uniformly by the third or fourth day of clinical signs.

b. *Dermal form.* Relatively mild. Partial anorexia; papular rash on tail, paws, and muzzle, with transition to dry crusts in 1-2 days; sometimes partial amputation of the tail and possibly also the paws; and deaths occurring rarely.

c. *Mixed form.* Symptoms were transient, lasting only two to three days. Suckling rats were most susceptible. Adults most often had the dermal form of the disease and survived (Marennikova et al., 1978b).

### *Pathology*

Lesions seen in the pulmonary form are severe interstitial pneumonia and pulmonary edema with serous or hemorrhagic pleural effusion. In addition to pox lesions and occasional spontaneous amputation of feet and tail, rats with the dermal form of the disease also had focal pneumonia and sometimes mucosal exanthema involving the mouth, nasopharynx, and rectum (Marennikova et al., 1978b).

Kraft et al. (1982) studied a group of rats received from Czechoslovakia via the USSR that had inapparent infection. They found desquamative lesions containing poxvirus virions in the nasal mucosa.

### *Diagnosis*

Definitive information is lacking. The hemagglutination inhibition test or enzyme-linked immunosorbent assay for mousepox might be useful. Virus isolation and characterization are essential.

### *Control*

Definitive information is lacking, but until proven otherwise, measures comparable to those used for mousepox should be employed. Great caution should be used when importing rodents from Eastern Europe and the USSR.

### *Interference with Research*

No data are available. Probably similar to mousepox in mice.

## ***Mycoplasma arthritidis***

### *Significance*

Uncertain. Subclinical infection may be very common in rats and mice.

### *Perspective*

*Experimental models of arthritis*: Most of the recent literature on this agent concerns laboratory models of arthritis produced by inoculating large doses of *Mycoplasma arthritidis* intravenously or into the footpad of rats and mice (Lindsey et al., 1978b; Cole and Cassell, 1979; Cole and Ward, 1979). It must be emphasized that these models are highly artificial and may have little relevance to the understanding of the host-parasite relationships in the natural infection.

*Natural infections in rats*: Natural infections of *M. arthritidis* in rats have been reported infrequently since 1938, with the organism having one of the following four roles:

a. Incidental infection has been reported (sometimes in association with *Mycoplasma pulmonis*) in various sites, including the nasopharynx (Ito et al., 1957; Ward and Cole, 1970; Stewart and Buck, 1975), middle ears (Preston, 1942; Stewart and Buck, 1975; Eamons, 1984), the lung (Cole et al., 1967), a paraovarian abscess (Preston, 1942), the submaxillary gland (Klieneberger, 1938), and multiple organs (Davidson et al., 1983).

b. Subclinical infection has been a complicating factor in studies of experimental arthritis (Pearson, 1959; Mielens and Rozitis, 1964; Cole et al., 1969).

c. As a contaminant of transplantable tumors *M. arthritidis* has caused polyarthritis and/or abscesses at the injection site in recipient rats (Woglom and Warren, 1938; Howell and Jones, 1963).

d. *M. arthritidis* has been a cause of spontaneous polyarthritis in wild (Collier, 1939) and laboratory (Findlay et al., 1939; Preston, 1942; Ito et al., 1957) rats.

Thus, the literature contains less than a dozen reports of natural arthritis due to *M. arthritidis* in rats, with the most recent such report appearing in 1969.

*Natural infections in mice*: Natural infections of *M. arthritidis* in mice were first reported in 1983 (Davidson et al., 1983). In that study the organism was isolated from the nasal passages, the conjunctiva, and the uterus and by laryngo-tracheo-bronchial lavage from approximately 10% of otherwise pathogen-free mice and rats housed in the same room. No gross or microscopic lesions attributable to *M. arthritidis* were found in either host.

### *Agent*

*M. arthritidis* is a bacterium, class Mollicutes, order Mycoplasmatales, family Mycoplasmataceae (sterol-requiring mycoplasmas). It is Gram negative, lacks a cell wall, pleomorphic, and may occur in filaments 2 to 30 μm long. It will grow on conventional horse serum-yeast extract mycoplasma medium, usually under facultatively anaerobic conditions at pH 7.8, 37°C, and 95% relative humidity. *M. arthritidis* requires arginine and usually produces "fried egg" appearance when grown on solid medium. For specific methods of cultural isolation, see Cassell et al. (1983a).

Determination of the species is based on biochemical and serologic tests (Razin and Freundt, 1984). The type strain is ATCC 19611 (NCTC 10162, PG6). Virulence factors of *M. arthritidis* have not been defined (Razin and Freundt, 1984). The organism can be preserved indefinitely by lyophilization or freezing at –70°C.

*Hosts*

Rats and mice are considered the natural hosts. A few isolates have been obtained from monkeys and humans, but their significance is unknown (Razin and Freundt, 1984).

*Epizootiology*

Current evidence suggests that subclinical (often noncultivable) infection occurs in many contemporary rats and mice, including cesarean-derived, barrier-maintained stocks (Thirkill and Gregerson, 1982; Davidson et al., 1983, Lindsey et al., 1986b). The preferred host sites and natural history of these infections are poorly understood.

*Clinical*

The infection is usually subclinical and noncultivable.

*Pathology*

Lesions usually are not present in subclinical infections (Davidson et al., 1983). The pathology of experimental arthritis due to *M. arthritidis* in rats and mice has been reviewed by Lindsey et al. (1978b).

*Diagnosis*

For rodent health surveillance the ELISA (Horowitz and Cassell, 1978; Cassell et al., 1981, 1983b) should be performed, followed by Immunoblot (Minion et al., 1984) on positive sera for differentiation of *M. arthritidis* and *M. pulmonis* antibodies. Adult breeding stock should be tested repeatedly by using the ELISA because only a few animals with subclinical infection usually seroconvert, and some do so only transiently. Few animals within a population may be infected, and very few organisms may be present in any host site. Isolation of the organism from such animals with subclinical infection may require culture of tissue homogenates from multiple organ sites, which is not practical in most instances (Cassell et al., 1983a). In the rare event of clinical arthritis, the organism should be cultured from joint exudates (Cassell et al., 1983a).

### *Control*

Definitive information is not available. However, major attention should be directed toward selection of *M. arthritidis*-free breeding stocks through intensive, repetitive testing by ELISA of small populations of breeders over many months, followed by strict barrier maintenance. If valuable stocks infected with *M. arthritidis* are to be rederived, it might be helpful to place breeders on an extended course of tetracycline treatment prior to cesarean derivation. Only known *M. arthritidis*-free stocks should be used as foster parents. The mode(s) of transmission are unknown.

### *Interference with Research*

Subclinical *M. arthritidis* infections can be activated to complicate experimental arthritis in rats (Pearson, 1959; Mielens and Rozitis, 1964; Cole et al., 1969).

*M. arthritidis* infection can cause spontaneous polyarthritis in rats (Collier, 1939; Findlay et al., 1939; Ito et al., 1957; Preston, 1942).

Transplantable tumors of rats can become contaminated with *M. arthritidis*, resulting in arthritis and/or abscesses at the injection site in recipients (Woglom and Warren, 1938; Klieneberger, 1939; Jasmin, 1957; Hershberger et al., 1960; Ward and Jones, 1962; Howell and Jones, 1963; Amor et al., 1964).

Experimental infections of rodents with *M. arthritidis* can be complicated by preexisting, latent infection with this mycoplasma (Thirkill and Gregerson, 1982).

Experimental infection of rats with *M. arthritidis* has been shown to increase susceptibility to experimental pyelonephritis (Thomsen and Rosendal, 1974).

Experimental infections of *M. arthritidis* in mice have been found to induce interferon production (Rinaldo et al., 1974; Cole et al., 1976b), activate T and B lymphocytes (Cole et al., 1977, 1981, 1982; Naot et al., 1977), suppress humoral and cellular immune responses (Kaklamanis and Pavlatos, 1972; Eckner et al., 1974; Cole et al., 1976a), and alter macrophage function (Dietz and Cole, 1982).

*M. arthritidis* is a frequent contaminant of rodent cell cultures (Barile, 1973).

## ***Streptobacillus moniliformis***

### *Significance*

Low.

*Perspective*

This organism was a common commensal of wild and laboratory rats (and an occasional pathogen of humans, mice, and other species) before the era of widespread cesarean derivation and barrier maintenance of laboratory rodents. There have been relatively few reports of the infection in the United States since 1960, including approximately a dozen cases of rat-bite fever in humans (Anderson et al., 1983).

*Agent*

*Streptobacillus moniliformis* is a bacterium of uncertain taxonomic position. It is a Gram-negative bacillus, which measures 0.1-0.7 × 1.0-5.0 μm, and occurs singly or in long, filamentous chains. It often has spherical, oval, fusiform, or club-shaped swellings. *S. moniliformis* requires serum, ascitic fluid, or blood for growth and is nonhemolytic. It is negative for catalase, oxidase, nitrate reduction, and indole production. *S. moniliformis* can form "cotton balls" or "fluff balls" in broth and can produce L-form variants (Savage, 1984).

Synonyms: *Streptothrix muris ratti, Nocardia muris, Actinomyces muris, Haverhilia multiformis, Asterococcus muris,* and many others.

*Hosts*

The natural host is the rat, with most common isolation sites being the nasopharynx, middle ear, respiratory tract, and subcutaneous abscesses (Freundt, 1959; Savage, 1972, 1984). Mice, guinea pigs, turkeys, humans, and others can contract the infection from rats, especially from rat bites (Harkness and Ferguson, 1982). In humans, cases resulting from bites have been referred to as "rat-bite fever" and cases occurring in milk-borne epidemics have been referred to as "Haverhill fever."

*Epizootiology*

The organism is a commensal of the nasopharynx in wild and conventionally reared laboratory rats (Strangeways, 1933; Klieneberger, 1935). It has not been reported from cesarean-derived, barrier-maintained rats or mice (Van Rooyen, 1936; Weisbroth, 1979).

Epizootic disease has occurred in laboratory mice (Levaditi et al., 1932; Mackie et al., 1933; Freundt, 1956) and wild mice (Williams, 1941) and is most likely to be seen in mice housed near infected rats (Freundt, 1959).

Transmission is by rat bites, aerosols, and fomites.

### *Clinical*

Rats harbor infection in the nasopharynx without clinical signs. The organism is not known to cause natural disease in rats.

In mice, early signs have included conjunctivitis, photophobia, cyanosis, diarrhea, anemia, hemoglobinuria, emaciation, and high mortality. In survivors septicemia apparently clears in a few weeks, but infection persists around joints for about 6 months (Savage et al., 1981). During the chronic phase of infection there may be diffuse swelling and reddening of limbs or tail, with the development of chronic arthritis, deformity and ankylosis, or amputation (ectromelia) at any stage in the evolution of joint disease. With the occurrence of spinal lesions, posterior paralysis, kyphosis, and priapism can occur. Abortions and stillbirths also have been reported (Levaditi et al., 1932; Mackie et al., 1933; Williams, 1941; Freundt, 1956, 1959; Sawicki et al., 1962).

In humans, the incubation period is usually 3 to 10 days, followed by abrupt onset of fever, chills, vomiting, headache, and myalgia. There is a maculopapular rash that is most pronounced on the extremities. Arthritis occurs in about two-thirds of cases, and other complications such as endocarditis and focal abscesses occur in some untreated cases. The recommended treatment is penicillin, administered for a minimum of 7 days (Roughgarden, 1965; Anderson et al., 1983).

### *Pathology*

In mice, the early lesions are those associated with septicemia, particularly focal necrosis of spleen and liver, splenomegaly, and lymphadenopathy. Subsequently, arthritis of varying stages and severity predominate (Lerner and Silverstein, 1957; Lerner and Sokoloff, 1959). There may be spontaneous amputation of limbs and tails (Levaditi et al., 1932; Mackie et al., 1933; Williams, 1941; Freundt, 1956, 1959).

### *Diagnosis*

Cultural isolation and identification of the organism (Martone and Patton, 1981) are essential, along with exclusion of other infectious agents and disease processes. Differential diagnosis should rule out mousepox and bacterial septicemias such as those caused by *Corynebacterium kutscheri* and *Salmonella enteritidis*.

### *Control*

Mice and rats from stocks that have been cesarean derived, barrier maintained, and regularly monitored for rodent pathogens by a comprehensive health surveillance program should be used. Housing mice and unmonitored rats in the same room should be avoided.

*Streptobacillus moniliformis* is considered rare in contemporary laboratory rats and mice. This is perhaps one of the most striking achievements of cesarean-derivation, barrier-maintenance methodology (Weisbroth, 1979).

*Interference with Research*

*S. moniliformis* is unlikely to be found to interfere with research results because it is rare in contemporary rodents. Nevertheless, it can cause high mortality in mice and is a serious zoonotic infection in people.

## COMMON ECTOPARASITES

The comprehensive text *Parasites of Laboratory Animals* (Flynn, 1973a), lists approximately 4 flea, 4 lice, 24 mite, and numerous tick parasites of mice and rats. However, an important distinction is made between the prevalence of ectoparasites among animals in nature and those in the laboratory. For laboratory populations, Flynn (1973a) lists as being common only four types of mite for mice (*Myobia musculi*, *Myocoptes musculinus*, *Radfordia affinis*, and *Psorergates simplex*) and one type of mite for rats (*R. ensifera*). Weisbroth (1982) states that *P. simplex* has not been reported in the past decade and can be regarded as rare. For the same reason *R. ensifera* can also be considered rare (unpublished observations of members of the ILAR Committee on Infectious Diseases of Mice and Rats). Thus, only three mites (*M. musculi*, *M. musculinus*, and *R. affinis*), all of which are parasites of mice, can be accepted as common ectoparasites in contemporary laboratory settings (Kunstyr and Friedhoff, 1980; Weisbroth, 1982).

### *Myobia musculi*

*Significance*

Moderate.

*Perspective*

*Myobia musculi* is considered the more pathogenic of the common mites of laboratory mice.

*Agent*

*Myobia musculi* is a fur mite, order Acarina. Adult *Myobia musculi*, which can be seen with a hand lens, appear pearly white and elongate (about twice as long as wide). Males and females have the same general appearance. The males measure 285-320 µm long × 145-175 µm wide. The females measure 400-500 µm long × 285-300 µm wide. The first pair of legs is very short, closely associated with the mouth parts, and modified for clasping hair. The second, third, and fourth pairs of legs have tarsi that end in a claw-like structure known as an empodium (Flynn, 1955, 1963e, 1973a).

### *Life Cycle*

The life cycle includes egg, larval, nymphal, and adult stages. The eggs are oval and about 200 µm long and are usually seen either attached to the base of hairs or inside mature females. Eggs hatch in about seven days, and completion of the entire life cycle requires about 23 days (Flynn, 1973a; Friedman and Weisbroth, 1977; Weisbroth, 1982).

### *Hosts*

Mice. Rarely, rats and other laboratory rodents.

### *Epizootiology*

Mites can be seen anywhere on the body but are most numerous alongside the hair bases and in the more densely furred areas (i.e., over the head and back). Transmission is by direct contact (Weisbroth, 1982).

The dynamics of mite populations on the host are very complex and are influenced by factors that include grooming, mouse strain susceptibility, and host immune responses. Athymic nude (*nu/nu*) and other furless mice are not susceptible to infestation (Weisbroth, 1982).

### *Clinical*

The general appearance of infested mice is not directly related to the size of the mite populations present. Infestations are commonly subclinical. Clinical signs include scruffiness, pruritis, patchy alopecia, self-trauma, ulceration of the skin, and pyoderma. Close inspection often reveals varying amounts of bran-like material (hyperkeratotic debris) and mites on the skin and around the base of the hairs (Csiza and McMartin, 1976; Weisbroth, 1982).

### *Pathology*

Mice of the C57BL strains and their congeneic sublines are particularly susceptible to severe skin disease caused by *M. musculi,* presumably because of their propensity to develop hypersensitivity to mites (Friedman and Weisbroth, 1975; Csiza and McMartin, 1976; Weisbroth et al., 1976; Weisbroth, 1982).

Lesions vary from mild to severe. Initially there is mild hyperkeratosis, but this often progresses to severe hyperkeratosis with fine bran-like material on the skin over virtually all of the body but particularly abundant over the dorsum, head, and shoulders. In more advanced cases, there is patchy alopecia and chronic, ulcerative dermatitis distributed most frequently asymmetrically in the shoulder and neck regions. Secondary bacterial infection commonly leads to suppurative and granulomatous inflammation. Hyperplasia of regional lymph nodes, splenic lymphoid hyperplasia, and increased serum immunoglobulins are common. Chronic infestation can cause secondary amyloidosis (Galton, 1963; Csiza and McMartin, 1976; Weisbroth et al., 1976; Weisbroth, 1982).

### *Diagnosis*

The diagnosis is made by demonstrating and identifying the mites, while excluding other causes of dermatitis such as fungi (ringworm) or *Staphylococcus aureus*. Mites can be demonstrated by using a stereoscopic microscope or hand lens to examine the pelage, particularly over the back and head. Alternatively, mice can be killed and placed either on black paper and left at room temperature or in tape-sealed Petri dishes and refrigerated for an hour. As the body cools, the mites leave it and can be collected from the paper or Petri dish. The mites are mounted under a coverslip on glass slides with immersion oil and identified microscopically on the basis of anatomic features (Flynn, 1955, 1963e, 1973a; Wagner, 1969; Weisbroth, 1982).

For preservation of mites, Hoyer's solution is recommended. Hoyer's solution is made by mixing the following, in sequence, at room temperature: 50 grams of distilled water, 30 grams of gum arabic, 200 grams of chloral hydrate, and 20 grams of glycerine (Flynn, 1963e).

### *Control*

Cesarean derivation and barrier maintenance are the most effective methods for eradication of mite infestations (Weisbroth, 1982). Treatment with insecticides is not recommended because they can alter experimental results.

### *Interference with Research*

Infestations of *M. musculi* have been found to cause secondary amyloidosis (Galton, 1963; Weisbroth, 1982). In addition, mite-infested mice should be considered undesirable for behavioral studies because behavioral patterns are likely to be altered by hypersensitivity to the mites.

### *Myocoptes musculinus* and *Radfordia affinis*

These two mites will not be discussed in detail because they are generally similar to *Myobia musculi* in morphology, epizootiology, life cycle, diagnosis, and control. *Myocoptes musculinus* causes lesions similar to but usually milder than those caused by *Myobia musculi*, whereas *Radfordia affinis* is not recognized as a significant pathogen. It must be emphasized that mite infestations of mice usually are due to more than one mite species. *M. musculinus* and *R. affinis* also are identified by characteristic morphologic features of the adults (Flynn, 1973a; Weisbroth, 1982).

#### *Interference with Research*

Mite infestations due to *M. musculinus* have been found to reduce the contact sensitivity of mice to oxazolone (Laltoo and Kind, 1979).

### Other Ectoparasites

Readers desiring more in-depth coverage and information on the less common species of ectoparasites of mice and rats should consult comprehensive reference works on the subject (Baker et al., 1956; Pratt and Littig, 1961; Pratt and Wiseman, 1962; Owen, 1972; Flynn, 1973a; Hsu, 1979; Weisbroth, 1982).

### *Staphylococcus aureus*

#### *Significance*

Low.

#### *Perspective*

This organism is considered one of the more important causes of naturally occurring skin lesions in mice and rats.

#### *Agent*

*Staphylococcus aureus* is a Gram-positive, coagulase-positive, coccus bacterium, family Micrococcaceae. It occurs in grape-like clusters, is facultatively anaerobic and usually produces yellow pigment when grown on blood agar. *S. aureus* produces many extracellular enzymes and toxins. It is one of the hardiest of non-spore-forming bacteria. Species subtypes are identified by bacteriophage typing and biochemical reactions (Oeding, 1983).

*Hosts*

Mice, rats, people, and many others.

*Epizootiology*

It commonly colonizes nasopharynx, lower digestive tract, fur, and skin of conventionally reared, as well as barrier-reared rodents. It can also be readily cultured from cages, room surfaces, and personnel.

The epizootiology of pathogenic types in animals is poorly understood. Human carriers may be an important source of infection for rodent colonies and vice versa (Blackmore and Francis, 1970).

Many rodent colonies have infection without overt disease. Pathogenesis probably is dependent on many factors including phage type(s) present, traumatic injuries of skin or mucosal surfaces, host factors, and sanitation.

*Clinical*

A variety of clinical syndromes have been attributed to *Staphylococcus aureus*, including the following:

a. *Ulcerative dermatitis in rats.* Intensely pruritic, moist eczematous lesions, usually 1-2 cm in diameter, occur on lateral surfaces of the shoulders and neck. Lesions appear to be initiated or aggravated by scratching with the ipsilateral rear foot. Pruritis associated with sialodacryoadenitis virus infections of Harderian or salivary glands may play a role (Ash, 1971; Fox et al., 1977b; Wagner et al., 1977).

b. *Ulcerative dermatitis in mice.* Moist eczematous lesions on face, neck, ears, and forelegs. In one facility 10-50% of VM/Dk mice were affected beginning around 8 months of age. The lesions were rarely seen in mice of several other strains in the facility (Taylor and Neal, 1980).

c. *Facial abscesses in immunocompetent mice.* Multiple abscesses and botryomycotic granulomas occur in deeper tissues of the face, including the orbital tissues, facial muscles, peridontium, and mandibles. In one facility the C57BL/6Bd strain was the most affected of several strains present. Another outbreak involved the BSVS strain (Shultz et al., 1973; Clarke et al., 1978).

d. *Orbital and facial abscesses in athymic (nu/nu) mice.* Purulent lesions of varying size occur commonly around the eyes and on the face (ILAR, 1976b).

e. *Tail lesions in rats.* Raised, yellow pustules occur on the proximal one-third of the tail, progressing to draining abscesses and sometimes sloughing of the tail (Hard, 1966).

f. *Preputial gland abscesses.* Preputial glands are firm and enlarged to a few millimeters in diameter. Many strains are affected, but C3H/HeN has the highest incidence (Needam and Cooper, 1976; Hong and Ediger, 1978a).

g. *Self-mutilation of penis.* Young male C57BL/6N mice develop this condition when first placed in cages with females for harem breeding. The sheath swells so that it can be impossible to protrude the penis. The penis of affected males may be mutilated severely so that the os penis often protrudes from the surface. Acute balanoposthitis is associated with accumulation of purulent exudate containing *S. aureus* in the sheath. Disease may be related to aggressive breeding activity of young males with traumatic injury of the penis (Hong and Ediger, 1978b; J. R. Lindsey, Department of Comparative Medicine, University of Alabama at Birmingham, unpublished).

h. *Traumatic pododermatitis in rats.* Exercise on circular activity wheels causes abrasions and lacerations with secondary staphylococcal pododermatitis of the hind feet (Morrow et al., 1977).

### *Pathology*

The primary mechanism of host defense against *S. aureus* is complement-mediated killing by polymorphonuclear leukocytes (Verhoef and Verbrugh, 1981; Quie et al., 1983). Thus, suppurative inflammation is a hallmark of *S. aureus* tissue invasion. In ulcerative dermatitis there is destruction of the epidermis, and the underlying dermis contains pustules, abscesses and, eventually, chronic or granulomatous inflammation. The other clinical syndromes are similar, differing mainly in location and stage of infection. Large numbers of organisms are usually present and can be demonstrated readily in Gram-stained sections or imprints.

Cell-mediated immunity can be important in host defense against *S. aureus* and in the pathogenesis of some rodent lesions associated with this agent. Experimentally delayed hypersensitivity to *S. aureus* can easily be induced in mice (Johnson et al., 1961; Taubler, 1968; Taubler and Mudd, 1968; Easmon and Glynn, 1975, 1977, 1979; Adlam and Easmon, 1983). Although not proven, it may be that hypersensitivity to *S. aureus* plays a role in the ulcerative dermatitis associated with this agent in mice and rats.

The preputial abscesses in C3H/HeN mice reported by Hong and Ediger (1978a) apparently result from ascending infection in the ducts of the preputial glands. Purulent exudate fills the ducts and glands and may dissect through the gland wall, resulting in subcutaneous abscesses in the pubic area. From the ventral surface these appear as small lumps (1-3 mm) underneath the skin. Organisms other than *S. aureus*, specifically, enteric bacteria, also have been observed to produce this lesion in C3H/HeN mice (J. R. Lindsey, Department of Comparative Medicine, University of Alabama at Birmingham, and J. E. Wagner, Veterinary Medical Diagnostic Laboratory, University of Missouri, Columbia, unpublished).

#### *Diagnosis*

The diagnosis of *S. aureus* is dependent upon isolation and identification of the organism and exclusion of other agents (e.g., dermatophytes and mites) as possible causes of lesions.

#### *Control*

General methods of control are improved sanitation, frequent sterilization of cages and other equipment, assurance of proper operation of cage washers, elimination of equipment that causes injury to the skin, and reduction in the number of animals per cage. In the case of self-mutilation of the penis in mice, reduction of the number of females per male in harems is helpful.

#### *Interference with Research*

Infections of *S. aureus* may require culling of breeders or may disrupt studies, particularly in older animals. Even more important may be alterations in host immune responses, e.g., it has been shown experimentally that injection of killed *S. aureus* into mice inhibits contact sensitivity to oxazolone by activating suppressor B cells (Benedettini et al., 1984). The occurrence of renal abscesses caused by *S. aureus* in rats has been observed following prolonged immunosuppression with corticosteroids (Simmons and Simpson, 1977).

### Dermatophytes

#### *Significance*

Low.

#### *Perspective*

Laboratory mice and rats occasionally have been found to serve as inapparent carriers of dermatophytes and, rarely, have been reported to have clinical dermatomycosis (ringworm or favus). Very few infected colonies have been incriminated as sources of dermatophyte infection for people (Dolan et al., 1958; MacKenzie, 1961; Brown and Suter, 1969; Refai and Ali, 1970; Kunstyr, 1980; Fox and Brayton, 1982).

### *Agent*

Fungi, class Deuteromycetes (Fungi Imperfecti), genera *Trichophyton* and *Microsporum*. *Trichophyton mentagrophytes* is the most common cause of inapparent infection and reported dermatomycosis in mice and rats. Other dermatophytes that have been isolated from the fur of mice and rats include *Trichophyton ajelloi, T. schoenleini, T. terrestre, Microsporum gallinae, M. gypseum,* and *M. cookei* (Georg, 1960; Dvorak and Otechenasek, 1964; Emmons et al., 1977; Weisbroth, 1979; Kunstyr, 1980; Fox and Brayton, 1982; Williford and Wagner, 1982).

### *Hosts*

Mice, rats, people, and numerous others (Georg, 1960).

### *Epizootiology*

Dermatophytes are not reported in cesarean-derived, barrier-maintained rodent stocks. Other animals and people probably are major reservoirs of infection for mice and rats. Organisms are parasites of keratin, i.e., hair and superficial layers of skin (Georg, 1960; Emmons et al., 1977).

### *Clinical*

Inapparent infections are thought to be more common than clinical disease, but both are rare (Dolan and Fendrick, 1959; Davies and Shewell, 1965; Feuerman et al., 1975; Fishman et al., 1976; Balsari et al., 1981). Clinical disease appears to have been observed in mice (Booth, 1952; Blank, 1957; Cetin et al., 1965; Reith, 1968; Fishman et al., 1976) far more frequently than in rats (Povar, 1965).

Lesions consist of irregularly defined areas of alopecia with a scaly to crusty appearance and occasional pustules at the edges. Lesions are most common on the head near the mouth and eyes, but can be seen anywhere on the body (Georg, 1960).

### *Pathology*

Uncomplicated lesions can be very subtle, with only thickening of the stratum corneum seen in sections stained with hematoxylin and eosin. Special stains such as periodic acid-Schiff or Gridley's fungus stain are valuable in demonstrating the organisms. Severe cases may have hypertrophy of the epidermis with varying degrees of acute and chronic inflammation in the dermis (Georg, 1960).

*Diagnosis*

For detection of asymptomatic carriers, the fur of several animals can be brushed while the animals are held over opened plates of culture medium and then the plates can be cultured for dermatophytes (Mackenzie, 1961). For clinical cases, hair can be plucked or skin scrapings can be taken from the periphery of lesions and mounted onto slides in 10% potassium hydroxide for visualization of hyphae and endospores. Definitive diagnosis is dependent on culture and identification of organisms by using Sabouraud's or other dermatophyte medium (Georg, 1960; Emmons et al., 1977).

*Control*

Where feasible, infected stocks should be destroyed and replaced by dermatophyte-free stock after thorough sterilization and disinfection of facilities and equipment. Cesarean derivation of valuable stocks may be desirable. Treatment of affected animals is not recommended.

For prevention of infection, barrier maintenance is effective. Rodents should be housed well away from laboratory animal species known to be more frequently infected, e.g., cats and dogs (Kunstyr, 1980).

Dermatophyte infections of mice and rats do not represent important zoonoses. The most common of these infections, *T. mentagrophytes* infection in mice, has been reported as a source of infection for humans in only six instances (Fox and Brayton, 1982), and these occurred in the 1950s and 1960s before cesarean-derivation and barrier-maintenance methods were in common practice.

*Interference with Research*

There are no known examples of dermatophyte infections interferring with research in contemporary mice and rats.

***Pasteurella pneumotropica***

*Significance*

Low.

*Perspective*

*1948-1950:* Jawetz (1948, 1950) and Jawetz and Baker (1950) published papers that seemed to implicate *Pasteurella pneumotropica* as an ubiquitous respiratory tract pathogen of major importance in mice.

*1973:* Moore et al. (1973) reported on a stock of gnotobiotic rats maintained in isolators and found that they were monocontaminated with *P. pneumotropica*, suggesting that the organism might normally inhibit the gastrointestinal tract.

*1974:* Jakab (1974) reported on the first in a series of studies in which mice experimentally infected with Sendai virus showed decreased clearance of intranasally inoculated *P. pneumotropica*. Although this and subsequent studies by Jakab and associates (Jakab, 1981) were entirely experimental, they possibly gave further impetus to the belief that *P. pneumotropica* is a respiratory pathogen.

*1980s:* More than 3 decades after the reports of Jawetz (1948, 1950) and Jawetz and Baker (1950) *P. pneumotropica* has not been incriminated as being responsible for outbreaks of respiratory disease in mice, i.e., their findings have not been confirmed in a natural outbreak. Perhaps their experimentally infected mice also had Sendai virus and/or *Mycoplasma pulmonis* infections. The gross and microscopic lesions they described were compatible with murine respiratory mycoplasmosis. Also, their mice were stated to have natural *Chlamydia trachomatis* infection and spontaneous pulmonary consolidation (Jawetz, 1950).

### *Agent*

*Pasteurella pneumotropica* is a Gram-negative, coccobacillus bacterium, family Pasteurellaceae, measuring $0.5 \times 1.2$ μm. It is nonhemolytic. Colonies on sheep blood agar are convex, measuring 0.5-1.5 mm at 24 hours, and gray or yellow in color. Oxidase, urease, and catalase are produced, and nitrate is reduced to nitrite (Carter, 1984).

### *Hosts*

Mice, rats, hamsters, guinea pigs, and many others.

### *Epizootiology*

*P. pneumotropica* can be isolated from a high percentage (up to 95%) of healthy animals in some colonies and from feces of gnotobiotic rats (Moore et al., 1973; Sparrow, 1976; Saito et al., 1978). It can be isolated from numerous organs: respiratory tract, oral cavity, intestine, uterus, urinary bladder, skin, and conjunctiva (Jawetz, 1948, 1950; Hoag et al., 1962; Heyl, 1963; Wheater, 1967; Kunstyr and Hartman, 1983). Transmission is probably by contact and fomites.

*Clinical*

This agent has been associated with a wide range of clinical manifestations and disease processes in laboratory rodents, including the following:

In mice:

a. Conjunctivitis (Wagner et al., 1969; Needham and Cooper, 1975)
b. Panophthalmitis (Weisbroth et al., 1969)
c. Dacryoadenitis (Wagner et al., 1969; Needham and Cooper, 1975)
d. Subcutaneous and cervical abscesses (Weisbroth et al., 1969; Wilson, 1976; Moore and Aldred, 1978)
e. Bulbourethral gland infections (Sebesteny, 1973)
f. Respiratory disease? (Hoag et al., 1962; Goldstein and Green, 1967; Brennan et al., 1969a,b; Saito et al., 1978)
g. Uterine infections (Hoag et al., 1962; Brennan et al., 1965; Blackmore and Casillo, 1972; Ward et al., 1978)
h. Otitis media (Harkness and Wagner, 1975)

In rats:

a. Ophthalmitis (Roberts and Gregory, 1980)
b. Conjunctivitis (Hill, 1974b; Young and Hill, 1974; Moore, 1979)
c. Subcutaneous abscesses (Van der Shaaf et al., 1970)
d. Mastitis (Hong and Ediger, 1978c)
e. Respiratory disease? (Burek et al., 1972)

*Pathology*

*P. pneumotropica* is an opportunist that most frequently causes lesions of the skin and adnexal structures. Lesions caused by *P. pneumotropica* usually are characterized by suppurative inflammation. Eye lesions of rats attributed to *P. pneumotropica* in past reports could have been caused by sialodacryoadenitis virus, with *P. pneumotropica* present merely as an opportunist or incidental inhabitant.

*Diagnosis*

Many colonies of mice and rats have *P. pneumotropica* infections of the upper respiratory tract, digestive tract, conjunctiva, and other sites but no demonstrable disease. Diagnostic efforts must discriminate between *P. pneumotropica* infection and *P. pneumotropica*-induced disease, and rule out other possible causative agents and disease processes.

*Pasteurella* spp., *Actinobacillus* spp., *Haemophilus* spp., and *Yersinia* spp., which are commonly found in mice and rats, give similar reactions in many biochemical tests. Therefore, extensive biochemical testing is required to accurately identify these organisms (Hooper and Sebesteny, 1974; Lentsch and Wagner, 1980; Simpson and Simmons, 1980; Ackerman and Fox, 1981; Kunstyr and Hartman, 1983; Carter, 1984; Wullenweber-Schmidt et al., 1988).

*Control*

Since this agent is usually an opportunist, control of important primary pathogens and other factors that compromise host defenses may be more important than efforts to control *P. pneumotropica* infection. Cesarean derivation and maintenance in a gnotobiotic isolator may be necessary to exclude the organism completely. Antibiotic therapy has been attempted in a few instances (Gray and Campbell, 1953; Moore and Aldred, 1978), but it has limited value.

*Interference with Research*

Lesions due to *P. pneumotropica* in the skin and adnexal tissues can interfere with research involving those organs.

## Mouse Papule Virus

*Significance*

Very low.

*Perspective*

Knowledge of this agent is limited to a single report in which a group of mice with skin lesions resembling those of mousepox was described (Kraft and Moore, 1961).

*Agent*

The agent is an unclassified virus. It is ether sensitive and heat labile and can pass through a filter of 450 nm pore size. Inclusions found in skin lesions were considered suggestive of poxvirus etiology. Sera from infected animals were negative by the hemagglutination test for antibodies to vaccinia virus. No isolates of the agent are available for further study (L. M. Kraft, Moffett Field, Calif., personal communication, 1985).

*Hosts*

Mice.

*Epizootiology*

Unknown.

*Clinical*

Papular skin lesions are characterized as areas of edema and hyperemia, with central indentation or dimple formation, randomly distributed over the body, including the feet and tail. Subsequently, there is keratinization and scab formation, followed by healing without scar formation. Lesions are most noticeable in nursing mice prior to the appearance of hair (Kraft and Moore, 1961).

*Pathology*

Raised papules are seen scattered over the entire body, particularly in neonatal mice before growth of hair. Microscopically, acidophilic, intracytoplasmic inclusions are present in the epidermis, and the dermis has variable infiltrates of neutrophils, lymphocytes, and histiocytes (Kraft and Moore, 1961).

*Diagnosis*

Diagnosis of a suspected occurrence of the disease should include isolation, characterization, and identification of the agent; fulfillment of Koch's postulates; and characterization of the clinical and pathological aspects of both the natural and experimental disease.

*Control*

Unknown.

*Interference with Research*

There are no known examples in which this agent interferes with research.

## Mouse Mammary Tumor Virus

### *Significance*

Infections of different mouse strains with variants of this agent provide a large assortment of valuable models for experimental viral carcinogenesis.

### *Perspective*

*1933:* Workers at the Jackson Laboratory (Little, Bittner, Green, and Murray) announced the discovery of a nonchromosomal influence of maternal origin that played a decisive role in the development of mouse mammary cancer (Gross, 1970).

*1936:* This "influence" was reported to be a virus transmitted through the mother's milk (Bittner, 1936; Visscher et al., 1942).

*1959:* DeOme et al. (1959) developed an assay for premalignant changes in the mouse mammary gland based on the outgrowth pattern of transplanted cells in mammary fat pads free of mammary rudiments.

*1974:* Lasfargues et al. (1974) successfully grew the virus in vitro.

*1976:* The ubiquity of the mouse mammary tumor virus (MMTV) provirus in cellular DNA of GR (substrain not given) mice was demonstrated through molecular hybridization studies (van Nie and Hilgers, 1976).

*1979:* Inbred strains of mice were shown to have different MMTV proviruses (Cohen and Varmus, 1979).

### *Agent*

MMTV is a medium-sized RNA virus, family Retroviridae. It is the prototype of a morphologically distinct subclass of retrovirus, type B, that is characterized by an eccentric location of the nucleocapsid within the viral envelope (Bernhard, 1958; Bentvelzen and Hilgers, 1980; Schlom, 1980).

Four major variants of the virus have been identified. MMTV-S (S for standard; the Bittner virus) is transmitted through the milk to nursing young and is highly oncogenic. MMTV-L (L for low oncogenic) is transmitted through germ cells and is weakly oncogenic. MMTV-P (P for pregnancy-dependent) is transmitted through both milk and germ cells and is highly oncogenic. MMTV-O (O for overlooked) is considered an endogenous virus in the genome of most mice (Bentvelzen and Hilgers, 1980; Medina, 1982).

*Hosts*

*Mus musculus* (laboratory and wild). Similar viruses have been reported in other species, including *Mus cervicolor, Mus cookii,* and *Mus caroli* (Bentvelzen and Hilgers, 1980; Teramoto et al., 1980).

*Epizootiology*

Mouse strains such as C3H, DBA/2, and A readily express MMTV-S, and the virus can be demonstrated in a variety of locations throughout the body, especially in mammary tissue and milk. Molecular studies indicate that other mouse strains have proviral copies in their cellular DNA (van Nie and Hilgers, 1976). MMTV proviruses can influence the incidence of malignancy, but most are cryptic, having no discernible effect (Traina-Dorge and Cohen, 1983).

Foster nursing experiments have demonstrated that transmission of MMTV-S occurs via ingestion of infected milk, and results in a high incidence of mammary tumors early in life (6-12 months) when the associated genetic and hormonal factors are also present (Bittner, 1936; Medina, 1982; Traina-Dorge and Cohen, 1983).

*Clinical*

Mammary tumors in female mice can be located on virtually any part of the body (ventral, lateral, and dorsal surfaces) from the chin to the pelvic region. A variable frequency of metastases to distant sites occurs, but the lungs are the most common site (Dunn, 1959; Medina, 1982).

*Pathology*

Current theory holds that the virus initially induces "hyperplastic alveolar nodules," which are preneoplastic lesions. The average latency period from infection to tumor expression is 6-9 months. The development of tumors is enhanced by administration of estrogen to male and female mice, forced breeding, and administration of carcinogens (e.g., 3-methylcholanthrene and 7,12-dimethylbenzanthracene). Glucocorticoid hormones appear to promote mammary tumor production through the induction of intracellular MMTV RNA (Ringold, 1983). Susceptibility to MMTV is controlled by host genetic factors, i.e., it is strain dependent (Medina, 1982; Michalides et al., 1983; Traina-Dorge and Cohen, 1983).

Mammary tumors usually are circumscribed, round to nodular, gray to white masses located in the subcutaneous tissue. They can become very large. Ulcerations and hemorrhages are common in large tumors. Most mammary tumors are adenocarcinomas of Dunn's histologic types A or B (Dunn, 1959). Type A tumors are characterized by uniform acini lined by a single layer of cuboidal cells, while type B tumors are variable in the extent of differentiation, but usually consist of irregular cords and sheets of cells. Other types include adenocarcinomas of types C, Y, L, and P; carcinomas with squamous cell differentiation; and carcinosarcomas. Other histologic types are rare (van Nie, 1967; Sass and Dunn, 1979).

Mice of many strains develop humoral and cellular immune responses to MMTV, indicating that mice infected early in life are not immunologically tolerant (Bentvelzen and Brinkhof, 1980).

### *Diagnosis*

Mouse mammary tumors appear as nodules or masses of varying size in the subcutaneous tissue. They are diagnosed and classified on the basis of histopathologic characteristics (Dunn, 1959; Sass and Dunn, 1979).

Detection and characterization of MMTV requires test procedures normally available only in specialized viral oncology laboratories. Some of the more common procedures are nucleic acid hybridization, immunologic assays for viral antigens, and bioassays for infectivity in different strains of mice (Medina, 1982). A better alternative for investigators whose studies require the presence or absence of MMTV or specific MMTV proviruses may be to obtain mice with the desired characteristics from either the National Institutes of Health (Dr. S. Potkay, Chief, Veterinary Resources Branch, Division of Research Services, Building 14A, Room 103, National Institutes of Health, Bethesda, MD 20205) or the National Cancer Institute (NCI) (Dr. J. G. Mayo, NCI-Frederick Cancer Research Facility, Biological Testing Branch, P.O. Box B, Frederick, MD 21701).

### *Control*

For most studies, control of MMTV is not required. The most practical method of control is through selection of mouse strains. Foster nursing on mouse strains that are free of the virus has been used to eliminate MMTV-S.

### *Interference with Research*

MMTV infection in mice is an extremely valuable model of mammary cancer, especially for studies of the interactions of the virus, hormones, genetics, and carcinogens. It is the only known animal model of virus-induced mammary cancer. The infection also can be a complicating factor in experimental carcinogenesis studies.

Concurrent infection of mice with the lactic dehydrogenase-elevating virus and MMTV-S reduces the incidence of virus-induced mammary tumors (Riley, 1966).

### Self-Mutilation Associated with Otitis Media

Harkness and Wagner (1975) reported on a single incident in which a small percentage of adult mice in a colony exhibited violent scratching of the external ears and adjacent tissues. Histologic sections of the external ears showed ulceration and acute inflammation of the ear pinnas, external canals, and adjacent tissues. The mice also had purulent otitis media from which *Mycoplasma pulmonis*, *Pasteurella pneumotropica*, and other agents were isolated. The skin condition was considered secondary to the otitis media.

## NONINFECTIOUS SKIN CONDITIONS IMPORTANT IN DIFFERENTIAL DIAGNOSIS

### Bite Wounds in Adult Mice and Rats

Fighting can be a serious problem in some strains of mice (Wimer and Fuller, 1966). It is usually worst among mature males but also occurs among females in some strains. Some of the most notorious fighters are mature males of the BALB/c, SJL/J, and HRS/J strains, which generally must be housed one per cage. Bite wounds can appear anywhere on the body, but they usually are most concentrated on the rump and lumbar regions, with few or none on the shoulders or head. The characteristic pattern of open and healing wounds along dorsal surfaces of the trunk is virtually diagnostic (Scott and Fredericson, 1951; Fredericson and Birnbaum, 1954).

Among male mice housed in groups, the submissive cage mates, which are bitten most frequently, often develop anemia and splenomegaly and have a much greater incidence of amyloidosis than do dominant males (Page and Glenner, 1972). In one colony of SW (Swiss Webster) mice, complication of bite wounds by group G streptococci reportedly caused necrotizing dermatitis and 35% mortality (Stewart et al., 1975).

Skin lesions caused by fighting also can occur in old male rats, but fighting among rats is usually of little consequence compared with that among mice. Housing in compatible groups or singly usually results in dramatic healing of bite wounds within a few days in both rats and mice.

### Bite Wounds in Weanling Mice

This syndrome was first reported in C3H/HeJ and C3HeB/FeJ mice, occurring usually at 5-8 weeks of age (Les, 1972). It was associated with the housing of weanling mice in groups of 40 per cage and sometimes affected all mice in a cage. Lesions varied from small red foci to encrusted excoriations up to 3 mm in diameter on the tail skin. Some tails became swollen, and the part distal to some lesions sloughed. As healing occurred, the lesions became small white scars readily visible on the tails of pigmented C3H mice. Koopman et al. (1984) have confirmed these observations for C3H/He mice.

A similar, if not identical, condition has been seen in weanling mice of the BALB/c strain (Cox et al., 1977). In addition to lesions on tails, these mice also had the lesions on their feet and ears. Using histologic methods, these investigators demonstrated that the dermis beneath the lesions regularly contained fragments of keratinized epithelium from the skin surface, suggesting that the skin lesions were bite wounds inflicted by cage mates. A major difference between C3H/He and BALB/c mice with this condition is that healing results in small but prominent white foci of scarring on the tails of pigmented C3H/He mice but leaves almost imperceptible scars on the tails of albino BALB/c mice.

The cause of this condition is unknown. Les (1972) and Koopman et al. (1984) have suggested that "social stress" plays a role. However, the cause may simply be hunger resulting from the sudden separation of weanlings from their dams, the simultaneous crowding of weanlings into large groups where access to food and water is limited, and/or poor palatability of food (e.g., due to hardness of the pelleted diet). Control is accomplished by housing smaller numbers of weanlings per cage (i.e., avoiding crowding). The major importance of the condition is that it be recognized as a distinct entity that can be readily differentiated from mousepox by clinical and pathological features.

### "Whisker-Trimming," "Hair-Nibbling," and "Barbering"

These are descriptive terms that have been applied to an assortment of patterns of alopecia associated with social behavior in mice. C57BL/6, C57BL/10, C3H, and SW mice have been the most studied, and heredity is thought to play a role. The dominant cage mate chews off the whiskers or hair of other cage mates giving the affected area a smoothly shaved appearance. The sites affected most are the whiskers and hair of the face, head, neck, and back. Usually, hair chewing occurs without injury to the underlying skin, although chronic hair chewing can result in thickening and increased pigmentation of the epidermis or even formation of foreign body granulomas in the dermis. If such chronically chewed mice are separated from the more dominant mouse, the regrowth of hair may be sparse and unpigmented, often with residual partial alopecia (Hauschka, 1952; Long, 1972; Thornburg et al., 1973).

## Muzzle Alopecia

Small patches of alopecia are located on the lateral surfaces of the muzzle. They can result from mechanical trauma associated with repeatedly inserting the muzzle through holes in the cage cover or between metal rods forming the food hopper (but is probably more often due to whisker-trimming by cagemates). Histologically, the affected skin may show hyperkeratosis, acanthosis, and mild inflammation (Litterst, 1974).

## Hair Growth Cycling Arrest

Mice are known to grow hair in distinct patterns or cycles (Borum, 1954; Chase, 1954; Chase and Eaton, 1959; Argyris, 1963). Occasionally, one may see an entire litter of runted mice about weaning age with complete loss of hair on the torso. A small tuft of hair remains at the base of the tail and normal-appearing hair is present on the head and legs. Such mice generally have severe systemic disease (e.g., mouse hepatitis virus infection) and, presumably, are experiencing a temporary arrest of normal hair growth cycling (J. R. Lindsey, Department of Comparative Medicine, University of Alabama at Birmingham, unpublished).

## "Ringtail"

This condition has been reported in mice (Nelson, 1960), laboratory rats (Njaa et al., 1957; Flynn, 1959; Totton, 1958), and the South African white-tailed hamster (Stuhlman and Wagner, 1971). It is characterized by the appearance of concentric rings around the tail, frequently followed by sloughing of all or part of the tail. The feet also may be swollen and reddened. The cause is thought to be environmental conditions of low (less than 40%) relative humidity and high (more than 80°F) temperature.

# 9

# Hemopoietic System

## Overview

The agents included in this section constitute a diverse assortment with very different host-parasite relationships. However, they do share some degree of commonality in pathogenetic mechanisms in that they all appear to have cell populations in the hemopoietic system as their chief target tissues.

Although lymphocytic choriomeningitis virus (LCMV) has traditionally been considered mainly a pathogen of the central nervous system, viremia and the immunologic responses of the host have central roles in pathogenesis, thus justifying its recognition as a pathogen of the hemopoietic system. The lactic dehydrogenase-elevating virus (LDV) causes persistent viremia, apparently replicates only in a small subset of macrophages, and through unknown mechanisms alters numerous immunologic functions and decreases the plasma clearance of lactic dehydrogenase isozyme V. Both *Haemobartonella muris* and *Eperythrozoon coccoides* are blood parasites. The murine leukemia viruses (MuLVs) are endogenous viruses found in all host cells of mice but cause hemopoietic neoplasms under appropriate conditions.

All of these agents have special importance in experimental oncology. MuLV-infected animals are frequently used as animal models for the study of viral carcinogenesis. The others, LCMV, LDV, *H. muris,* and *E. coccoides,* are notorious as inadvertent contaminants of transplantable tumors and other test systems, in which they frequently alter research results. In addition, LCMV infection has importance as a zoonosis.

## Lymphocytic Choriomeningitis Virus

### *Significance*

Lymphocytic choriomeningitis virus (LCMV) is a highly significant zoonotic infection of laboratory personnel who work with transplantable rodent tumors (particularly in hamsters) and rodent cell lines (Biggar et al., 1976; Pike, 1979), and of owners of pet hamsters (Parker et al., 1976). The virus also has importance as an unwanted contaminant that can alter research results of in vitro and in vivo rodent test systems (see below) and for the experimental study of virus-host interactions (Lehmann-Grube et al., 1983).

### *Perspective*

Lymphocytic choriomeningitis virus (LCMV) has been recognized as an important zoonotic agent and indigenous rodent pathogen for about five decades (Hotchin, 1971b). Traditionally, mice have been considered the primary source of LCMV infection. However, since 1960 three epidemics of LCMV infection involving at least 236 human cases have occurred in the United States, and all have been associated with Syrian hamsters, either as laboratory animals bearing transplantable tumors or as pets (Gregg, 1975). Because of the unique host-parasite relationship of LCMV infection in mice, experimental infections in mice have been used extensively as models for the investigation of such diverse phenomena as virus-specific immunological tolerance, virus-induced T-cell-mediated immunopathology, virus-induced immune complex disease, in vivo viral interference, and activation of natural killer cells (Lehmann-Grube et al., 1983).

### *Agent*

LCMV is an RNA virus, family Arenaviridae, genus *Arenavirus*. LCMV is the type species of the genus. Other members of this genus include Lassa virus and the Tacaribe Complex (Amapari, Junin, Latino, Machupo, Parana, Pichinde, Tacaribe, and Tamiami Viruses). The LCMV strains used most widely for experimental purposes are WE, E-350, and CA 1371 (Lehmann-Grube, 1982; Matthews, 1982).

LCMV and other members of the genus *Arenavirus* have unique ultrastructural characteristics. The virions are pleomorphic, have a diameter of 50-300 nm (mean, 110-130 nm), and consist of a membranous envelope with surface projections surrounding an interior containing granules (host ribosomes that measure 20-25 nm in diameter) instead of a defined core. Virus particles bud from plasma membranes of infected cells and can form large intracytoplasmic inclusions (Murphy and Whitfield, 1975; Rawls and Buchmeier, 1975; Rawls and Leung, 1979).

LCMV and other members of the genus *Arenavirus* are highly sensitive to lipid solvents, detergents, and disinfectants such as formaldehyde. Infectivity is rapidly lost at pH values below 5.5 and above 8.5 (Biggar et al., 1976; Rawls and Leung, 1979).

LCMV can be propagated in a wide range of mammalian cells, but BHK-21, L, and Vero cells are most commonly used (Rawls and Leung, 1979; Matthews, 1982).

### *Hosts*

Wild mice (*Mus musculus*) are the principal reservoir hosts, but laboratory mice and Syrian hamsters also serve as important natural hosts. Humans, monkeys, dogs, rabbits, guinea pigs, rats, and chickens are also susceptible (Wenner, 1948; Hotchin, 1971b; Ackerman, 1973; Forster and Wachendorfer, 1973; Gregg, 1975; Skinner et al., 1977; Smith et al., 1984b). LCMV also utilizes numerous cell lines as laboratory hosts, including transplantable tumor lines (Biggar et al., 1976) and tissue culture cell lines (van der Zeijst et al., 1983).

### *Epizootiology*

Infections of LCMV are generally thought to be very common in wild *M. musculus* (Ackerman, 1973). Of 1,795 house mice trapped in West Germany, 65 (3.6%) were found to be infected (Ackerman, 1973). Following the discovery of LCMV in laboratory mice at a research institute in England, the infection was diagnosed in 51 (67%) of 76 wild mice trapped in the vicinity (Skinner et al., 1977).

Natural LCMV infections have been reported in only about five colonies of laboratory mice (Traub, 1935; Findlay et al., 1936; Lepine and Sautter, 1936; Skinner and Knight, 1969; Smith et al., 1984b). Sato and Miyata (1986) surveyed laboratory mice in Japan for anti-LCMV antibodies using an indirect fluorescent antibody (IFA) test, and found seropositives in 3 (2.2%) of 152 specific-pathogen-free mice and 30 (5.6%) of 539 conventional mice.

Although hamsters infected with LCMV were found to be widely dispersed in the United States in recent years, those infections were traced to a single hamster breeder and a nearby laboratory supplying investigators with transplantable hamster tumors (Gregg, 1975). One can only conclude that past health monitoring procedures for hamsters and transplantable hamster tumors have been inadequate and that the spread of LCMV infection can be extremely insidious.

Only infected mice and hamsters are known to transmit the virus. Both species can have chronic infections, with high concentrations of virus shed in urine, saliva, and milk. The portals of entry are probably mucus membranes and broken skin. Vertical (transovarian and/or transuterine) transmission is known to occur in mice and is considered 100% efficient for mice born to infected dams. Vertical transmission is also thought to occur in hamsters but has not been definitively proved. Once introduced into a population of mice, the infection can spread to all members of that population (Traub, 1939; Skinner and Knight, 1971; Parker et al., 1976; Lehmann-Grube, 1982).

*Clinical*

Clinical signs in mice vary greatly, depending on the strain of virus, strain of mouse, and age of mice at the time of infection, but the following two forms of natural LCMV infection are generally recognized:

a. *Persistent tolerant infection.* This form results when infection is acquired in utero or within a few days after birth. There is lifelong viremia and shedding of virus. Transient runting can occur during the first 3 weeks of life. Thereafter, the mice appear normal but can have modest growth retardation. At 7-10 months of age, immune complex glomerulonephritis occurs and is associated with emaciation, ruffled fur, hunched posture, ascites, and some deaths (Hotchin, 1962; Pollard and Sharon, 1973; Traub, 1973; Lehmann-Grube, 1982).

b. *Nontolerant (acute) infection.* This form occurs when infection is acquired after the first week of life (after the development of immunocompetence). Viremia occurs, but there is no shedding of virus. The outcome is either death within a few days or weeks, or recovery with elimination of the virus. Most of the available data on this form of infection have been obtained from experimental inoculation of the virus intracerebrally, subcutaneously, intraperitoneally, or intravenously (not the normal routes). However, depending on the mouse strain, natural infections of LCMV in adult mice can range from inapparent to severe disease with high mortality. Considering that few natural outbreaks have been reported in mice, asymptomatic infections in adults may be the most common (Hotchin, 1962; Hotchin and Benson, 1963; Skinner et al., 1977).

Natural infections in hamsters are generally considered subclinical (Forster and Wachendorfer, 1973; Bowen et al., 1975). However, Parker et al. (1976) studied experimental LCMV infections in hamsters and reported that hamsters with persistent viremia developed progressive glomerulonephritis and had reduced litter sizes. They also observed runting in some congenitally infected animals.

In humans, the usual clinical manifestations are those of flu-like disease, with fever, headache, myalgia, nausea, vomiting, sore throat, and photophobia being the major symptoms. Occasionally, rash, diarrhea, cough, lymphadenopathy, orchitis, delirium, or amnesia occurs. Unless physicians are alerted to the possibility of LCMV infection, the disease is frequently diagnosed as influenza, mononucleosis, herpes encephalitis, or tuberculous meningitis (Biggar et al., 1976).

*Pathology*

Experimentally, the type and degree of LCMV-induced disease in mice have been shown to be greatly influenced by the virus strain, dose, and route of inoculation; mouse strain and age; and other factors (Parker et al., 1976; Lehmann-Grube, 1982). However, there are two types of natural disease that are dependent on the age of the mouse at the time of infection:

a. *Persistent tolerant infection.* Infection occurs in utero or shortly after birth; lifelong viremia and virus shedding occur. These mice are not tolerant in the classical sense but have a kind of split tolerance in that T-cell activity is suppressed while B-cell activity is not. Specifically, there is diminution of LCMV-specific, major histocompatibility complex class I restricted cytotoxic T-lymphocyte activity, but unabated generation of LCMV-specific B-cell responses with production of high titers of antibodies to all LCMV polypeptides (Francis et al., 1987). Infectious virus circulates bound to LCMV-specific IgG and complement. These complexes accumulate in the renal glomeruli, choroid plexus, and, to a lesser degree, in synovial membranes, in blood vessel walls, and beneath the epidermis of the skin to cause late-onset disease that becomes apparent clinically around 7-10 months of age (Hotchin and Collins, 1964; Oldstone and Dixon, 1967, 1969, 1970; Kajima and Pollard, 1970; Buchmeier and Oldstone, 1978; Oldstone et al., 1980, 1983; Lehmann-Grube et al., 1983; Moskophidis and Lehmann-Grube, 1984). T-lymphocytes of the helper subset (Thy-1.2$^+$, Lyt-2$^-$, L3T4$^+$) are persistently infected with LCMV (Tishon et al., 1988). There is generalized lymphoid hyperplasia and perivascular accumulation of lymphocytes and plasma cells in all visceral organs (Pollard and Sharon, 1969, 1973). Interferon is thought to have a central role in the development of immune complex disease (Riviere et al., 1980; Ronco et al., 1980; Jacobson et al., 1981; Saron et al., 1982; Woodrow et al., 1982).

b. *Nontolerant (acute) infection.* Infection is acquired after the development of immunocompetence. Viremia occurs but there is no shedding of virus. If the mouse recovers from the acute disease, virus is eliminated from the blood and tissues in weeks or months (Hotchin, 1971a). Almost all of the data on this type of infection have been obtained from mice infected experimentally by the intracerebral, intraperitoneal, intravenous, or subcutaneous route. After intracerebral inoculation of LCMV, the predominant lesions are meningoencephalitis and hepatitis with large infiltrates of lymphocytes (Lillie and Armstrong, 1945; Collins et al., 1961; Rodriguez et al., 1983). When the virus is given by the other routes, there is multifocal hepatic necrosis and generalized lymphocytolysis of T and B cells with fibrinoid necrosis by four to five days. In survivors, regeneration of lymphoid organs commences on about day 9 (Mims and Tosolini, 1969; Lehmann-Grube and Lohler, 1981; Lohler and Lehmann-Grube, 1981). Both the morphologic lesions and elimination of the virus in the nontolerant infection are due to cell-mediated immune responses involving *H-2*-restricted cytotoxic T lymphocytes (Zinkernagel and Doherty, 1973, 1975, 1979; Doherty et al., 1974) and, possibly, natural killer cells (Welsh, 1978; Welsh and Doe, 1980). T-lymphocytes of the cytotoxic-suppressive subset (Lyt-$2^+$) are thought to be particularly important in elimination of the virus (Moskophidis et al., 1987). LCMV-infected mice can be protected from disease by numerous immunosuppressive regimens (Lehmann-Grube, 1982). Athymic (*nu/nu*) mice inoculated with the virus at 3 to 6 weeks of age do not develop disease but have persistent viremia (Christoffersen et al., 1976; Christoffersen and Bro-Jorgensen, 1977; Ronco et al., 1981).

LCMV infection in hamsters appears to have a pathogenesis similar to that in mice, but far less is known about the infection in hamsters. Hamsters with congenital LCMV infection and hamsters inoculated with the virus as newborns develop persistent viremia and viruria through three months of age. After that time half of them clear the virus and remain healthy; the others maintain the viremia and viruria and develop chronic glomerulonephritis and generalized chronic vasculitis presumably due to immune complex disease. Adult hamsters inoculated with LCMV develop viremia and viruria but clear the virus in three to six months without becoming diseased (Parker et al., 1976).

### *Diagnosis*

Serologic methods are the most practical procedures for routine diagnosis, but bleeding and processing of blood from an animal suspected of LCMV infection should be done with care because of the likelihood of viremia. The methods of choice are the IFA, micro plaque-reduction test for neutralizing antibody, and enzyme-linked immunosorbent assay. The IFA is particularly useful for rapid diagnosis early in the course of infection, while the micro plaque-reduction test is considered best for chronic infection. The complement fixation test is considered relatively insensitive and is not recommended (Hotchin and Sikora, 1975; Kimmig and Lehmann-Grube, 1979; Lehmann-Grube et al., 1979; Ivanov et al., 1981; Smith et al., 1984b).

The mouse antibody production (MAP) test can be used in testing transplantable tumors and other biologic materials for contamination with LCMV (Rowe et al., 1959a, 1962). Alternatively, virus isolations in tissue cultures followed by detection of LCMV antigen by using immunofluorescence (Hotchin and Sikora, 1975), or direct examination by immunofluorescence methods of tissues suspected of having LCMV infection (Wilsnack and Rowe, 1964) can be useful in selected instances.

### *Control*

The most practical method of control is to obtain mice and hamsters only from populations shown by regular health surveillance testing to be free of LCMV and to maintain them in a barrier facility that excludes wild rodents. Such stocks should also be retested at regular intervals to reconfirm their LCMV-free status. In addition, all biologic materials such as transplantable tumors coming into the facility must be pretested and shown to be free of the virus before experimental use. Periodic testing of animals receiving such materials is also desirable (Rowe et al., 1962; Collins and Parker, 1972; Bowen et al., 1975).

Once LCMV infection is diagnosed in mice, hamsters, a transplantable tumor, or other biologic materials, the entire stock should be destroyed and incinerated. Animal cages and other equipment should be removed and autoclaved. Animal rooms should be fumigated with either formalin [40% formaldehyde in water, sprayed on all room surfaces at 35.7 ml/$m^3$ (1 ml/$ft^3$)] or paraformaldehyde [10.7 g/$m^3$ (0.3 g/$ft^3$) vaporized in a high-temperature silicone fluid at 96°C (205°F)] and allowed to remain vacant for 7-10 days (Biggar et al., 1976).

Cesarean derivation of animal stocks is of no value because of transovarian or transuterine infection (Hotchin, 1962; Skinner and Knight, 1971; Parker et al., 1976; Lehmann-Grube, 1982).

### *Interference with Research*

LCMV infection is an important zoonotic infection that can result in fatality or have serious complications such as meningitis, orchitis, arthritis, and alopecia (Lewis et al., 1965; Baum et al., 1966; Hirsch et al., 1974; Bowen et al., 1975; Biggar et al., 1976; Pike, 1979).

LCMV has been a frequent contaminant of biologic materials used in research, including the following:

a. Transplantable tumors of mice (DeBuryn, 1949; Stewart and Haas, 1956; Haas, 1960; Molomut and Padnos, 1965; Molomut et al., 1965; Collins and Parker, 1972; Bhatt et al., 1986), hamsters (Lewis et al., 1965; Baum et al., 1966; Bowen et al., 1975; Gregg, 1975; Biggar et al., 1976), and guinea pigs (Nadel and Haas, 1955; Jungeblut and Kodza, 1963).

b. Tissue culture cell lines (Lehmann-Grube et al., 1969; van der Zeijst et al., 1983).

c. Virus stocks, including leukemia viruses (Collins and Parker, 1972), distemper virus (Dalldorf, 1939), rabies virus (Wiktor et al., 1965), and mouse poliomyelitis virus (Wenner, 1948).
d. Toxoplasma gondii sublines (Grimwood, 1985).

LCMV infection has an inhibitory effect on tumor induction due to polyomavirus (Hotchin, 1962), Rauscher virus (Youn and Barski, 1966), and mammary tumor virus (Padnos and Molomut, 1973) in mice, and transplantable leukemias in guinea pigs (Nadel and Haas, 1955; Jungeblut and Kodza, 1963) and mice (Padnos and Molomut, 1973).

LCMV infection in mice causes induction of natural killer cell activity early in the infection and proliferation of virus-specific cytotoxic T lymphocytes in chronic infection (Zinkernagel and Doherty, 1975, 1979; Welsh, 1978; Welsh and Doe, 1980; Pfau et al., 1982).

LCMV infection causes severe depression of humoral and/or cellular immunity in mice (Mims and Wainwright, 1968; Lehmann-Grube et al., 1972; Bro-Jorgensen and Volkert, 1974; Bro-Jorgensen et al., 1975; Guttler et al., 1975; Thomsen et al., 1982; Wu-Hsieh et al., 1988).

LCMV infection delays rejection of skin (Lehmann-Grube et al., 1972) and tumor (Guttler et al., 1975) allografts.

LCMV infection increases susceptibility of mice to ectromelia virus (Mims and Wainwright, 1968) or *Eperythrozoon coccoides* (Seamer et al., 1961) infection.

LCMV infection increases susceptibility of mice to bacterial endotoxin (Hotchin, 1962; Barlow, 1964).

LCMV infection increases susceptibility of mice to x-irradiation (Bro-Jorgensen and Volkert, 1972).

LCMV infection abrogates the naturally occurring insulin-dependent diabetes mellitus of BB rats, presumably by suppressing autoimmune mechanisms causing the disease (Dyrberg et al., 1988; Schwimmbeck et al., 1988).

## Lactic Dehydrogenase-Elevating Virus

### *Significance*

Lactic dehydrogenase-elevating virus is highly significant for research involving transplantable tumors, viral oncology, immunology, and serial passage of infectious agents in mice. It has low significance for many studies using mice.

### *Perspective*

In studies to develop a method for early detection of cancer, Riley and Wroblewski (1960) found that a 5- to 10-fold increase in serum lactate dehydrogenase (LDH) occurred in mice following inoculation with Ehrlich carcinoma cells. Riley et al. (1960) demonstrated that this effect was due to a transmissible agent, lactic dehydrogenase-elevating virus (LDV), which was associated with his transplantable mouse tumors. Subsequently, Riley (1968) showed that more than 50 transplantable mouse tumors were contaminated with LDV, and evidence from many other laboratories (Notkins, 1965; Riley, 1974; Rowson and Mahy, 1975) further incriminated this virus as a major variable in tumor immunobiology.

### *Agent*

LDV is an RNA virus, family Togaviridae, presently assigned to an unnamed genus that includes hog cholera, bovine diarrhea, equine arteritis, and simian hemorrhagic fever viruses (Brinton, 1982; Matthews, 1982; Rowson and Mahy, 1985). Virions are enveloped and average 50-55 nm in diameter. The nucleocapsid is approximately 30-35 nm in diameter. Maturation of virions occurs by budding from cytoplasm into intracytoplasmic vesicles (Brinton, 1982; Rowson and Mahy, 1985).

Antigenic diversity between the various isolates of LDV is poorly understood because the virus-antibody complexes that are present in infected mice interfere with conventional serum neutralization tests. Limited studies with heterologous antibody produced in rats or rabbits suggest that there are at least two serologically distinct strains (Bailey et al., 1965b; Cafruny and Plagemann, 1982; Rowson and Mahy, 1985).

LDV can be propagated in primary tissue cultures of mouse origin, including spleen, bone marrow, embryo fibroblast, and peritoneal exudate cells. However, virus production in such cultures generally declines after the first week, an effect thought to be due to the depletion of permissive macrophages. This effect can be largely eliminated by adding 10% L-cell-conditioned medium which provides a macrophage growth factor (Brinton, 1982; Rowson and Mahy, 1985).

LDV is inactivated by lipid solvents, detergents, and acid pH. The virus can be stored indefinitely in plasma at –70°C, but not at 4°C. Virus-infected plasma or feces retains infectivity for only about 24 hours at room temperature (Brinton, 1982).

### *Host*

Mice (*Mus musculus*). The virus does not replicate in rats, hamsters, guinea pigs, rabbits, or in cell cultures from them (Notkins, 1965; Brinton, 1982; Rowson and Mahy, 1985).

*Epizootiology*

LDV has been isolated from wild mice in Australia (Pope, 1961), Europe (Rowson, 1963; Georgii and Kirschenhofer, 1965; Field and Adams, 1968), and the United States (Pope and Rowe, 1964). Wild mice presumably serve as reservoir hosts.

LDV infection is not likely to be seen in breeding colonies of laboratory mice, but is very likely to occur in mice used in certain types of experiments if appropriate preventive measures are not followed. Transmission occurs most readily during experimental procedures such as mouse-to-mouse passage of contaminated tumors, cells, or serum, or use of the same needle to inoculate multiple mice. Experimentally, any parenteral route is effective (Notkins, 1965).

Although mice infected with LDV shed the virus in feces, urine, saliva, and milk, the virus titer in these excretions declines sufficiently after the first week of infection that the risk of transmission to other mice is subsequently relatively low. A similar pattern also holds for transplacental transmission. Dams infected during gestation can have a high percentage of infected progeny, but dams infected one week before mating or a few days after parturition have relatively few infected progeny. Fighting (bite wounds) increases transmission between cage mates (Notkins and Scheele, 1963; Plagemann et al., 1963; Crispens, 1964; Notkins, 1965).

*Clinical*

LDV infection results in lifelong viremia in which the virus is complexed to antiviral antibody, but clinical signs do not occur (Rowson and Mahy, 1985). The exception to this general rule is the flaccid paralysis seen in C58 (strain designation incompletely given) and AKR strain mice with age-dependent polioencephalomyelitis caused by LDV at 5 months of age or older (see below).

*Pathology*

After infection the LDV titer in the mouse's serum reaches $10^{10}$-$10^{11}$ median infectious doses ($ID_{50}$) 12-14 hours after infection, drops to $10^7$ $ID_{50}$/ml by 72-96 hours, and drops further to $10^5$ $ID_{50}$/ml by about 2 weeks, when the titer stabilizes for life. The virus replicates in macrophages so that virus titers in spleen, lymph nodes, liver, and thymus are similar to those in serum (Notkins, 1965).

The activity of plasma LDH begins to rise about 24 hours after infection, peaks at an 8- to 11-fold increase above normal at 72-96 hours after infection, and then gradually declines over the next three months but remains significantly elevated for life. SJL/J mice are unique in that they experience a 15- to 20-fold increase in serum LDH, a recessive trait of this strain (Crispens, 1971, 1972; Inada and Mims, 1987). The increase in LDH is due to decreased clearance of only one of five isozymes of LDH, LDH V (Plagemann et al., 1963; Warnock, 1964). Several other plasma enzymes are increased in activity but to a lesser degree than LDH (Notkins, 1965; Brinton, 1982).

The virus replicates only in a small subpopulation of macrophages, the specific identity of which remains in question. Initially, considerable evidence seemed to implicate the Ia positive macrophage as the susceptible cell (Inada and Mims, 1984, 1985a,b, 1987). More recently, it has been shown that macrophages with a trypsin-sensitive receptor (Ia antigen is not trypsin-sensitive) are the permissive subpopulation (Kowalchyk and Plagemann, 1985; Buxton et al., 1988). SJL/J mice apparently have more of these cells than other strains of mice (Inada and Mims, 1987). Cytopathic effects have been seen in vitro in these cells. The virus replicates for one cell cycle only, unless the specific subpopulation of macrophages is replenished. After infection these cells have impaired antigen-presenting capacity and do not trigger memory T cells (Isakov et al., 1982a,b; Stueckemann et al., 1982a,b). Acute infection also causes rapid, transient interferon production (Evans and Riley, 1968; DuBuy et al., 1973), which is associated with enhanced Fc and complement receptor activity of macrophages (Lussenhop et al., 1982).

During the first few days of infection, there is necrosis of the thymus-dependent regions of lymphoid tissues throughout the body (Hanna et al., 1970a,b; Profitt et al., 1972) and lymphocytopenia (Riley, 1968). Thymus weight decreases by 40% but returns to normal or above normal weight by seven days after infection. These changes in lymphoid tissues are abrogated by adrenalectomy prior to LDV infection (Profitt and Congdon, 1970; Santisteban et al., 1972; Brinton, 1982).

In the first few weeks of infection there is depression of cellular immunity, as evidenced by the longer survival of skin allografts (Howard et al., 1969) and increased tumor growth (Michaelides and Schlesinger, 1974); these functions gradually return to normal after weeks or months.

Antigenic challenge by T-cell-dependent antigens within 24 hours of LDV infection leads to enhanced humoral responses, while challenge three weeks or longer after infection leads to diminished responses (Mergenhagen et al., 1967; Riley et al., 1975; Isakov et al., 1982c). A similar enhanced response during early infection has been reported for a T-cell-independent antigen, but diminution of the response in chronic infection did not occur, suggesting defective T-cell function (Michaelides and Simms, 1980). Mice infected with LDV produce high blood levels of anti-LDV IgG antibodies that remain high for a year or longer (Coutelier et al., 1986).

Circulating antigen-antibody complexes are produced by four weeks post infection. These complexes partially neutralize the virus, but it is still infectious. Complexes are deposited in glomeruli but produce only a mild membranous glomerulopathy. Protective antibody is not produced (Notkins et al., 1968; Porter and Porter, 1971).

LDV infection causes overt disease in mice of the C58 and AKR strains when they are immunosuppressed, either naturally during the aging process or experimentally by the administration of cyclophosphamide or x-irradiation. Mice of the C58 strain are more susceptible than those of the AKR strain. Beginning at five months of age C58 mice lose Lyt-1,2 cells, and the process reaches completion around 1 year of age, rendering them susceptible to age-dependent polioencephalomyelitis upon infection with LDV. Motor neurons in the anterior horn of the spinal cord are infected with LDV (Contag et al., 1986), resulting in neuronal destruction, mononuclear infiltration, and microglial proliferation in the gray matter of the cord. Clinically, there is flaccid hind limb paralysis. Polygenic inheritance of susceptibility, possibly involving the *H-2* complex, has been proposed (Duffey et al., 1976; Martinez, 1979; Martinez et al., 1980; Nawrocki et al., 1980; Bentley et al., 1983). When other mouse strains are given cyclophosphamide prior to inoculation with LDV, a wide range of different nervous system lesions is produced (Stroop and Brinton, 1983).

### *Diagnosis*

Diagnosis of LDV infection usually is based on the finding of increased levels of LDH activity in the plasma of mice. Screening of transplantable tumors, virus inocula, and other preparations for LDV contamination is done by injecting an aliquot into LDV-free mice and performing the LDH assay on plasma or serum 72-96 hours later (Notkins, 1965; Collins and Parker, 1972; Brinton, 1982). The diagnosis of LDV infection is based on the occurrence of an 8- to 11-fold increase in LDH activity in blood plasma within the period of 72-96 hours. Only pathogen-free mice should be used for this purpose as it has been reported that prior infection with mouse hepatitis can delay the increase in LDH for five days or more (Dillberger et al., 1987b). Different bleeding techniques also can affect plasma LDH activity levels (Dillberger et al., 1987a). Plasma may be stored at room temperature for 24 hours without affecting activity (Dillberger et al., 1987a). LDV can be propagated in primary cultures of mouse tissues, but virus isolation is not practical for most diagnostic purposes (Brinton, 1982).

### *Control*

LDV can be eliminated from tumors by passage of tumor cells in a rodent species other than the mouse or by maintenance of tumor cells in tissue culture (Plagemann and Swim, 1963, 1966; Notkins, 1965). LDV can be eliminated from stocks of murine plasmodia by separating parasitized erythrocytes from the mononuclear leukocytes that serve as host cells for LDV and vigorously washing the parasitized erythrocytes before passaging them in pathogen-free mice (Parke et al., 1986).

LDV-free animals can be derived from known contaminated stocks by selection of animals with normal plasma LDH concentration or by cesarean derivation. The risk of vertical and horizontal transmission from an infected dam is far greater during early stages (week one) of the infection (Notkins, 1965).

LDV infection is not likely to be encountered in mice from commercial barrier breeding facilities.

*Interference with Research*

Riley (1974) has aptly described LDV as "the benign modifier of body chemistry." Although LDV affects mainly the immune system and concentrations of certain enzymes in the plasma, its potential for altering research data is enormous and complex. It is extremely subtle because infection is subclinical throughout life. Its effects on many biologic endpoints can differ dramatically with time after infection (e.g., one week after infection versus weeks or months after infection). In addition, subtle interactions with other agents can occur (e.g., immunosuppression caused by LDV can alter defenses against other infectious agents).

LDV infection causes an 8- to 11-fold increase in plasma LDH and a two- to three-fold increase in several other plasma enzymes (Brinton, 1982).

LDV infection can enhance or suppress growth of transplantable mouse tumors. In general, tumor growth is enhanced early after LDV infection (because of depressed cellular immunity) and is influenced less during chronic infection. Some examples include Ehrlich ascites tumor (Bailey et al., 1965a), MOPC-315 plasmacytoma (Michaelides and Schlesinger, 1974), Gardner lymphoma (Speckman and Riley, 1975), and a chemically induced fibrosarcoma (Henderson et al., 1979).

LDV infection results in the altered incidence and behavior of spontaneous virus-induced neoplasms, including the Bittner mammary tumor (Riley, 1966) and murine sarcoma virus (Turner et al., 1971; McDonald, 1983). LDV infection has been reported to suppress the development of pulmonary adenomas in response to urethan (Theiss et al., 1980) and carcinogenesis caused by vinyl chloride-vinyl acetate (Brinton and Brand, 1977).

LDV infection does not alter the development of spontaneous reticulum cell sarcoma and lymphatic leukemia in SJL/J, AKR/Cu, and AKR/J mice, and does not influence carcinogenicity of methylcholanthrene or benzanthracene (Isakov et al., 1981).

LDV infection causes delayed allograft rejection in mice (Howard et al.,

1969), prevents development of experimental allergic encephalomyelitis in mice (Inada and Mims, 1986), and prevents the occurrence of autoimmune disease in NZB and (NZB × NZW)$F_1$ mice (Oldstone and Dixon, 1972).

LDV infection causes elevation of serum gamma globulin levels and increased humoral antibody responses during early infection (Notkins et al., 1966; Mergenhagen et al., 1967; Riley et al., 1975; Michaelides and Simms, 1980; Isakov et al., 1982c) and a reduced humoral response during chronic infection (Michaelides and Simms, 1980).

LDV is a polyclonal lymphocyte activator during the early stages of infection (Michaelides and Simms, 1980).

LDV inhibits carbon clearance (Notkins and Scheele, 1964; Mahy et al., 1965) and reduces the plasma clearance of injected asparaginase (Riley et al., 1970).

LDV infection greatly enhances the severity of *Eperythrozoon coccoides* infection; the dual infection results in severe hemolytic anemia (Riley, 1964; Fitzmaurice et al., 1974). It exacerbates murine malaria caused by *Plasmodium yoelii* (Henderson et al., 1978) and increases susceptibility to experimental *Listeria monocytogenes* infection (Bonventre et al., 1980).

An Ehrlich ascites tumor was found to induce interferon and enhance natural killer cell activity when injected into mice, and both effects were traced to LDV contamination (Koi et al., 1981). Interferon induction occurred after injection of a mouse monoclonal antibody into mice, and the cause was shown to be LDV contamination (Nicklas et al., 1988).

## *Haemobartonella muris*

### *Significance*

*Haemobartonella muris* has little significance for most experimental uses of rats. It has high significance for studies involving rat-to-rat passage of materials (e.g., transplantable tumors or inocula for experimental blood parasite infections).

### *Perspective*

Since Mayer (1921) discovered this agent as a complicating factor in studies of experimental *Trypanosoma brucei* infection in rats, it has occasionally been rediscovered by unwary experimentalists. In 1960 Sacks and co-workers (Sacks and Egdahl, 1960; Sacks et al., 1960) rediscovered it as a "filterable hemolytic anemia agent," and it was correctly identified later by Moore et al. (1965). Thus, this usually subclinical infection of rats and contaminant of biologic materials from rats can be a subtle complication of research.

### *Agent*

*Haemobartonella muris* is a bacterium, order Rickettsiales, family Anaplasmataceae. It is Gram negative; cocci (100-500 nm in diameter), diplococci, or slender rods (100 nm in diameter × 300-700 nm in length); obligately parasitic and occurs in indentations on the erythrocyte surface or in vacuoles within erythrocytes and, rarely, free in plasma. It is not cultivable outside the host. Growth in the host is inhibited by arsenicals and tetracyclines (Ristic and Kreier, 1984).

Viability is rapidly lost after 0.5 hour at 37°C, 6-8 hours at 25°C, and 24-48 hours at 4°C. It can be preserved indefinitely in 10% dimethyl sulfoxide stored in liquid nitrogen (Ristic and Kreier, 1984).

### *Hosts*

Rats. Possibly mice and hamsters (Ristic and Kreier, 1984).

### *Epizootiology*

Natural transmission is by the spined rat louse *Polyplax spinulosa* (Crystal, 1958, 1959a,b). Transplacental and oral transmission have been suggested (Weinman, 1944), but definitive proof of both possibilities is lacking (Crystal, 1958, 1959a,b; Owen, 1982).

Transmission is readily accomplished by injecting biologic materials (e.g., blood, transplantable tumors, tissue homogenate) contaminated with the agent via parenteral routes. Thus, inadvertent transmission during experimental procedures constitutes an important source of infection.

### *Clinical*

Infection can persist throughout life without clinical signs, unless it is activated by natural or experimental immunosuppression.

During active disease, signs can include anemia, pallor, dyspnea, weight loss, and hemoglobinuria. A hemogram can reveal anemia, reticulocytosis, increased IgG and IgM, reduced plasma proteins, increased clotting time, and terminal hyperphosphatemia (Kessler, 1943; Kessler and Zwemer, 1944; Baker et al., 1971; Finch and Jonas, 1973; Cox and Calaf-Iturri, 1976; Lindsey et al., 1978b).

### *Pathology*

In natural infections there are no lesions, and parasitemia cannot usually be detected by examination of stained blood smears. Active disease is characterized by anemia, hemoglobinuria, splenomegaly, and parasitemia (Baker et al., 1971).

*Diagnosis*

Activation of infection by splenectomy followed by demonstration of parasitemia can be used to diagnose the infection in individual animals. Alternatively, rats known to be free of *Haemobartonella muris* and other pathogens can be splenectomized and then injected parenterally with transplantable tumor homogenates, pooled blood from groups of rats, or other test materials, followed by attempts to demonstrate parasitemia (Baker et al., 1971; Cassell et al., 1979).

Animals that are several months of age are more susceptible than young rats to severe disease following splenectomy. After splenectomy or injection of the test material into previously splenectomized rats, parasitemia usually appears in 2-6 days, the erythrocyte count may drop to less than one million/$mm^3$, and death may ensue because of a hemolytic crisis (Baker et al., 1971; Cassell et al., 1979).

In blood smears stained by the Giemsa or Romanowsky methods, organisms appear as coccoid, dumbbell, or long rod forms on erythrocytes. Transmission electron microscopy can be used for confirmation (Tanaka et al., 1965). Organisms must be differentiated from the basophilic stippling that is common in rodent erythrocytes (Griesemer, 1958; Baker et al., 1971; Cassell et al., 1979).

*Control*

Cesarean derivation and barrier maintenance apparently have been very successful in eliminating the infection from breeding colonies. *Polyplax splinulosa* must be controlled.

Rat tumors, cells, and other biologic materials to be passaged in rats should be screened to ensure the absence of the agent (Baker et al., 1971). Organic arsenicals and tetracyclines are reported to eliminate the organism from hosts with either latent or active infection (Ristic and Kreier, 1984).

*Interference with Research*

Because of their usual clinically silent character, *H. muris* infections may be extremely subtle causes of variability in certain biologic responses. Infection has been shown to do the following:

a. Reduce the half-life of erythrocytes (Rudnick and Hollingsworth, 1959).

b. Modulate the course of experimental malaria (Hsu and Geiman, 1952) and trypanosomiasis (Marmorston-Gottesman and Perla, 1930).

c. Enhance phagocytic activity, e.g., clearance of intravenously injected carbon (Elko and Cantrell, 1968).

d. Increase the rejection rate of transplantable tumors (Sacks et al., 1960).

e. Cause fulminant hemolytic anemia in recipient rats given *H. muris*-contaminated transplantable tumors (Sacks and Egdahl, 1960; Sacks et al., 1960).

Subclinical *H. muris* infections are activated by the ablation of splenic phagocytes by methods including splenectomy (McCluskie and Niven, 1955; Scheff et al., 1956), injection of anti-rat spleen serum (Pomerat et al., 1947; Thomas et al., 1949), intravenous injection of ethyl palmitate (Stuart, 1960; Finch and Jonas, 1973), injection of Polonium-210 (Scott and Stannard, 1954), and whole body x-irradiation (Rekers, 1951; Scott and Stannard, 1954; Berger and Linkenheimer, 1962). Also, latent infections can be activated by experimental infections of *Plasmodium* sp. (Hsu and Geiman, 1952).

### *Eperythrozoon coccoides*

#### *Significance*

*Eperythrozoon coccoides* has little significance for most experimental uses of mice. This agent is highly significant for studies involving mouse-to-mouse passage of materials such as transplantable tumors or inocula for experimental blood parasite infections.

#### *Perspective*

This is an agent that is subject to occasional rediscovery by investigators who passage biologic materials in mice without monitoring for contaminating pathogens. A classic example is the work of Stansly and co-workers (Stansly et al., 1962; Ansari et al., 1963), who were attempting to demonstrate an oncogenic virus by passaging in mice splenic filtrates from leukemic mice. They described a filterable agent and named it the spleen weight increase factor or SWIF, only to learn later that they had rediscovered *Eperythrozoon coccoides* (Stansly and Neilson, 1965).

Demonstration that *E. coccoides* infection enhances the disease caused by mouse hepatitis virus infection in mice and separation of these two indigenous agents by Gledhill and associates (Gledhill and Andrewes, 1951; Niven et al., 1952; Gledhill and Dick, 1955; Gledhill et al., 1955; Gledhill, 1961) are important historical landmarks in the field of laboratory animal disease.

### *Agent*

*Eperythrozoon coccoides* is a bacterium, order Rickettsiales, family Anaplasmataceae. It is a Gram-negative, coccoid organism, measuring 350-500 nm in diameter. It is obligately parasitic, and occurs loosely attached to erythrocytes and free in blood plasma. It grows in embryonated hen's eggs. Growth in the host is inhibited by neoarsphenamine and tetracyclines (Kreier and Ristic, 1968; Ristic and Kreier, 1984).

*E. coccoides* readily passes coarse bacterial filters. It has an unusually low specific gravity, and is not completely sedimented by centrifugation of infected plasma at 100,000 × *g* for 1 hour. It is inactivated rapidly by disinfectants and drying. Freezing (–70°C) preserves its infectivity, while 37°C for 3 hours destroys its infectivity (Stansly and Neilson, 1966; Baker et al., 1971).

### *Hosts*

Mice. Possibly rats, hamsters, and rabbits (Ristic and Kreier, 1984).

### *Epizootiology*

*Polyplax serrata*, the mouse louse, is considered the main vector; it transmits the infection mechanically (Berkenkamp and Wescott, 1988). Transmission by oral, intranasal, and transplacental routes has been suspected but not proved. The infection persists throughout life (Baker et al., 1971).

Reliable data on prevalence of *E. coccoides* in contemporary mouse stocks are lacking. The agent is most likely to be encountered in conventionally reared stocks of mice that have not been cesarean derived and maintained by barrier methods (Baker et al., 1971).

Inadvertent transmission in biologic materials (such as transplantable tumors, inocula for passage of experimental parasitic infections, blood plasma, and cell-free filtrates) rather than natural transmission poses the greatest threat in modern research (Baker et al., 1971; Lindsey et al., 1978b; Iralu and Ganong, 1983).

### *Clinical*

Natural and experimental infections of *E. coccoides* usually are inapparent.

### *Pathology*

The spleen weight increases to three-four times normal by post infection day seven, reduces to one and one-half to two times normal by day 21, and persists at this latter size at least until day 42. Microscopically, there are increased erythroid elements in the enlarged spleen and increased fixed macrophages in the spleen and liver (Thurston, 1955; Baker et al., 1971; Cox and Calaf-Iturri, 1976; Lindsey et al., 1978b).

### *Diagnosis*

Detection of subclinical *E. coccoides* infection is usually by splenectomy to produce active infection, followed by demonstration of the agent in peripheral blood. Following splenectomy, persistently infected mice can develop massive parasitemia within 2-4 days, but it can be surprisingly short-lived (a few to 24 hours). Thus, detection of the organism may require frequent examination of blood (e.g., every 6 hours). The preferred approach is to splenectomize several pathogen-free mice. These mice are then inoculated intraperitoneally or intravenously with test material that is to be monitored for the infection (e.g., pooled blood or spleen from mice of a colony suspected of having latent infection, transplantable tumors, antisera, cell lines). Peripheral blood is examined for the organism every 6 hours for four days. The organism can be demonstrated in peripheral blood by light microscopic examination of stained blood smears, electron microscopy, acridine orange, and indirect fluorescent antibody (IFA) test. In Giemsa- or Romanowsky-stained blood smears, organisms appear as distinctive ring forms on erythrocytes and free in plasma. IFA is particularly useful for detecting small numbers of organisms (Berkenkamp and Wescott, 1988). The organism must be differentiated from the basophilic stippling that is common in rodents (Tanaka et al., 1965; Baker et al., 1971).

### *Control*

Cesarean derivation followed by barrier maintenance (including ectoparasite control) are thought to be effective, but definitive data are lacking. Treatment with neoarsphenamine or tetracycline can be useful in selected situations. The most important approach is to prescreen tumors and other biologic materials to be passaged in mice to ensure the absence of the agent (Baker et al., 1971).

### *Interference with Research*

*E. coccoides* infection has been shown to cause the following:

a. Suppress interferon production in mice during the first 3 weeks after infection (Glasgow et al., 1971, 1974).

b. Exacerbate concurrent infections of mouse hepatitis virus (Niven et al., 1952; Nelson, 1953; Gledhill and Dick, 1955; Gledhill et al., 1955; Gledhill and Niven, 1957), lymphocytic choriomeningitis virus (Seamer et al., 1961), or lactate dehydrogenase-elevating virus (Arison et al., 1963; Riley, 1964; Riley et al., 1964).

c. Reduce pathogenicity of concurrent infection by *Plasmodium* sp. (Peters, 1965; Ott and Stauber, 1967).

d. Increase phagocytic activity in mice (Gledhill et al., 1965).

e. Increase susceptibility of mice to bacterial endotoxins (Gledhill and Niven, 1957).

The agent can be a common contaminant of inocula used to perpetuate experimental blood parasite infections in mice (Peters, 1965; Ott and Stauber, 1967; Iralu and Ganong, 1983).

Subclinical infection can be activated by whole body x-irradiation (Berger and Linkenheimer, 1962) or splenectomy (Marmorston, 1935).

## Murine Leukemia Viruses

### *Significance*

This large group of genetically related viruses, referred to collectively as the murine leukemia viruses (MuLVs), has provided a wide range of model systems for studies of the molecular biology, virology, genetics, pathology, immunopathology, and experimental chemotherapy of leukemias.

### *Perspective*

The discovery of the MuLVs was linked historically to the development of inbred strains of mice, many of which were selected for their susceptibility or resistance to MuLV (Heston, 1974, 1975). Furth et al. (1933) developed the mouse strain AKR, which has a high incidence of leukemia. Furth (1946) later showed that thymectomy prevented the leukemia in these mice. In 1951, Gross (1951a,b) demonstrated that when cell-free filtrates of leukemic tissues from a strain of mouse now known as AKR were injected into infant C3H/Bi mice, leukemia was successfully transmitted. This led to the discovery of numerous strains of MuLVs in transplantable murine tumors, including those described by Graffi (1957), Friend (1957), Schoolman et al. (1957), Moloney (1960), Rauscher (1962), and Tennant (1962). Gross (1959) and Lieberman and Kaplan (1959) demonstrated that radiation-induced lymphoid tumors of mice also contained MuLVs. Subsequently, MuLVs were studied extensively by using both in vivo and in vitro systems, which contributed many of the modern concepts of viral oncology, such as the oncogene theory (Huebner and Todaro, 1969) and the role of reverse transcriptase (Baltimore, 1970). In no instance, however, have the basic mechanisms of leukemogenesis been fully explained (Furmanski and Rich, 1982).

### *Agents*

The MuLVs are RNA viruses, family Retroviridae, subfamily Oncovirinae, genus type C oncovirus group, subgenus mammalian type C oncovirus, species murine leukemia and sarcoma viruses. Related viruses infecting mammalian hosts include baboon type C oncovirus; bovine leukosis virus; feline sarcoma and leukemia viruses; gibbon ape leukemia virus; guinea pig type C oncovirus; porcine type C oncovirus; rat type C oncovirus; woolly monkey sarcoma virus; and, more recently, the human T-cell lymphotropic virus (HTLV), currently referred to as the human immunodeficiency virus (HIV) (Lieber and Todaro, 1975; Poiesz et al., 1981; Matthews, 1982).

Like other members of the Retroviridae, MuLVs have a spherical, enveloped virion measuring 80-100 nm in diameter with glycoprotein surface projections of approximately 8 nm in diameter. The genome is a dimer of linear, positive-sense, single-stranded RNA. Genetic information for production of infectious progeny consists of three genes: *gag,* which codes for nonglycosylated virion proteins; *pol,* which codes for reverse transcriptase; and *env,* which codes for envelope glycoproteins. The *env* glycoproteins are responsible for type specificity, while the major internal *gag* protein defines group (subgenus) specificity (Matthews, 1982).

Numerous strains of MuLV have been recognized. Strains usually are designated by their discoverer's name(s) or by symbols assigned by the original investigators. Different strains of MuLVs have 80% genetic homology and are very prone to undergo mutation or recombination. They are generally classified on the basis of their host range (infectivity) for tissue culture cells. The host range is probably determined by the *env* gene product, gp70 protein. The ecotropic (or mouse tropic) MuLVs replicate only in mouse cells. However, the replication of MuLVs in cells of different mouse strains is restricted by the *Fv-1* locus. The xenotropic strains grow only on nonmurine cells, e.g., mink, rabbit, human, and duck. Amphotropic strains replicate in both mouse and nonmurine cells. Polytropic [or dualtropic or mink cell focus (MCF)] strains grow on mouse and nonmurine cells but differ from amphotropic strains by serologic neutralization. The amphotropic strains occur mainly in wild mice. The dualtropic strains are laboratory-derived recombinant viruses (Steeves, 1974; Hartley et al., 1977; Famulari, 1983; Risser et al., 1983; Goff, 1984).

### *Hosts*

Laboratory and wild *Mus musculus* are considered the natural hosts. Experimentally, leukemias have been induced by the inoculation of MuLV into neonatal mice, rats, and hamsters (Steeves, 1974).

*Epizootiology*

There are two distinct phases in the life cycle of the type C oncoviruses. In one phase, the virus genome exists as DNA integrated in the host cell genome (the so-called provirus), where it is replicated and transmitted to all daughter cells along with the host cell genome. In the second phase, complementary RNA sequences are synthesized from the DNA provirus and packaged in extracellular virions for transmission to other host cells. In the target cells there is reverse transcription of the RNA genome into DNA and integration of the DNA into the host cell genome (Bishop and Varmus, 1975; Lilly and Mayer, 1980).

The endogenous type C oncoviruses are integrated in the DNA of the host's sex cells and are transmitted vertically as Mendelian traits. All laboratory and wild *M. musculus* are thought to harbor endogenous type C oncoviruses. Horizontal transmission is inefficient but can occur by transfer of virus in saliva, sputum, urine, feces, or milk or by intrauterine infection. The exogenous type C oncoviruses, of which the Friend, Moloney, and Rauscher strains are prototypes, are laboratory variants that have been derived from transplantable tumors and are known to become integrated only in the DNA of somatic cell lines (Lieber and Todaro, 1975; Lilly and Mayer, 1980).

*Clinical*

Despite the fact that all mice have endogenous MuLVs, leukemias and related malignancies occur naturally in only 1-2% of most strains (Furmanski and Rich, 1982). In contrast, AKR mice have a high incidence of spontaneous thymic lymphoma, reaching 90% by 9 months of age. In affected mice, the most common signs are dyspnea (due to thymic lymphoma), peripheral lymphadenopathy, or abdominal enlargement (Squire et al., 1978).

*Pathology*

The mechanisms of MuLV expression (replication) and leukemogenesis are extremely complex. The MuLVs are a collection of viruses that are related in genetic sequence but that have diverse patterns of host range and tissue tropism. All mouse strains have MuLV genomes (proviruses) for ecotropic and xenotropic viruses at different loci in their genomes. Mouse strains with a low incidence of leukemia (BALB/c, A/J, C3H/He, and CBA/J) have single ecotropic proviruses at a few nonallelic chromosomal loci, while mouse strains with a high incidence of leukemia (AKR, C58, C3H/Fa) have multiple ecotropic proviruses at nonallelic chromosomal loci. The chromosome number and precise location of these loci is strain dependent. Mouse strains with a high incidence of leukemia spontaneously express high titers of ecotropic MuLV in all organs early in life, and these persist throughout life. In contrast, mouse strains with a low incidence of leukemia express only low titers of virus. Expression of the viral genomes in mice with a low incidence of leukemia, however, can be induced by chemical carcinogens, radiation, and other stimuli. The complex mechanisms by which endogenous MuLVs induce leukemia, in mouse strains with either a low or high incidence of leukemia, appear to involve the expression and interaction of multiple MuLV genomes of both ecotropic and xenotropic viruses through such processes as recombination, DNA transfection, and transcomplementation (Furmanski and Rich, 1982; Morse and Hartley, 1982; Famulari, 1983; Risser et al., 1983; Goff, 1984). Host susceptibility is influenced by a number of mouse genes including those of the *Fv-1, Fv-2, In, nu,* and *hr* loci and the *Ir* locus of the major histocompatibility complex (Lilly and Pincus, 1973; Heiniger et al., 1974; Steeves and Lilly, 1977; Lilly and Mayer, 1980; McCubrey and Risser, 1982; Meruelo and Bach, 1983).

The mouse leukemias are, with few exceptions, actually lymphomas because they are predominantly solid tumors of lymphocytes or other hematopoietic cells. The spontaneous tumors in mice are mainly of two types. The majority of those occurring before 1 year of age are thymic lymphomas, while the predominant type seen in older mice is histiocytic (reticulum cell) lymphomas (Dunn, 1954; Squire et al., 1978; Della Porta et al., 1979).

The classification scheme and morphologic descriptions of the spontaneous and experimentally induced hemopoietic neoplasms reported by Dunn (1954), with minor modification, serve as the standard for diagnosis. This family of neoplasms includes thymic lymphomas, nonthymic lymphomas, histiocytic (reticulum cell) lymphomas, lymphatic leukemias, granulocytic leukemias, erythroleukemia, plasma cell tumors, and mast cell tumors (Dunn, 1954; Squire et al., 1978; Della Porta et al., 1979).

The incidence of spontaneous hemopoietic neoplasms occurring in mice has been the subject of numerous investigations. For comparative data and references on many strains of mice, the reader is referred to the tabulated information given by Squire et al. (1978) and Furmanski and Rich (1982).

### *Diagnosis*

The diagnosis of spontaneously occurring hemopoietic neoplasms in the mouse is usually made on the basis of morphologic features in histologic sections (Dunn, 1954; Squire et al., 1978; Della Porta et al., 1979). Tumor cell types also can be determined by analysis of cell surface antigens (Old and Stockert, 1977). The isolation and characterization of MuLVs require specialized techniques usually available only in research laboratories dedicated to viral oncology. However, MuLV type and group specificity can be determined by immunofluorescence of fixed cells by use of an appropriate panel of type- or group-specific antisera (Matthews, 1982).

### *Control*

All mice probably have vertically transmitted endogenous MuLV proviruses as an integral part of their genomes; this is true even for mice that are otherwise considered germfree (Kajima and Pollard, 1965). Horizontal transmission can occur but is considered inefficient (Furmanski and Rich, 1982). Therefore, control measures are not usually considered useful unless mice are being infected experimentally with high doses of MuLV, in which case the infected mice should be isolated from uninfected control mice.

### *Interference with Research*

Although all mice have endogenous MuLVs, their presence probably has little significance for most research purposes in which mice are used. MuLV expression and the associated occurrence of neoplasms, however, can present competing endpoints in some studies, e.g., studies of the aging processes in various organs. Thus, an awareness of spontaneous tumors in different strains of mice or the induction of tumors by specific test chemicals can be useful in the design of some experiments. Also, active MuLV infection can cause suppression of humoral and cellular immunity without clinically obvious disease (Specter et al., 1978).

# 10

# Central Nervous System

## Overview

There are only two infectious agents that are considered primary pathogens of the central nervous system. Theiler's murine encephalomyelitis virus only rarely causes clinical disease in mice. *Encephalitozoon cuniculi*, a common pathogen in rabbits, has been reported in mice and rats only a few times and has not been observed to cause clinical disease in the latter species. Both agents have been encountered as contaminants of rodent cell cultures.

## Theiler's Virus

### *Significance*

Low. Theiler's virus probably is rare as a natural infection of contemporary mice and rats.

### *Perspective*

Theiler's murine encephalomyelitis virus (TMEV) infection in mice resembles poliomyelitis virus infection in humans. However, there are few reported instances of natural disease caused by TMEV in mice (Theiler, 1934, 1937, 1941; Theiler and Gard, 1940a; Thompson et al., 1951) and only one in rats (McConnell et al., 1964). The major importance of TMEV is that experimental infections in mice provide valuable models of poliomyelitis-like infection (Theiler, 1941; Gard, 1943) and virus-induced demyelinating disease (Dal Canto and Lipton, 1975; Lipton, 1975; Lipton and Dal Canto, 1979a,b).

### *Agent*

TMEV is a RNA virus, family Picornaviridae, genus *Enterovirus*. Other members of this genus include polioviruses, coxsackieviruses, and enteroviruses. Strains of TMEV are divided into two groups based on pathogenicity for mice and in vitro growth characteristics. The small-plaque strains are Theiler's original (TO) and similar strains (DA, WW, $TO_4$, Yale, and BeAn 8386). These produce small plaques in L929 cells, are relatively avirulent, cause chronic demyelinating disease in mice, do not hemagglutinate human erythrocytes, and are not readily cultivated in embryonating eggs. The large-plaque strains are FA, GDVII, and others that produce large plaques in L929 cells, are highly virulent for mice, may or may not hemagglutinate human erythrocytes, and grow readily in eggs (Lipton, 1980). The MHG strain was isolated from rats (Hemelt et al., 1974). All strains are antigenically related in the cross-neutralization, hemagglutination inhibition, and complement fixation tests (Hemelt et al., 1974).

The virus particles are naked icosahedral nucleocapsids, measuring 20-30 nm in diameter, and have a single-stranded RNA genome. The virions contain four major structural polypeptides: VP1, VP2, and VP3, each with a molecular weight of 27,000-58,000, and VP4, with a molecular weight of 6,000. In the large-plaque strains, VP1 is slightly heavier than in the less virulent small-plaque strains (Stroop and Baringer, 1981; Downs, 1982, Matthews, 1982).

TMEV can be propagated in several continuous cell lines, but BHK-21 cells are most commonly used (Lipton, 1978a). TMEV is rapidly inactivated by heating at 50-55°C for 30 minutes and by treatment with 50% acetone or alcohol, but not by treatment with ether (Theiler and Gard, 1940a).

### *Hosts*

Laboratory mice (Downs, 1982) and rats (McConnell et al., 1964).

### *Epizootiology*

Natural TMEV infection has been reported most frequently in laboratory mice (Downs, 1982) and on one occasion in laboratory rats (McConnell et al., 1964), but not in wild *Mus musculus* (Downs, 1982). The prevalence of TMEV infection in mice has been reported to be 5% of commercial barrier breeding colonies (Lindsey et al., 1986a) and 62% of other mouse populations (Parker, 1980) in the United States. The prevalence of TMEV infection in laboratory rats is unknown; however, one survey found 44% of laboratory rats in the United States to be serologically positive (Parker, 1980). Unfortunately, these data probably overestimated the true prevalence of TMEV as they were obtained by use of the hemagglutination inhibition (HAI) test, known to give false positive results for TMEV (Kraft and Meyer, 1986; Van Der Logt, 1986).

In naturally infected mice the virus occurs at a low titer in the intestinal mucosa, intestinal contents, feces, and less frequently, in the mesenteric lymph nodes. Transmission is by the fecal-oral route. In infected colonies housed in ordinary shoe-box cages, the infection is usually acquired between 3 and 6 weeks of age and most animals eventually become infected. Virus has been demomstrated in the feces of an individual mouse for only 53 days and persistent infection of the intestinal tract is considered unlikely (Olitsky, 1940; Theiler and Gard, 1940b; Lipton and Rozhon, 1986).

### *Clinical*

Natural infections in mice are usually inapparent and, presumably, caused by less virulent wild-type strains of TMEV resembling TO. Clinical disease is a rare occurrence, appearing at a rate of only 1 in 4,000-10,000 infected animals. Affected mice have flaccid paralysis of one or both rear legs but otherwise appear normal. There is little or no mortality (Theiler, 1934, 1937; Olitsky, 1940; Theiler and Gard, 1940a).

One epizootic in mice has been reported to be due to a highly virulent strain of TMEV resembling GDVII (Thompson et al., 1951). Signs included circling, rolling, hyperexcitability, convulsions, tremors, weakness, or flaccid paralysis of hind legs in some mice, and high mortality (62% of 240 mice). The outbreak occurred in a mouse room where GDVII was being used experimentally and sanitation was admittedly poor.

The MHG strain of TMEV was originally isolated from three adult rats with natural disease consisting of circling, incoordination, tremors, and torticollis (McConnell et al., 1964).

### *Pathology*

Natural disease in mice results from the rare occurrence of viremia, i.e., dissemination of virus from the intestine to the spinal cord and brain. This occurs most frequently around 6-10 weeks of age. The predominant lesion is poliomyelitis, with necrosis and neuronophagia of ventral horn cells and nonsuppurative inflammation composed primarily of lymphocytes. Little if any secondary demyelination is seen in the natural disease. TMEV can be isolated from the lesions for at least 1 year (Theiler, 1934, 1937; Theiler and Gard, 1940a; Lipton and Dal Canto, 1979a).

A variety of neurologic disease models has been developed by using different strains of TMEV, routes of virus inoculation, and strains of mice. These models resemble the natural disease very little because large doses of virus are usually inoculated intracerebrally. In general, the large-plaque strains (FA or GDVII) produce acute encephalitis and death in weanling mice only 4-5 days after inoculation (Theiler and Gard, 1940a). In contrast, the intracerebral inoculation of the small-plaque strains (TO, DA, WW, and others) causes an acute poliomyelitis after an incubation period of a few weeks, followed by persistent viral infection with varying degrees of chronic demyelination and remyelination after a few months, with the latter processes resembling multiple sclerosis in man (Dal Canto and Lipton, 1975, 1979, 1980, 1982; Lipton, 1975; Penney and Wolinsky, 1979; Brahic et al., 1981; Stroop et al., 1981; Rodriguez et al., 1983; Dal Canto and Barbano, 1984; Lipton et al., 1984). SJL/J, SWR, and DBA/2 mice are highly susceptible to chronic demyelination, whereas A, C57BL/6, C57BL/10 and DBA/1 mice are resistant (Lipton and Dal Canto, 1976b, 1979b; Lipton and Rozhon, 1986). Susceptibility to demyelination can be prevented by immunosuppressive regimens of cyclophosphamide or antilymphocyte serum (Lipton and Dal Canto, 1976a), is influenced by the H-2D region and is associated with TMEV-specific delayed-type hypersensitivity (Clatch et al., 1985), suggesting that it is immune mediated.

*Diagnosis*

The HAI test with GDVII antigen and human type O erythrocytes has been the standard procedure for serologic screening of mouse stocks for many years (Lahelle and Horsfall, 1949; Fastier, 1950, 1951). It is essential that the HAI test be performed at 4°C to avoid false-positive results. Even so, the HAI probably still gives a significant proportion of false positives, and the enzyme-linked immunosorbent assay is now considered the test of choice (Kraft and Meyer, 1986; Van Der Loft, 1986). The complement fixation and serum neutralization tests may also be useful for some purposes, such as comparisons of the antigenic relatedness of TMEV strains (Downs, 1982). The mouse antibody production (MAP) test can be used for screening biologic materials for the presence of virus (Rowe et al., 1959, 1962).

Definitive diagnosis is usually made by isolation of virus from spinal cords or brains of mice with clinical disease, but it is also possible to isolate virus from the intestinal contents of mice with asymptomatic infection (Downs, 1982). The virus can be propagated in several continuous cell lines (Sturman and Tamm, 1966; Hemelt et al., 1974; Lipton, 1978a,b), but BHK-21 cells are most commonly used (Lipton and Dal Canto, 1979b).

*Control*

The most practical method of control is to obtain mice from breeding populations that have been shown to be free of the infection by serologic testing, followed by barrier maintenance and regular testing to reconfirm their TMEV-free status.

TMEV infection has been eliminated from valuable mouse stocks by foster nursing infant mice on TMEV-free mice or rats (von Magnus and von Magnus, 1948; Dean, 1951). Also, the isolation and quarantine of individual breeding pairs with subsequent selection of TMEV negative progeny have been successful eliminating the infection (Lipman et al., 1987). Cesarean derivation is effective but usually is not justified.

### *Interference with Research*

There are a few examples in the literature in which indigenous TMEV infections in mice have interfered with studies of unrelated viruses in mice (Theiler and Gard, 1940a; Melnick and Riordan, 1947; Thompson et al., 1951).

## ***Encephalitozoon cuniculi***

### *Significance*

*Encephalitozoon cuniculi* has low significance for most studies. It is highly significant for studies involving passage of transplantable tumors and other materials in mice and rats.

### *Perspective*

*1923:* Levaditi et al. (1923a,b, 1924) discovered this organism in the brains of rabbits with encephalitis and named it *Encephalitozoon cuniculi*. In subsequent years it was found to be ubiquitous in laboratory rabbits and only occasionally present in laboratory rodents and other species (Shadduck and Pakes, 1971).

*1953-1969:* During this period *E. cuniculi* was incriminated as a cause of interference with research in which mice and rats were used. A syndrome characterized by hepatosplenomegaly and attributed to an ascites hepatitis agent was observed following the intraperitoneal passage of tissues in mice (Lackey et al., 1953; Morris et al., 1956; Jordan and Mirick, 1965a,b). It was later shown to be due to *E. cuniculi* (Nelson, 1962, 1967; Weiser, 1965; Arison et al., 1966). *E. cuniculi* was found to contaminate transplantable tumors resulting in altered experimental results in mice (Arison et al., 1966) and rats (Petri, 1965, 1966, 1967, 1968, 1969). Also, during this period the genus name was temporarily changed to *Nosema* (Shadduck and Pakes, 1971).

*1969:* Shadduck (1969) reported the first successful in vitro cultivation of *E. cuniculi;* he used rabbit choroid plexus cells.

*1972:* Hunt et al. (1972) demonstrated transplacental transmission of the organism in rabbits.

*1973-1988:* A large number of serologic tests were developed for diagnosis of *E. cuniculi* infection (see below).

### *Agent*

*Encephalitozoon cuniculi* is a protozoan, order Microsporidia. *Nosema cuniculi,* and *Nosema muris* are synonyms for *E. cuniculi.* Mature spores are oval, 1.5 × 2.5 μm, occur intracellularly, and are not surrounded by a cyst wall. Spores are Gram positive, argyrophilic, variably acid fast, and have a periodic acid-Schiff-positive granule at one pole. Spores stain dark magenta or purple with Goodpasture's carbol fuchsin and stain poorly with hematoxylin and eosin (Perrin, 1943b; Weiser, 1965; Shadduck and Pakes, 1971; Wilson, 1979).

It has been grown successfully in tissue cultures of several cell lines (Shadduck, 1969; Bismanis, 1970; Cox and Pye, 1975; Waller, 1975; Shadduck and Geroulo, 1979).

### *Hosts*

Rabbits, mice, rats, hamsters, guinea pigs, dogs, nonhuman primates, humans, and many other mammals (Perrin, 1943a; Lainson et al., 1964; Petri, 1969; Shadduck and Pakes, 1971; Margileth et al., 1973; Shadduck et al., 1978; Zeman and Baskin, 1985).

### *Epizootiology*

*E. cuniculi* is considered ubiquitous in rabbits. Surveys of prevalence suggest that most rabbit colonies are infected (Koller, 1969; Flatt and Jackson, 1970; Cox and Pye; 1975; Waller, 1977; Lyngset, 1980) unless they have been specifically rederived to exclude this infection (Cox et al., 1977; Bywater and Kellett, 1978). Prevalence within infected colonies has ranged from 15 to 76% (Shadduck and Pakes, 1971). Rabbits undoubtedly provide the major source of infection for mice and rats in research facilities.

Prevalence of the organism in contemporary mouse and rat stocks is not known but is thought to be very low in comparison to that in rabbits. In a recent serologic survey in the United Kingdom, Gannon (1980a) found that 1 of 17 mouse colonies and 2 of 12 rat colonies were infected.

Transmission in most animals is primarily horizontal by the orofecal route (Wilson, 1979). Organisms are shed in the urine and ingested by another host. Transmission in rabbits is both vertical (Hunt et al., 1972) and horizontal (Shadduck and Pakes, 1971; Cox et al., 1979). In mice, horizontal transmission is known to occur between cagemates, but transplacental transmission has not been demonstrated (Liu et al., 1988). Studies of transmission in rats have not been done.

### *Clinical*

Natural infections usually are inapparent.

### *Pathology*

In rats and rabbits the classic lesion of *E. cuniculi* infection in the brain is a meningoencephalitis with multifocal granulomatous inflammation. Activated macrophages form so-called glial nodules in response to the agent. These nodules can have necrotic centers or appear as solid sheets of cells. With special stains, the organisms can be seen in compact masses within cyst-like spaces in individual cells or scattered in the glial nodules. Varying numbers of lymphocytes and plasma cells are seen in the meninges and around vessels. The brain lesions in mice are similar, except for the lack of the granulomatous foci (Perrin, 1943b; Yost, 1958; Innes et al., 1962; Attwood and Sutton, 1965; Shadduck and Pakes, 1971; Shadduck et al., 1979; Majeed and Zubaidy, 1982).

The organism also occurs intracellularly in the renal tubular epithelium with or without the presence of an inflammatory response, and in the renal tubular lumens. In chronic infections focal destruction of tubules and replacement by fibrous connective tissue results in small pits on the cortical surface (Yost, 1958; Flatt and Jackson, 1970). Lesions in organs other than the kidney and brain are less consistent (Shadduck and Pakes, 1971).

Strain differences in susceptibility to experimental infection have been documented. Strains BALB/c, A/J, and SJL are resistant to experimental infection; strains C57BL/10, DBA/2, and AKR show intermediate susceptibility; and strains C57BL/6, DBA/1, and 129/J are very susceptible (Niederkorn et al., 1981). MRL/MpJ– *lpr*/*lpr* mice are no more susceptible than MRL/MpJ– +/+ mice (Liu and Shadduck, 1988).

Experimental infection of euthymic mice results in chronic nonlethal infection, whereas infection of athymic (*nu*/*nu*) mice leads to death in a few weeks, suggesting that resistance is T-cell dependent (Gannon, 1980b; Niederkorn et al., 1981; Schmidt and Shadduck, 1983). Infection of immunocompetent mice results in transient augmentation of natural killer cell activity in spleen (Niederkorn et al., 1983) and lung (Niederkorn, 1985).

The intraperitoneal inoculation of *E. cuniculi,* as in the passage of contaminated transplantable tumors, results in ascites in mice (Nelson, 1962, 1967; Arison et al., 1966; Petri, 1969).

Disseminated disease caused by *E. cuniculi* has been reported in a severely immunocompromised human infant (Margileth et al., 1973).

### Diagnosis

Several serologic tests have been developed for diagnosis of the infection in rabbits, including an indirect immunofluorescent antibody (IFA) test (Chalupsky et al., 1973; Jackson et al., 1973; Cox and Pye, 1975; Cox and Gallichio, 1978), India ink immunoreaction (Waller, 1977; Kellett and Bywater, 1978), complement fixation (Wosu et al., 1977), immunoperoxidase (Gannon, 1978), indirect microagglutination (Shadduck and Geroulo, 1979), enzyme immunoassay (Cox et al., 1981), and enzyme-linked immunosorbent assay (Beckwith et al., 1988). However, only the IFA and immunoperoxidase tests have been used in surveying mouse and rat colonies (Gannon, 1980a). Serologic testing is superior to other methods for the screening of colonies.

Other methods used for diagnosis include detection of parasites in urine (Goodman and Garner, 1972; Pye and Cox, 1977), demonstration of typical lesions and organisms in tissue sections (Petri and Schiodt, 1966; Koller, 1969; Flatt and Jackson, 1970), and an intradermal skin test (Pakes et al., 1972). In rabbits, results of the intradermal test correlate well with the presence of brain lesions caused by the organism (Pakes et al., 1984b).

### Control

Although transplacental transmission occurs, serologic testing of adult animals with selection of *E. cuniculi*-free breeding stocks can be used successfully for eradicating the infection in rabbits (Cox et al., 1977; Bywater and Kellett, 1978), and possibly could be useful for doing so in mice and rats.

Cesarean derivation, barrier maintenance, and improved sanitation of mouse and rat stocks appear to have been effective in reducing the prevalence of *E. cuniculi* in these species in recent decades. Mice and rats should not be housed near rabbits unless the rabbits are known to be free of *E. cuniculi*.

### Interference with Research

The histologic changes caused by *E. cuniculi* infection in the brain and kidneys can complicate the interpretation of lesions in studies requiring histopathology (Bender, 1925; Frenkel, 1956; Waksman and Adams, 1956; Innes et al., 1962; Attwood and Sutton, 1965; Howell and Edington, 1968; Shadduck and Pakes, 1971; Gannon, 1980a; Majeed and Zubaidy, 1982; Ansbacher et al., 1988).

*E. cuniculi* can contaminate transplantable tumors and alter host responses during their passage in mice (Arison et al., 1966), rats (Petri, 1965, 1966, 1967, 1968, 1969), and hamsters (Meiser et al., 1971).

Mice experimentally infected with *E. cuniculi* have reduced humoral antibody titers to sheep erythrocytes and reduced proliferative spleen cell responses to mitogens (Niederkorn et al., 1981; Didier and Shadduck, 1988), and altered natural killer cell activity (Niederkorn et al., 1983; Niederkorn, 1985). Altered humoral immune responses due to *E. cuniculi* infection also have been reported in rabbits (Cox, 1977; Cox and Gallichio, 1978; Waller et al., 1978).

# 11

# Genitourinary System

### Overview

Only three agents cause primary infections of the genitourinary tract in mice and rats. *Leptospira interrogans* serovar *ballum*, an agent that causes renal infection, has been reported on a few occasions in laboratory mice. *Mycoplasma muris*, an anaerobic mycoplasma, has been isolated from the vaginas of mice in a single colony. Natural infections of *M. pulmonis* also occur in the genital tract of female rats. LEW rats are highly susceptible to severe genital (as well as respiratory) disease due to *M. pulmonis*, and this is characterized by purulent endometritis or pyometra, salpingitis, and perioophoritis. Similar genital lesions attributable to *M. pulmonis* are rare in rats of other strains (see discussion of this agent on pp. 42-48 for references).

### ***Leptospira interrogans*** **serovar** ***ballum***

#### *Significance*

*Leptospira interrogans* serovar *ballum* has limited significance as a naturally occuring infection.

#### *Perspective*

Although its prevalence in contemporary stocks of mice is probably low, *Leptospira interrogans* serovar *ballum* has been reported as an indigenous infection in a few colonies of laboratory mice in the United States and Europe. Several clinical cases of leptospirosis have occurred in personnel who worked in these colonies (Alexander, 1984).

### *Agent*

*Leptospira interrogans* serovar *ballum* is a bacterium, order Spirochaetales, family Leptospiraceae. Members of the genus *Leptospira* are Gram negative, motile, helicoidal rods, measuring 0.1 × 6.0-12.0 μm. They are visible by dark-field illumination and phase-contrast microscopy. Parasitic members of the genus belong to the species *L. interrogans*, which is subdivided into approximately 180 serovars by cross-agglutination and agglutinin-adsorption tests. *L. interrogans* serovar *ballum* is one of many that occurs naturally in wild rodents (Johnson and Faine, 1984; Alexander, 1985).

Transmission of leptospiras is in part dependent on contamination of and survival in the environment. Conditions of moisture, warmth (25°C), and neutral pH favor survival. Leptospiras are inactivated by dessication, pH below 6.2 or above 8.0, and common disinfectants (Turner, 1967).

The methods of cultivation, identification, and serologic testing for leptospiral organisms are highly specialized and usually are performed by specialty laboratories (Sulzer and Jones, undated; Turner, 1968, 1970). Specimens from human patients are usually submitted through county and state departments of public health to the Centers for Disease Control, Atlanta, Georgia. Specimens from animals can be submitted to state veterinary diagnostic laboratories or to the National Animal Disease Laboratory, Ames, Iowa.

### *Hosts*

Wild mice are considered the primary reservoir hosts of *L. interrogans* serovar *ballum* for laboratory mice and people (Yager et al., 1953; Stoenner and Maclean, 1958; Hathaway et al., 1983; Alexander, 1984). However, wild rodents are considered the most important natural hosts of leptospiral organisms in general and have been found to be infected with numerous serovars of *L. interrogans*. Wild rats are considered the primary reservoir hosts of *L. interrogans* serovar *icterohemorrhagiae* for humans and other species (Turner, 1967; Feigin and Anderson, 1975).

### *Epizootiology*

Natural infections of *L. interrogans* serovar *ballum* in colonies of laboratory mice have been reported on several occasions (Stoenner and

Maclean, 1958; Boak et al., 1960; Kappeler et al., 1961; Barkin et al., 1974; Alexander, 1984). In addition, *L. interrogans* serovar *ballum* infection has been found in pet mice on one occasion (Friedmann et al., 1973).

There are two phases of infection: the septicemic and leptospiruric phases. During the latter phase the organisms occur in the renal tubules and are shed in the urine, contaminating the bedding and food. The organisms infect new hosts through skin abrasions, the nose, the mouth, or the conjunctiva (Turner, 1967). Bites have been associated with transmission of *L. interrogans* serovar *ballum* to people in some cases (Stoenner and Maclean, 1958; Boak et al., 1960; Kappeler et al., 1961; Barkin et al., 1974).

### *Clinical*

Natural infections of *L. interrogans* serovar *ballum* in mice are subclinical (Stoenner et al., 1959).

Clinical manifestations in personnel who contracted *L. interrogans* serovar *ballum* from infected mice have included fever, chills, headache, myalgia, and orchitis (Stoenner and Maclean, 1958; Boak et al., 1960; Kappeler et al., 1961; Friedmann et al., 1973; Barkin et al., 1974).

### *Pathology*

There are no descriptions of lesions associated with *L. interrogans* serovar *ballum* infection in mice. During the leptospiruric phase the organism can be demonstrated in renal tubules by using histologic sections stained by silver impregnation methods such as Warthin-Starry (Friedmann et al., 1973).

### *Diagnosis*

The most common diagnostic method is serology in which the microscopic agglutination test with live antigen is used. Definitive diagnosis requires isolation and serologic identification of the organism (Alexander, 1985; Sulzer and Jones, undated). These procedures are best performed by laboratories that specialize in these methods (see above).

### *Control*

Cesarean-derivation and barrier-maintenance methods are thought to be effective. Stoenner et al. (1959) claimed to have eliminated *L. interrogans* serovar *ballum* from a colony of mice by feeding them a pelleted diet containing 1 kg of chlortetracycline hydrochloride per ton for 10 days. On the seventh day of treatment the mice were transferred to autoclaved cages with water bottles that had been autoclaved.

### *Interference with Research*

*L. interrogans* serovar *ballum* infection in mice has not been shown to alter the results of experimentation. However, it represents a serious zoonosis and is unacceptable in experimental animals.

## ***Mycoplasma muris***

### *Significance*

The prevalence of *Mycoplasma muris* in mice is unknown.

### *Perspective*

*M. muris* is an anaerobic mycoplasma of a previously unrecognized species that was recently isolated from the vaginas of mice in a single laboratory (McGarrity et al., 1983).

### *Agent*

*Mycoplasma muris* is a bacterium, class Mollicutes, order Mycoplasmatales, family Mycoplasmataceae (sterol-requiring mycoplasmas). *M. muris* is a recently described, new species of mycoplasma. It is a strict anaerobe that grows only on SP-4 medium (not on standard horse serum and yeast extract medium suitable for other rodent mycoplasmas), and hydrolyzes arginine. It hemadsorbs to guinea pig erythrocytes and is serologically distinct from all other known mycoplasmas (McGarrity et al., 1983).

### *Host*

Mice.

### *Epizootiology*

*M. muris* has been isolated only from the vagina of pregnant RIII strain mice in one laboratory. Its prevalence in other strains and populations of mice is unknown.

### *Clinical*

*M. muris* has not been associated with clinical disease.

### *Pathology*

No data are available.

### *Diagnosis*

The only method available for diagnosis currently is culturing with SP-4 medium under strict anaerobic conditions. No data are available on the use of other methods such as the mycoplasma enzyme-linked immunosorbent assay for diagnosis of this infection (McGarrity et al., 1983).

### *Control*

No data are available. The agent presumably can be eliminated by cesarean derivation and barrier maintenance.

### *Interference with Research*

Unknown.

# 12

# Multiple Systems

## Overview

The agents considered in this group appear to affect multiple systems. However, this may simply reflect the present lack of understanding of these host-parasite relationships. Included in the group are three parvoviruses (Kilham rat virus, H-1 virus, and minute virus of mice), polyoma virus, and the hantaviruses. The hantaviruses are a group of closely related viruses that occur primarily in wild rodents but that also have been found in laboratory rats, mainly in Japan and Europe. Some of the hantaviruses cause serious zoonotic infections in people.

## Kilham Rat Virus

### *Significance*

There are few reports of natural disease or interference with research due to this virus, but its high prevalence in rats and propensity for damaging populations of replicating cells in vivo and in vitro make it a significant pathogen.

### *Perspective*

Kilham rat virus (KRV)* was discovered by Kilham and Olivier (1959) during attempts to isolate a suspected oncogenic virus from rats with ex-

*NOTE: Kilham and Olivier (1959) named this virus "Rat Virus (RV)" and that is its official taxonomic name (Siegl et al., 1985). In this publication we have chosen to use the more distinctive name Kilham Rat Virus (KRV), which is commonly used in the United States.

perimental tumors (a *Cysticercus fasciolaris*-induced sarcoma in F344 rats and a transplantable leukemia in OM rats). In subsequent years research with this agent emphasized molecular biology of the virus (Tattersall and Cotmore, 1986) and experimental animal models for producing lesions such as cerebellar hypoplasia (Kilham and Margolis, 1975; Margolis and Kilham, 1975) while relatively little attention was given to understanding the natural history and pathogenesis of KRV in rat colonies (Jacoby et al., 1987).

*Agent*

KRV is a single-stranded DNA virus, family Parvoviridae, genus *Parvovirus*. KRV is the type species of the genus (Siegl et al., 1985). It is synonymous with rat virus (RV) and parvovirus r-1. Approximately a dozen strains of the virus have been isolated (Tattersall and Cotmore, 1986). The virion is non-enveloped, and measures 18-30 nm in diameter. The genus *Parvovirus* presently contains 13 distinct serotypes, three of which occur in rodents: KRV, H-l virus, and Minute Virus of Mice. Serotyping is based on the neutralization (NT), complement fixation (CF), and hemagglutination inhibition (HAI) tests (Jacoby et al., 1979; Tattersall and Cotmore, 1986). KRV can be propagated in primary rat embryo, 324K, and BHK-21 cells (Jacoby et al., 1979, 1987).

Parvoviruses are remarkably resistant to environmental conditions. Infectivity is retained after heating at 80°C for 2 hours or 40°C for up to 60 days. They also are resistant to dessication, pH 2 to 11, chloroform, ether, and alcohol (Toolan, 1968; Jacoby et al., 1979; Tattersall and Cotmore, 1986).

*Hosts*

Laboratory and wild rats (*Rattus norvegicus*) are the natural hosts. Syrian hamsters and several other species have been infected experimentally (Kilham, 1966; Jacoby et al., 1979; Tattersall and Cotmore, 1986).

*Epizootiology*

KRV is a common natural infection of wild and laboratory rats. Kilham (1966) found antibodies to KRV in 40% to 62% of wild rats at four different locations near Hanover, New Hampshire, and in 89% of a population of laboratory rats. More recent serological surveys of laboratory rats reported prevalences of 44% (Lindsey et al., 1986a) and 71% (Parker, 1980) in the United States, 74% in Canada (Lussier and Descoteaux, 1986), 60% in the United Kingdom (Gannon and Carthew, 1980), and 32% in West Germany (Kraft and Meyer, 1986).

Transmission of KRV is primarily by the horizontal route, either through direct contact or fomites. Contaminated fomites are probably important because parvoviruses are extremely stable to dessication. The efficiency of horizontal transmission may depend on strain of virus and age at which rats are infected. Virus has been reported to be shed in urine, feces, milk, and nasal secretions (Lipton et al., 1973; Kilham and Margolis, 1974a,b; Robinson et al., 1974; Tattersall and Cotmore, 1986; Jacoby et al., 1987, 1988). Rats infected by the oronasal route at two days of age transmitted the virus to cagemates for 10 weeks, whereas rats infected at 4 weeks of age were able to infect their cagemates for only 3 weeks post infection (Jacoby et al., 1988). Transplacental infection has been suggested (Kilham and Margolis, 1966, 1969; Robey et al., 1968; Novotny and Hetrick, 1970), but its occurrence has been questioned on the basis of more recent experimental data (Tattersall and Cotmore, 1986; Jacoby et al., 1988). Persistent infection has been shown to occur for up to 14 weeks in rats infected as infants (Paturzo et al., 1987).

KRV has been shown to persistently infect a number of cultured cell lines (Kilham et al., 1968; Wozniak and Hetrick, 1969; Lum, 1970; Bass and Hetrick, 1978) and to be a frequent contaminant of transplantable tumors (Kilham and Olivier, 1959; Lum and Schreiner, 1963; Kilham and Moloney, 1964; Tattersall and Cotmore, 1986). Thus contaminated cells and tumors are important sources of KRV infection.

### *Clinical*

Natural infections nearly always are subclinical. Clinical disease is a rare event, and few examples have been reported (Kilham and Margolis, 1966; Coleman et al., 1983).

Natural disease due to KRV was observed in 13-day pregnant rats by Kilham and Margolis (1966). They reported increased numbers of uterine resorption sites in the dams and runting, ataxia, cerebellar hypoplasia, and jaundice in pups from several litters. KRV was isolated from the pups, as well as from tissues, feces, and milk of the dams.

Spontaneous deaths, scrotal cyanosis, abdominal swelling, dehydration, and other signs of severe illness occurred in juvenile and 7-week-old male rats within 2 weeks after these animals were added to a colony of adult rats that were serologically positive for KRV (Coleman et al., 1983)

### *Pathology*

KRV infects actively replicating (S-phase) cells and thus, has a predilection for proliferating and growing tissues. Also, productive infection is always lytic and thus, infection usually leads to cell destruction (Margolis et al., 1971; Tattersall and Cotmore, 1986). For these reasons, the major pathologic effects of KRV infection would be expected to occur during fetal development and early life. Although the number of reports is small, this has been borne out in natural infections. Although transplacental infection is probably not important as a mode of transmission (Jacoby et al., 1988), fetal deaths and teratologic effects have been attributed to KRV in a few instances (Kilham and Margolis, 1966; Jacoby et al., 1979). Natural infections of KRV also have been the cause of severe disease in rats from birth to 9 weeks of age. The findings in this group have included stunting, cerebellar hypoplasia, jaundice, and hemorrhagic infarction with thrombosis in multiple organs (including brain, spinal cord, testes, and epididymis). Amphophilic intranuclear inclusions occurred in the endothelium and other cells of affected organs (Coleman et al., 1983). Focal necrosis, hypertrophy and vacuolar degeneration of hepatocytes, cholangitis, and biliary hyperplasia can occur in the liver (Kilham and Margolis, 1966; Jacoby et al., 1979; Coleman et al., 1983). Hemorrhagic encephalopathy was reported to occur in one group of naturally infected adult LEW rats following the administration of 100-150 mg/kg of cyclophosphamide (El Dadah et al., 1967).

Experimental infections of KRV, in which large doses of virus were inoculated by unnatural routes, have been used in developing a large array of experimental animal models (reviewed by Kilham and Margolis, 1975; Margolis and Kilham, 1975). These have included models of teratologic effects (Kilham and Ferm, 1964), cerebellar hypoplasia (Margolis and Kilham, 1968; Margolis et al., 1971), hepatitis (Bergs and Scotti, 1967; Margolis et al., 1968), and hemorrhagic encephalopathy (Cole et al., 1970; Margolis and Kilham, 1970; Nathanson et al., 1970; Baringer and Nathanson, 1972) in rats, and of cerebellar hypoplasia, "mongolism," and periodontal disease in Syrian hamsters (Kilham, 1961a,b; Baer and Kilham, 1962a,b, 1964; Toolan, 1968; Lipton and Johnson, 1972).

*Diagnosis*

Serologic methods are used for routine health monitoring. The enzyme-linked immunosorbent assay (Singh and Lang, 1984) and the indirect fluorescent antibody test are considered most sensitive, but do not discriminate between infections due to different serotypes of parvoviruses in rats (i.e., KRV or H-1 virus). The HAI, CF, and NT tests are used for serotype discrimination (Cross and Parker, 1972; Tattersall and Cotmore, 1986).

For the diagnosis of natural disease outbreaks due to KRV, virus serology, demonstration of typical pathologic lesions, and virus isolation should be carried out (Coleman et al., 1983). The virus can be propagated in primary rat embryo, 324K, and BHK-21 cells (Jacoby et al., 1979, 1987).

*Control*

The most practical approach to control of KRV infection is to obtain only rats demonstrated to be free of the virus by regular serologic monitoring. Also, transplantable tumors, cell lines, and virus stocks should be tested for KRV infection by the mouse antibody production (MAP) test before being brought into an animal facility (Rowe et al., 1959a).

For those breeding colonies that have the infection, the most practical solution may be to eliminate the colony and repopulate with KRV-free stock. To eliminate the infection from valuable breeding stocks of rats, cesarean derivation should be successful because transplacental transmission is not considered important (Jacoby et al., 1987, 1988; Paturzo et al., 1987). Alternatively, it might be possible to isolate individual breeding pairs of rats from KRV-infected populations in separate containment devices such as filter-top cage systems, with subsequent selection of seronegative progeny as breeders (Lipman et al., 1987; Weir et al., 1987).

*Interference with Research*

Although transplacental transmittal is generally considered unimportant, early work did suggest such transmission (Kilham and Margolis, 1966). If transplacental transmittal does occur, KRV infection might interfere with studies of fetal development and might have teratogenic effects.

KRV can contaminate transplantable tumors (Kilham and Olivier, 1959; Lum and Schreiner, 1963; Kilham and Moloney, 1964; Tattersall and Cotmore, 1986) and rat cell tissue cultures (Dawe et al., 1961; Wozniak and Hetrick, 1969; Lum, 1970; Bass and Hetrick, 1978; Jacoby et al., 1979).

KRV has been reported to suppress the development of leukemia due to Moloney virus (Bergs, 1969).

KRV infection has been reported to alter in vitro lymphocyte responses (Campbell et al., 1977a,b) and cytotoxic lymphocyte activity (Darrigrand et al., 1984).

Inapparent KRV infection can be exacerbated to cause clinical disease by immunosuppression (El Dadah et al., 1967).

KRV infection has been reported to induce interferon production in vivo (Kilham et al., 1968).

## H-1 Virus

*Significance*

Although quite prevalent in contemporary rat stocks, this virus is not known to cause natural disease and has been shown to interfere with research in very few instances. It has been found useful for producing a few experimental infection models in animals.

*Perspective*

MVM was isolated from a human tumor cell line (HEp-1) after it had been passaged in rats (Toolan et al., 1960; Toolan, 1961), and therefore, the virus was probably of rat origin (Tattersall and Cotmore, 1986). Like Kilham rat virus, H-1 virus has been used to produce experimental malformations of the central nervous system, skeleton and teeth, particularly in rats and hamsters (reviewed by Toolan, 1968; Kilham and Margolis, 1975; Margolis and Kilham, 1975). The natural history of H-1 virus in rat populations has been studied very little.

*Agent*

H-1 virus is a single-stranded DNA virus, family Parvoviridae, genus *Parvovirus*. The virion is non-enveloped and measures 18-30 nm in diameter. Approximately five strains of H-1 virus have been characterized (Jacoby et al., 1979; Tattersall and Cotmore, 1986). The genus *Parvovirus* presently contains 13 distinct serotypes, three of which occur in rodents: H-1 virus, Kilham rat virus and Minute Virus of Mice. Serotyping is based on the neutralization (NT), complement fixation (CF) and hemagglutination inhibition (HAI) tests (Tattersall and Cotmore, 1986). Parvoviruses can be propagated in primary rat embryo, 324K, and BHK-21 cells (Jacoby et al., 1979, 1987). They are remarkably resistant to environmental conditions. Infectivity is retained after heating at 80°C for 2 hours or 40°C for up to 60 days. They also are resistant to dessication, pH 2 to 11, chloroform, ether, and alcohol (Toolan, 1968; Jacoby et al., 1979; Tattersall and Cotmore, 1986).

*Hosts*

Laboratory and wild rats (*Rattus norvegicus*) are the natural hosts. Syrian hamsters and several other species have been infected experimentally (Kilham, 1966; Kilham and Margolis, 1975; Margolis and Kilham, 1975; Tattersall and Cotmore, 1986).

---

*NOTE: This virus was designated "H-1" by Toolan (1961, 1968), and this is its official taxonomic name (Siegl et al., 1985). The virus is also commonly called Toolan H-1 virus in the United States.

### Epizootiology

H-1 virus is a common natural infection of wild and laboratory rats. Kilham (1966) found antibodies to KRV in none to 100% of wild rats at four different locations near Hanover, New Hampshire, and in 80% of a population of laboratory rats. More recent serological surveys of laboratory rats have given prevalences of 11% (Lindsey et al., 1986a) and 52% (Parker, 1980) in the United States, 71% in Canada (Lussier and Descoteaux, 1986), and 27% in West Germany (Kraft and Meyer, 1986).

The epizootiological characteristics of H-1 virus infection in rat colonies are generally assumed to be similar to those of Kilham rat virus infection which has been investigated much more extensively (Robey et al., 1968; Lipton et al., 1973; Kilham and Margolis, 1974a,b; Robinson et al., 1974; Tattersall and Cotmore, 1986; Jacoby et al., 1987, 1988). Transmission is primarily horizontal, and virus is shed in urine, feces, nasal secretions, and milk. Transplacental infection in rats has been demonstrated only after parenteral inoculation of pregnant dams (Kilham and Margolis, 1969). Viral persistence and latency have not been adequately studied (Tattersall and Cotmore, 1986).

### Clinical

Clinical signs have not been reported to occur in natural infections of H-1 virus.

### Pathology

Natural infections of H-1 virus are not known to cause disease.

As with other rodent parvoviruses, H-1 virus infection requires replicating (S-phase) cells and productive infection is always lytic (Margolis et al., 1971; Margolis and Kilham, 1975; Tattersall and Cotmore, 1986). Because of these basic virus-host relationships, experimental infections of fetal and infant hamsters and rats with H-1 virus have provided models of disease including cerebellar hypoplasia, runting, "mongolism," bone and tooth abnormalities, and multiple organ malformations (Toolan, 1960, 1968; Ferm and Kilham, 1964, 1965; Margolis and Kilham, 1968, 1975; Kilham and Margolis, 1975).

### Diagnosis

The diagnosis of H-1 infection is usually made during health surveillance testing as natural infections are inapparent. The enzyme-linked immunosorbent assay and indirect fluorescent antibody test are usually used for initial screening, followed by either the HAI, CF, or NT tests for discriminating between H-1 virus and Kilham rat virus infections (Cross and Parker, 1972; Tattersall and Cotmore, 1986). For virus isolation primary rat embryo, 324K, and BHK-21 cells can be used (Jacoby et al., 1979, 1987).

*Control*

The same measures as recommended for Kilham rat virus should be effective in the control of H-1 virus.

*Interference with Research*

It may be possible for H-1 virus to alter the results of studies concerned with fetal development or teratogenesis (Kilham and Margolis, 1969); but this has not been reported to occur as a result of natural infection.

H-1 virus has been reported to cause hepatocellular necrosis in infected rats when they are subjected to liver injury by hepatotoxic chemicals, parasitism, or partial hepatectomy (Ruffolo et al., 1966; Kilham et al., 1970).

H-1 virus infection has been found to inhibit experimental tumor induction by adenovirus 12 (Toolan and Ledinko, 1968) and dimethylbenzanthracene (Toolan et al., 1982) in hamsters.

## Minute Virus of Mice

*Significance*

The significance of minute virus of mice (MVM) is uncertain. It has little significance for most studies, but may be highly significant for studies involving mouse transplantable tumors, leukemias, and in vitro immunoassays.

*Perspective*

MVM was first recognized as a contaminant in a stock of mouse adenovirus by Hartley and Rowe (1960). It was later described and named by Crawford (1966), and further characterized by Crawford et al. (1969). Subsequently, it was identified as a prevalent indigenous infection in mouse colonies (Parker et al., 1970b), and as one of the most common contaminants of mouse leukemia virus stocks and transplantable tumors (Collins and Parker, 1972). Two strains of the virus MVM(p) and MVM(i) have been of particular interest to molecular biologists (Ward and Tattersall, 1982; Tattersall and Cotmore, 1986).

*Agent*

MVM is a single-stranded DNA virus, family Parvoviridae, genus *Parvovirus*. The genus *Parvovirus* presently contains 13 distinct serotypes, three of which occur in rodents: MVM, H-1 virus, and Kilham rat virus. Serotyping is based on the neutralization (NT), complement fixation (CF), and hemagglutination inhibition (HAI) tests (Siegl et al., 1985; Mengeling et al., 1986; Tattersall and Cotmore, 1986).

The virion of MVM measures 26 nm in diameter, has an icosahedral capsid with 32 capsomeres, and is non-enveloped. The complete nucleotide sequence of the genome is 5081 nucleotides long. The genome encodes for three proteins that make up the viral capsid, VP-1, VP-2, and VP-3, plus two nonstructural proteins, NS-1 and NS-2 for which the function is uncertain (Ward and Tattersall, 1982; Astell et al., 1983; Cotmore et al., 1983; Cotmore and Tattersall, 1986).

Recognized strains of MVM include MVM(CR), the original strain of Crawford (1966); MVM(p), the prototype strain derived by plaque purification from MVM(CR); MVM(i), the immunosuppressive variant discovered by Bonnard et al. (1976); MVM-890; and CZ-7 (Tattersall and Cotmore, 1986). Two strains have been studied extensively, MVM(i) and MVM(p). MVM(i) grows lytically in mouse T-lymphocytes (thus, sometimes referred to as the lymphotropic strain), inhibits various functions mediated by T-lymphocytes in vitro, and is restricted in fibroblasts. MVM(p) grows in mouse fibroblasts (the fibrotropic strain), is restricted in T-lymphocytes, and does not inhibit T-lymphocyte functions (McMaster et al., 1981; Spalholz and Tattersall, 1983; Tattersall and Bratton, 1983). The nucleotide sequences of the genomes of both MVM(p) (Astell et al., 1983) and MVM(i) (Sahli et al., 1985) have been determined. The genomic organization of the two strains is identical but there are 29 amino acid differences in their putative viral gene products (Sahli et al., 1985). Both the lymphotropic and fibrotropic determinants have been found to map to the same 237-nucleotide sequence within the coding region of the virus structural gene (Gardiner and Tattersall, 1988b).

MVM can be propagated in A9 fibroblast, 324K (SV40 transformed human newborn kidney), and EL4 mouse T-cell lymphoma cells, and rat and mouse embryo tissue cultures (Parker et al., 1970a; Gardiner and Tattersall, 1988a).

Parvoviruses are remarkably resistant to environmental conditions. Infectivity is retained after heating at 80°C for 2 hours or 40°C for up to 60 days. They also are resistant to dessication, pH 2 to 11, chloroform, ether, and alcohol (Toolan, 1968; Tattersall and Cotmore, 1986).

*Hosts*

Laboratory and wild mice (*Mus musculus*) are the natural hosts (Tattersall and Cotmore, 1986).

*Epizootiology*

MVM is a common infection of wild and laboratory mice. Parker et al. (1970b) found 76 (20%) of 390 sera from wild *Mus musculus* trapped in Florida, Georgia, Maryland, and Indiana to be positive for MVM by the HAI test; positives were found in mice from all four states. In laboratory mice Parker et al. (1970b) found serological evidence of the infection in 38 (86%) of 44 conventional colonies, three (38%) of eight "specific pathogen-free" colonies, and none of five germfree mouse colonies. More recent surveys of laboratory mice have given prevalences for colonies infected with MVM of 73% (Lindsey et al., 1986) and 81% (Parker, 1980) in the United States, 50% in Canada (Lussier and Descoteaux, 1986), 33% in West Germany (Kraft and Meyer, 1986), and 3% in France (Van Der Logt, 1986).

MVM is also a common contaminant of mouse leukemia virus stocks and transplantable tumors. In one study, Parker et al. (1970b) found 79 (40%) of 195 mouse leukemias and transplantable tumors to be contaminated. Later, Collins and Parker (1972) demonstrated MVM in 151 (32%) of 465 mouse leukemia virus stocks and transplantable tumors. In the latter study, MVM ranked second to lactic dehydrogenase-elevating virus in occurrence as a viral contaminant.

MVM is highly contagious. Virus is shed in the urine and feces. Fomites such as contaminated food and bedding are particularly important because the virus is very resistant to environmental conditions. Nasal-oral contact is also effective in transmission but aerosols are probably not important because uninfected mice in cages eight inches away from infected mice do not become infected. Maternal antibody is protective until 6 to 8 weeks of age but most mice in infected colonies become infected by two or three months of age. Transplacental infection is not considered important (Parker et al., 1970b).

*Clinical*

Natural infections are inapparent (Parker et al., 1970b).

*Pathology*

Natural infections of MVM are not known to produce disease (Parker et al., 1970a,b; Ward and Tattersall, 1982; Tattersall and Cotmore, 1986).

Experimental infections of MVM(CR) in fetal and neonatal mice, rats, and hamsters produce lesions such as runting, cerebellar hypoplasia, and periodontal disease (Kilham and Margolis, 1970, 1971; Baer and Kilham, 1974). However, the lesions due to MVM(CR) are relatively mild by comparision to the lesions produced experimentally by Kilham rat virus or H-1 virus (Kilham and Margolis, 1975; Margolis and Kilham, 1975).

*Diagnosis*

Serologic methods are used for routine health surveillance. The enzyme-linked immunosorbent assay and the immunofluorescent antibody test are considered most sensitive (Tattersall and Cotmore, 1986). Mice of the MRL/MpJ strain are reported to give frequent false positive HAI test results for MVM (Jonas, 1984). Transplantable tumors and other biologic materials from mice can be screened by the mouse antibody production (MAP) test (Rowe et al., 1959) and/or virus isolation (deSouza and Smith, 1989). The HAI, CF, and NT tests can be used in situations where discrimination between MVM, Kilham rat virus, and H-1 virus infection is desired (Cross and Parker, 1972; Tattersall and Cotmore, 1986).

*Control*

MVM can be eliminated from stocks of mice by cesarean derivation, but elimination of infected mice followed by replacement with MVM-free mice is often more practical. Maintenance of MVM-free mice can be difficult because the virus is highly contagious. Adherence to strict barrier procedures is required. Careful attention to the exclusion of wild mice and prompt elimination of MVM-infected stocks of laboratory mice in other parts of the facility are essential. Regular serologic monitoring of all mouse subpopulations must be practiced for early detection (Parker et al., 1970b).

Infection can become established in a colony through introduction of contaminated transplantable tumors, virus stocks, and other biologic materials that are passaged in mice. All such materials should be monitored for MVM and other infectious agents before admission to a facility (Rowe et al., 1959; Parker et al., 1970b; de Souza and Smith, 1989).

*Interference with Research*

Direct evidence that wild type MVM in contemporary mouse stocks interferes with research is lacking. However, it is clear that MVM is a common contaminant of mouse leukemia virus stocks, transplantable tumors, hybridomas, and other cell lines (Parker et al., 1970a; Collins and Parker, 1972;

de Souza and Smith, 1989). Thus, it seems highly probable that studies involving these materials are at times compromised because of inadvertent MVM contamination.

Considerable evidence that MVM can interfere with research has come from studies of MVM(i), a single variant of the virus that may or may not occur as a natural infection in contemporary mice. MVM(i) grows lytically in cytotoxic T-lymphocyte clones, abrogates cytotoxic T-lymphocyte responses, suppresses T-lymphocyte mitogenic responses and suppresses T helper-dependent B-lymphocyte responses, in vitro (Bonnard et al., 1976; Herbermann et al., 1977; Engers et al., 1981; McMaster et al., 1981; Tattersall and Cotmore, 1986).

The intramuscular inoculation of MVM(p) into mice suppresses the growth of Ehrlich ascites tumor cells given intraperitoneally (Guetta et al., 1986).

A parvovirus serologically related to MVM has been reported as a contaminant of calf serum (Nettleton and Rweyemamu, 1980).

## Polyoma Virus

### *Significance*

Polyoma virus has limited significance as a naturally occurring infection of mice likely to interfere with research. Its major importance has been for use in experimental model systems, including in vivo viral carcinogenesis (Eddy, 1982), in vitro transformation of cells (Topp et al., 1980), and certain aspects of human polyoma virus infection (Shah and Christian, 1986).

### *Perspective*

*1953:* Gross (1953a,b) and Stewart (1953) independently observed sarcomas in mice that had been inoculated with extracts of murine leukemia virus.

*1957:* Stewart et al. (1957) demonstrated that polyoma virus (which had caused the sarcomas in the 1953 study described above) replicates in tissue culture.

*1958:* Eddy et al. (1958) discovered that inoculation of the virus into newborn hamsters led to tumor induction with a shorter latent period than in mice.

*1961:* Wild mice were shown to have a high prevalence of polyoma virus infection (Rowe, 1961; Rowe et al., 1961).

*1972:* The virus was found to be a common contaminant of transplantable murine tumors and stocks of murine leukemia viruses (Collins and Parker, 1972).

*Agent*

Polyoma virus is a DNA virus, family Papovaviridae, genus *Polyomavirus*. Mouse polyoma virus is the type species of the genus. It is related to K virus, simian virus 40, rabbit kidney vacuolating virus, and others. The virion is spherical, measures 44 nm in diameter, and icosahedral. It hemagglutinates guinea pig, hamster, sheep, and human O erythrocytes at 4°C. It can be propagated in primary cultures of mouse embryo or mouse kidney, and in 3T3 and 3T6 mouse fibroblasts. It is highly resistant to environmental conditions and to physical and chemical agents (Eddy, 1982; Shah and Christian, 1986).

*Host*

Wild and laboratory mice (*Mus musculus*) are the natural hosts. Wild mice serve as reservoir hosts (Rowe, 1961).

*Epizootiology*

The prevalence of polyoma virus infection is poorly understood. The virus has been demonstrated to occur focally in populations of wild mice (Rowe et al., 1959b, 1961) and to occur in colonies of laboratory mice in the United States, Europe, and Japan (Rowe et al., 1959b; Parker et al., 1966), primarily in colonies housed in close proximity to experimentally infected mice (Parker et al., 1966). It is not likely to be seen in mice from commercial barrier breeding facilities in the United States.

The virus is highly contagious. It is shed in urine, saliva, and feces, but excreted in higher titer and for a longer periods of time in urine. In persistently infected dams, the titer of virus in the kidney increases during late pregnancy (McCance and Mims, 1979). The virus has a propensity for airborne dissemination and intranasal infection. Transmission occurs readily within and between cages in the same room. Contaminated feed and bedding can be important sources of infection. Transplacental transmission can occur but only if mice are infected during gestation (Rowe et al., 1958; Rowe, 1961; McGarrity et al., 1976; McCance and Mims, 1977; McGarrity and Dion, 1978).

The respiratory tract is generally accepted as the natural route of infection of mice with polyoma virus as smaller amounts of virus are required to establish the infection by this route than by the alimentary route (Rowe et al., 1959a, 1960). Dubensky et al. (1984) used an *in situ* hybridization technique to follow the pattern of infection after intranasal infection of neonatal mice. Primary replication of the virus occurred in the nasal mucosa, submaxillary salivary glands, and lungs. This was followed by a systemic phase in which viral replication predominated in lung and liver, and also occurred in kidney and colon around six days post infection. The lungs, kidney, and colon appeared to be the main portals for exit of the virus.

### *Clinical*

Natural infections are usually inapparent (polyoma virus-induced tumors have not been reported in naturally infected immunocompetent mice). Tumors caused by the virus occur more readily in immunocompromised hosts (Eddy, 1982; Rubino and Walker, 1988).

Athymic (*nu*/*nu*) mice given heterotransplants of human tumors contaminated with the virus have been reported to develop a syndrome characterized by wasting and paralysis of the rear legs and tail (Sebesteny et al., 1980; McCance et al., 1983).

### *Pathology*

Morphologic lesions, including polyoma virus-induced tumors, usually are not found in naturally infected mice (Eddy, 1982).

In experimental infection, factors that favor tumor formation include infection at a very young age, inoculation of very large doses of the virus, inoculation of the virus directly into tissues (i.e., use of either the subcutaneous, intravenous, or intracerebral routes), and immunosuppression of the host (Shah and Christian, 1986). Experimental inoculation of the virus into adult mice does not result in tumor induction because an efficient immune response prevents virus-transformed cells from growing to form tumors. A polyoma tumor-specific transplantation antigen (TSTA) is induced in the early phase of polyoma virus infection prior to DNA synthesis, and protection from tumor development is T-cell-dependent and directed toward this antigen (Allison, 1980; Ito, 1980; Eddy, 1982; Ramquist et al., 1988).

In neonatal mice inoculated with high doses of virus, transformed cells multiply to numbers that cannot be controlled effectively by the immature immune system. Tumors appear around 2-3 months and most develop by 4-7 months postinoculation. Infection of neonates can be prevented by maternal antibody in infected colonies (Ito, 1980; Eddy, 1982; Shah and Christian, 1986).

Pleomorphic salivary gland tumors are the most common lesions occurring in experimentally infected neonatal mice. Sarcomas and carcinomas of the kidney, subcutis, mammary gland, adrenal gland, bone, cartilage, blood vessels, and thyroid also occur. Many are transplantable to syngeneic hosts. Strains of mice differ in their susceptibilities, with those of C57BL and

C57BR/cd lineage being among the most resistant and athymic (*nu/nu*) mice being the most susceptible (Eddy, 1982).

Athymic (*nu/nu*) mice heterotransplanted with a human tumor contaminated with polyoma virus have been reported to show progressive weight loss and flaccid paralysis of the rear legs and tail. The brain and spinal cord had multifocal demyelination associated with virus particles in the cytoplasm and nuclei of oligodendroglia. The disease was attributed to primary destruction of oligodendroglia by the virus. Intracytoplasmic and intranuclear inclusions also were present in epithelium of the bronchi, ureters, and renal pelvis (Sebesteny et al., 1980; McCance et al., 1983). Subsequent investigations of this syndrome by Harper et al. (1983) gave a different explanation. Most of their *nu/nu* mice inoculated with polyoma virus developed vertebral tumors resulting in compression of the spinal cord, and they concluded that the lesions in the nervous system occurred secondarily.

Malignant tumors also occur following experimental inoculation of polyoma virus into neonatal hamsters, rats, guinea pigs, mastomys, and ferrets. Newborn rabbits develop benign tumors that subsequently regress. Infections in these species and in mice are extremely important animal models of virus-induced tumors (Barthold and Olson, 1974; Eddy, 1982; Shah and Christian, 1986).

### *Diagnosis*

The enzyme-linked immunosorbent assay and the hemagglutination inhibition test are commonly used in routine health monitoring. The mouse antibody production (MAP) test can be used for screening tumor lines and other biologic materials (Rowe et al., 1959a,b, 1961). Tissue sections can be examined for presence of the virus using an immunoperoxidase test for the major capsid polypeptide (Gerber et al., 1980) or *in situ* DNA hybridization (Dubensky et al., 1984). Virus isolation using primary mouse embryo or mouse kidney cultures, or 3T3 or 3T6 mouse fibroblasts can be useful in selected situations (Shah and Christian, 1986).

### *Control*

Control of polyoma virus is not likely to be a problem except in those animal facilities where mice are given experimental infections of the virus, transplantable tumors or other biological materials contaminated with the virus are introduced into the facility, or wild mice gain access to the facility and transmit the infection to laboratory mice. Once established in a mouse facility, the infection can spread rapidly to adjacent rooms. If experimental infections of polyoma virus are to be carried out in a facility, rigorous containment measures such as the use of plastic film isolators may be necessary to prevent spread of the infection (McGarrity et al., 1976; Eddy, 1982). Transplantable tumors and other biologic specimens should be screened for the virus before entry into an animal facility.

Cesarean derivation and barrier maintenance are considered very effective in eliminating the virus because transplacental transmission probably is of little or no importance in natural infections (McCance and Mims, 1977). However, more practical methods such as isolation and quarantine of individual breeding pairs with subsequent selection of seronegative progeny or removal of neonates and fostering them on polyoma virus-free dams should be effective (Lipman et al., 1987). Strict isolation of virus-free mice from polyoma virus-infected stocks and exclusion of wild mice are essential for preventing reinfection. Laminar flow units and filter-top cages are helpful in reducing the spread of infection in laboratories in which the agent is used experimentally (McGarrity et al., 1976).

### *Interference with Research*

Polyoma virus can complicate research by contaminating tumor lines, stocks of other viruses, and other biologic materials that are passaged in mice (Collins and Parker, 1972).

Polyoma virus-contaminated tumors can cause paralysis and wasting in athymic (*nu*/*nu*) mice (Sebesteny et al., 1980; McCance et al., 1983) due to vertebral tumors and compression of the spinal cord (Harper et al., 1983).

Neonatal mice from naturally infected colonies can be refractory to experimental infection with polyoma virus because of maternal antibody (Eddy, 1982).

Mice subjected to neonatal thymectomy later developed parotid gland tumors because the colony had inadvertently become infected with polyoma virus (Law, 1965).

## Hantaviruses

### *Significance*

The genus *Hantavirus* includes several recently recognized viruses from different regions of the world (LeDuc, 1987). Some of these agents have caused persistent, subclinical infections in laboratory rats (and other rodents introduced into laboratories), resulting in serious illness in research personnel (Kawamata et al., 1980, 1987; Tsai, 1987a). The most important human pathogen in the group, Hantaan virus, has been called "the most significant zoonotic pathogen of laboratory rodents since the discovery of lymphocytic choriomeningitis virus" (Johnson, 1986).

*Perspective*

In the period from the early 1940s to the early 1970s there were recognized across Eurasia a large assortment of clinical syndromes in humans, most commonly referred to as hemorrhagic fevers (H. W. Lee et al., 1979). These included hemorrhagic nephrosonephritis in Russia, recognized around 1944 (Smorodintsev, 1959), epidemic hemorrhagic fever (EHF) in China, recognized about 1942-1944 (H. W. Lee et al., 1979), nephropathia epidemica (NE) in Scandinavia (Myhrman, 1951; Lahdevirta, 1971), Korean hemorrhagic fever (KHF) in Korea (Smadel, 1953; Earle, 1954), EHF in Eastern Europe (Gajdusek, 1962), and EHF in Japan (Tamura, 1964).

During the Korean War thousands of cases of KHF, a syndrome often characterized by acute high fever, shock, hemorrhage, and renal failure, occurred in United Nations' forces and attracted worldwide attention (Smadel, 1953; Earle, 1954; Tsai, 1987b). H. W. Lee et al. (1978) isolated the causative agent of KHF from the field mouse, *Apodemus agrarius*, and named it Hantaan virus (H. W. Lee et al., 1981). Following the discovery of successful cell cultures for Hantaan virus (French et al., 1981; Kitamura et al., 1983), a large number of Hantaan-related viruses were isolated and assigned to the genus, *Hantavirus* (McCormick et al., 1982; White et al., 1982; Schmaljohn and Dalrymple, 1983).

Naturally infected laboratory rats have been the source of *Hantavirus* infections in research personnel in Japan (Umenai et al., 1979; Kawamata et al., 1980, 1987), Belgium (Van Ypersele de Strihou, 1979; Desmyter et al., 1983), the United Kingdom (Lloyd et al., 1984), and France (Dournon et al., 1984). In Japan alone, at least 126 human cases and one death have occurred (Kawamata et al., 1987). As of 1987, hantaviruses still had not been eradicated from all animal facilities in Japan (Kawamata et al., 1987). Wild rodents brought into the laboratory have caused human infections of hantaviruses in Korea (H. W. Lee and Johnson, 1982) and Russia (Tsai, 1987a).

*Agents*

The agents are single-stranded RNA viruses, family Bunyaviridae, genus *Hantavirus*. This is a new genus based on morphological, genetic, antigenic, and physiochemical similarities (McCormick et al., 1982; White et al., 1982; Hung et al., 1983; Schmaljohn and Dalrymple, 1983; Schmaljohn et al., 1983, 1985). Collectively, they have been grouped together by the World Health Organization as the viruses of hemorrhagic fever with renal syndrome (HFRS) in humans (W.H.O., 1983). Hantaan virus, the cause of KHF, is the prototype member of the genus. Thus far the genus has not been separated into species but several strains of hantaviruses have been isolated: Hupei-I from a patient with EHF in China; SR-11 from a laboratory rat associated with an EHF outbreak in Japan; Tchoupitoulas from a wild Norway rat in New Orleans, La.; Hallnas-I and Puumala from *Clethrionomys glareolus* trapped in areas where NE occurs in Sweden and Finland, respectively; and Prospect Hill-I from *Microtus pennsylvanicus* in Frederick, Md.; Girard Point from a Norway rat trapped near Philadelphia, Pa.; and others (Schmaljohn and Dalrymple, 1983; Schmaljohn et al., 1983, 1985; LeDuc et al., 1984; Childs et al., 1985; Goldgaber et al., 1985; LeDuc et al., 1985a).

In addition to *Hantavirus*, genera within the Bunyaviridae are *Bunyavirus* (prototype, Bunyamwera virus), *Nairovirus* (prototype, Crimean/Congo hemorrhagic fever virus), *Phlebovirus* (prototype, Sandfly fever virus), and *Uukuvirus* (prototype, Ukuniemi virus). The five genera are serologically, morphologically, and biochemically distinct. The Bunyaviridae are generally spherical, measure 80-120 nm in diameter, have surface projections 5-10 nm in length that are anchored in a lipid bilayered envelope, and have a genome of single-stranded RNA consisting of three segments (Martin et al., 1985).

Hantaan virus virions include round particles that measure 98 nm in diameter and oval particles that measure 110 × 173 nm in length. Negatively stained virions have an enveloped surface with a square grid-like pattern. The virus is stable at pH 7.0-9.0 but is inactivated at pH 5.0. It is relatively stable at 4-20°C but is inactivated rapidly at 37°C. It can be stored at –60°C (H. W. Lee, 1982; Martin et al., 1985). It can be grown in A-549 and Vero E6 cells (H. W. Lee, 1982; Schmaljohn et al., 1983).

### *Hosts*

The natural hosts of all hantaviruses appear to be small mammals, primarily rodents. Multiple species may serve as hosts in a given geographical area, and the strain of virus and likelihood of causing disease in man vary from region to region. Thus far, there are about five dominant virus-rodent-human disease (if known) associations: (i) Hantaan virus—the field mouse *Apodemus agrarius*—KHF in Korea (H. W. Lee, 1982; H. W. Lee et al., 1978) and the severe form of EHF in China (Song et al., 1983); (ii) Puumala virus—the bank vole *Clethrionomys glareolus*—NE in Eastern Europe and Scandinavia (Lahdevirta, 1971; Chumakov et al., 1981; Lahdevirta et al., 1984; Yanagihara et al., 1985a); (iii) Urban and laboratory rat viruses—*Rattus norvegicus* —moderate disease in people, mostly in Asia but occasionally in Europe (Umenai et al., 1979; Van Ypersele de Strihou, 1979; H. W. Lee and Johnson, 1982; H. W. Lee et al., 1982; Desmyter et al., 1983; Kitamura et al., 1983; Dournan et al., 1984; Lloyd et al., 1984; Kawamata et al. 1987); (iv) Girard Point and other viruses from North and South America—*Rattus norvegicus*—no disease recognized in humans although serological evidence of infection has been found (LeDuc et al.,

1984, 1985a; Childs et al., 1985, 1988; Tsai, 1985; Yanagihara et al., 1985b); and (v) Prospect Hill virus—the meadow vole *Microtus pennsylvanicus*—no disease recognized in people (LeDuc et al., 1984).

### *Epizootiology*

Hantaviruses are transmitted to humans from persistently infected rodents and other small mammals. In laboratory settings, this has usually been from laboratory rats or their tumors to people. The major mode of transmission is respiratory infection by aerosols of urine, feces, and saliva containing infectious virus. Animal contact is not necessary as many visitors to infected animal facilities have contracted the infection. Animal bites can transmit the infection but appear to be of relatively minor importance (LeDuc, 1987; Tsai, 1987a).

Reservoir hosts of Hantaan virus show no clinical signs, but the virus appears in their lungs about ten days after infection and subsequently appears in the urine and saliva. Peak virus shedding occurs about three weeks after infection, but virus can be detected in the lungs for six months and occasionally for up to two years. Aerosols are the main method of transmission (H. W. Lee, 1982; W.H.O., 1983; Morita et al., 1985). The epizootiology of other *Hantavirus* infections is poorly understood.

Although hantaviruses appear to be worldwide in distribution, it should be emphasized that human disease due to these agents has been reported only in Europe and Asia. Serologic surveys of rats and other small mammals have given evidence of *Hantavirus* infections in many areas of the world where disease due to hantaviruses is not known to occur, including North and South America (P. W. Lee et al., 1981b; LeDuc et al., 1984, 1985a; Childs et al., 1985, 1987a,b; Tsai, 1985).

### *Clinical*

Reservoir hosts remain asymptomatic during infection (H. W. Lee, 1982; W.H.O., 1983).

The clinical severity of *Hantavirus* infections in people varies according to geographic distribution of virus strains and, possibly, to other factors. KHF caused by Hantaan virus ranges from severe to mild. The incubation period is usually 2-3 weeks. Signs include fever, headache, muscular pains, hemorrhages (cutaneous petechiae or ecchymoses, hemoptysis, hematuria, hematemesis, melena), and proteinuria (Earle, 1954; Giles et al., 1954; Sheedy et al., 1954). About 20% of patients develop shock, severe hemorrhages, and renal failure (the "hemorrhagic fever with renal syndrome"). Mortality can be 5-10% (H. W. Lee, 1982; W.H.O., 1983).

Cases of NE in human patients in Scandinavia tend to be relatively mild, have few hemorrhagic features, and show a mortality of less than 0.5%. There is acute onset of fever, headache, nausea, and vomiting followed in 3-6 days by proteinuria, oliguria, hematuria, and thrombocytopenia. Oliguria persists only a few days and is followed by polyuria. Most patients recover within three weeks (W.H.O., 1983; Lahdevirta et al., 1984).

### *Pathology*

Lesions have not been observed in reservoir hosts infected with hantaviruses. Lungs and other tissues may contain large amounts of virus without morphologic lesions (H. W. Lee et al., 1981; P. W. Lee et al., 1981a; H. W. Lee, 1982; Kurata et al., 1983; LeDuc et al., 1984).

Characteristic lesions in human patients that die of KHF are retroperitoneal edema; diffuse myocardial hemorrhage in the right atrium of the heart; severe congestion, hemorrhage, and necrosis in the renal medulla; and hemorrhage and necrosis in the anterior lobe of the pituitary gland (Lukes, 1954).

Mice and rats have been used for studies of experimental Hantaan virus infections. This virus is fatal for newborn mice (P. W. Lee et al., 1981a; Kurata et al., 1983; Yamanouchi et al., 1984; Nakamura et al., 1985).

### *Diagnosis*

Laboratory rats and biological materials such as transplantable tumors from laboratory rats constitute the greatest concern, particularly those from Eurasian sources. Since *Hantavirus* infections in rodents are inapparent, the diagnosis is most likely to be made through health surveillance. The recommended serological tests for this purpose are indirect fluorescent antibody test, enzyme-linked immunosorbent assay, and hemagglutination inhibition. Non-infectious antigen should be used and care should be taken to work with animals and blood products in a biological safety cabinet. P3 conditions are needed for working with unconcentrated virus in small amounts (Johnson, 1988).

For testing transplantable tumors and other biologic materials for *Hantavirus* contamination, the rat antibody production (RAP) test is recommended. Use 6-week-old pathogen-free rats; they should be prebled (to obtain control serum) and blood for serological testing should be collected 6 weeks after inoculation. Again, it is necessary that P3 containment conditions be maintained because the virus is excreted in urine and feces (Johnson, 1988).

Rats of the LOU strain and the transplantable plasmacytomas from that strain, which originated from a colony in Belgium, have been found to be infected with a member of the genus *Hantavirus*, and a number of personnel contracted this infection in Belgium and the United Kingdom (van Ypersele de Strihou, 1979; Desmyter et al., 1983; Lloyd et al., 1984). Therefore, rats and tumors from these lines should be screened before use. A large number of rat cell lines maintained by the American Type Culture Collection in Rockville, Md., have been tested and found to be free of hantaviruses (LeDuc et al., 1985b). Also, LOU rats obtained by the National Institutes of Health from the University of Louvain in Belguim have been tested and found free of these viruses (Johnson, 1986).

The hantaviruses can be isolated and propagated in A-549 and Vero E6 cells (French et al., 1981; H. W. Lee, 1982; Kitamura et al., 1983; Schmaljohn et al., 1983; Yamanishi et al., 1983). Again, P3 conditions should be maintained.

### *Control*

The best approach is to prevent *Hantavirus* infections by obtaining only animals, transplantable tumors, and other biologic materials that have been tested and found to be free of the infection. Also, contamination of rodent stocks by wild rodents must be prevented.

Laboratory rodent stocks found to be infected with a *Hantavirus* should be destroyed and replaced with pathogen-free stock (W.H.O., 1983; HFRS, 1988). Although not proven to be effective, cesarean derivation has been recommended for eliminating the infection in valuable genetic stocks (Johnson, 1986; HFRS, 1988).

### *Interference with Research*

The hantaviruses are important zoonoses (Johnson, 1986; Tsai, 1987b).

# Part III
# Indexes to Diagnosis and Research Complications of Infectious Agents

# Introduction

Part III is intended to serve as an index for diagnostic problem solving in situations for which infectious agents of mice and rats may be responsible. Three index categories, clinical signs, pathology, and research complications, have been listed in alphabetical order. When a problem suspected of being caused by an infectious agent is encountered, one or more of these lists should be consulted to identify quickly the most likely causative agent(s). One should then consult the information in Part II on the most likely candidate agents to narrow the list of possible causes and to devise further testing to make the definitive diagnosis. Once the precise cause(s) is known, specific corrective measures can be implemented.

# Clinical Signs

Abdominal Enlargement
- Kilham rat virus
- Lymphocytic choriomeningitis virus
- Murine leukemia viruses

Abortions and Stillbirths
- *Streptobacillus moniliformis*

Abscesses
- Cervical
  - *Klebsiella pneumoniae*
  - *Pasteurella pneumotropica*
  - *Streptococcus pyogenes*
- Facial, orbital, and tail
  - *Staphylococcus aureus*
- Preputial gland
  - *Pasteurella pneumotropica*
  - *Staphylococcus aureus*

Alopecia
- (see Dermatitis and Alopecia)

Amputations, Necrotic, of Limbs or Tails
- *Corynebacterium kutscheri*
- Ectromelia virus
- *Mycoplasma arthritidis*
- Poxvirus(es) in rats
- Ringtail
- *Streptobacillus moniliformis*

Annular Constrictions of Tail
- Ringtail

Anorexia
- *Corynebacterium kutscheri*
- Ectromelia virus
- *Klebsiella pneumoniae*
- Poxvirus(es) in rats

Ataxia
- Kilham rat virus

Athymic (*nu*/*nu*) Mice, More Susceptible than Immunocompetent Mice to:
- *Chlamydia trachomatis*
- *Encephalitozoon cuniculi*
- *Giardia muris*
- Mouse cytomegalovirus
- Mouse hepatitis virus
- *Pneumocystis carinii*
- Pneumonia virus of mice

Polyoma virus
Sendai virus
*Spironucleus muris*
*Staphylococcus aureus*
*Syphacia* sp.

Athymic (*nu/nu*) Mice, Equally or Less Susceptible than Immunocompetent Mice to:
*Bacillus piliformis*
K virus
Lymphocytic choriomeningitis virus
*Mycobacterium avium-intracellulare*
*Mycoplasma pulmonis*
Reovirus-3
*Streptococcus pneumoniae*

Athymic (*nu/nu*) Mice, Not Susceptible to:
*Myobia musculi*
*Myocoptes musculinus*

Birth Weight Reduced
*Salmonella enteritidis*
Sendai virus

Cervical Edema
Sialodacryoadenitis virus

Chattering (Mice)
*Chlamydia trachomatis*
*Mycoplasma pulmonis*
Sendai virus

Circling (or Rolling)
Kilham rat virus
*Mycoplasma neurolyticum* (experimental)
*Pseudomonas aeruginosa*
*Streptobacillus moniliformis*
Theiler's virus

Conjunctivitis
Ectromelia virus
*Pasteurella pneumotropica*
*Salmonella enteritidis*
Sialodacryoadenitis virus
*Staphylococcus aureus*
*Streptobacillus moniliformis*

Convulsions
Theiler's virus

Corneal Ulceration
Sialodacryoadenitis virus

Cyanosis
*Chlamydia trachomatis*
*Haemobartonella muris*
*Salmonella enteritidis*
*Streptobacillus moniliformis*

Deaths, High Mortality (greater than 50%) Possible
*Bacillus piliformis*
*Citrobacter freundii* (Biotype 4280)
Ectromelia virus
Mouse hepatitis virus (infant mice)
Poxvirus(es) in rats
*Salmonella enteritidis*
*Streptobacillus moniliformis*
Theiler's virus

Deaths in Neonates
Mouse hepatitis virus
Sendai virus

Deaths Unlikely (in uncomplicated infections)
*Aspicularis tetraptera*
*Encephalitozoon cuniculi*
*Entamoeba muris*
*Eperythrozoon coccoides*
*Giardia muris*
Hantaviruses
H-1 virus
*Hymenolepis nana*
K virus
Lactic dehydrogenase-elevating virus
Minute virus of mice
Mouse adenoviruses
Mouse cytomegalovirus
Mouse thymic virus
*Mycobacterium avium-intracellulare*
*Mycoplasma arthritidis*

- *Mycoplasma collis*
- *Mycoplasma muris*
- *Mycoplasma neurolyticum*
- *Pasteurella pneumotropica*
- *Pneumocystis carinii*
- Pneumonia virus of mice
- Polyoma virus
- *Pseudomonas aeruginosa*
- *Radfordia affinis*
- Rat coronavirus
- Rat rotavirus-like agent
- Sialodacryoadenitis virus
- *Spironucleus muris*
- *Syphacia* sp.
- Theiler's virus
- *Tritrichomonas muris*

Deaths, Usually Low Mortality
- *Corynebacterium kutscheri*
- *Haemobartonella muris*
- Kilham rat virus
- Lymphocytic choriomeningitis virus
- Mouse hepatitis virus
- Mouse rotavirus
- *Mycoplasma pulmonis*
- *Salmonella enteritidis*
- Sendai virus
- *Streptococcus pneumoniae*

Dehydration (see Diarrhea)

Dermatitis and Alopecia
- Due to Infectious Agents
  - Dermatophytes (fungi)
  - Ectromelia virus
  - Mouse papule virus
  - *Myobia musculi*
  - *Myocoptes musculinus*
  - *Pasteurella pneumotropica*
  - *Staphylococcus aureus*
- Due to Noninfectious Causes
  - Bite (fight wounds)
  - Hair growth arrest
  - Muzzle alopecia
  - "Whisker trimming" ("hair nibbling," "barbering")

Diarrhea
- *Bacillus piliformis*
- *Citrobacter freundii* (Biotype 4280)
- *Giardia muris* (evidence uncertain)
- Mouse hepatitis virus (infant mice)
- Mouse rotavirus (infant mice)
- Reovirus-3 (evidence uncertain)
- *Salmonella enteritidis*
- *Spironucleus muris* (evidence uncertain)

Draining Superficial Lymph Nodes
- *Klebsiella pneumoniae*
- *Streptococcus pyogenes*

Dyspnea
- *Chlamydia trachomatis*
- Cilia-associated respiratory bacillus
- *Corynebacterium kutscheri*
- *Haemobartonella muris*
- Murine leukemia virus
- *Mycoplasma pulmonis*
- Sendai virus
- *Streptococcus pneumoniae*

Emaciation
- Lymphocytic choriomeningitis virus
- *Salmonella enteritidis*
- *Streptobacillus moniliformis*

Facial Abscesses
- *Staphylococcus aureus*

Facial Edema
- Ectromelia virus

Gestation Prolonged
- Sendai virus

Growth Retardation
- Cilia-associated respiratory bacillus
- *Citrobacter freundii* (Biotype 4280)
- *Hymenolepis nana*
- Kilham rat virus
- Lymphocytic choriomeningitis virus
- *Mycoplasma pulmonis*

Rat rotavirus-like agent
Reovirus-3 (evidence uncertain)
Sendai virus
Sialodacryoadenitis virus

Head Tilt
*Mycoplasma pulmonis*
*Pseudomonas aeruginosa*
Theiler's virus

Hemoglobinuria
*Haemobartonella muris*
*Streptobacillus moniliformis*

Hunched Posture
(see Reluctance to Move)

Hyperexcitability
Theiler's virus

Inapparent Infections (Agents that usually cause subclinical or latent infections under natural conditions)
*Aspicularis tetraptera*
*Bacillus piliformis*
*Corynebacterium kutscheri*
Dermatophytes
*Encephalitozoon cuniculi*
*Entamoeba muris*
*Eperythrozoon coccoides*
*Giardia muris*
*Haemobartonella muris*
Hantaviruses
*Hymenolepis nana*
K virus
Kilham rat virus
*Klebsiella pneumoniae*
Lactic dehydrogenase-elevating virus
*Leptospira interrogans* serovar *ballum*
Lymphocytic choriomeningitis virus
Minute virus of mice
Mouse adenoviruses
Mouse cytomegalovirus
Mouse hepatitis virus
Mouse mammary tumor virus
Mouse rotavirus

Jaundice
Kilham rat virus
Mouse hepatitis virus (athymic mice)
Reovirus-3 (evidence uncertain)

Keratoconus
Sialodacryoadenitis virus

Kyphosis
*Streptobacillus moniliformis*

Litter Size Reduced
Kilham rat virus
*Salmonella enteritidis*
Sendai virus

Lymphadenopathy
Cervical
*Klebsiella pneumoniae*
*Streptococcus pyogenes*
Peripheral
Murine leukemia viruses
*Myobia musculi*
*Myocoptes musculinus*

Mastitis
*Pasteurella pneumotropica*

Ocular Discharge
Sialodacryoadenitis virus

Pallor (Anemia)
*Haemobartonella muris*
*Streptobacillus moniliformis*

Panophthalmitis
*Pasteurella pneumotropica*

Papular Rash
Ectromelia virus
Poxvirus(es) in rats

Paralysis of Rear Legs
Lactic dehydrogenase-elevating virus (in C58 and AKR mice)
Polyoma virus [in athymic (*nu/nu*) mice]

*Streptobacillus moniliformis*
Theiler's virus

Photophobia
Sialodacryoadenitis virus
*Streptobacillus moniliformis*

Pododermatitis
*Staphylococcus aureus*

Polypnea
Cilia-associated respiratory bacillus
*Corynebacterium kutscheri*
*Mycoplasma pulmonis*
*Streptococcus pneumoniae*

Priapism
*Streptobacillus moniliformis*

Pruritis
Dermatophytes (fungi)
*Myobia musculi*
*Myocoptes musculinus*
*Staphylococcus aureus*

Rectal Prolapse
*Citrobacter freundii* (Biotype 4280)
*Syphacia* sp. (evidence uncertain)

Reluctance to Move (Animals often sit in hunched posture and have ruffled coats)
*Bacillus piliformis*
*Chlamydia trachomatis*
Ectromelia virus
Lymphocytic choriomeningitis virus
*Mycoplasma pulmonis*
*Salmonella enteritidis*

Respiratory Rales
Cilia-associated respiratory bacillus
*Corynebacterium kutscheri*
*Mycoplasma pulmonis*
*Streptococcus pneumoniae*

Ruffled Hair Coat
(see Reluctance to Move)

Runting
(see Wasting Syndrome)

Scrotal Cyanosis
Kilham rat virus

Self-Mutilation of Penis
*Staphylococcus aureus*

Skin Ulceration
Dermatophytes (fungi)
*Myobia musculi*
*Myocoptes musculinus*
*Staphylococcus aureus*

Sneezing
*Klebsiella pneumoniae*
*Mycoplasma pulmonis*
Sialodacryoadenitis virus

Snuffling
Cilia-associated respiratory bacillus
*Mycoplasma pulmonis*
Sendai virus
Sialodacryoadenitis virus
*Streptococcus pneumoniae*

Stunted Growth
(see Growth Retardation)

Subcutaneous Mass
Mouse mammary tumor virus

Swelling (Edema)
Feet and tail
Ectromelia virus
Poxvirus(es) of rats
Ringtail
*Streptobacillus moniliformis*
Neck
Sialodacryoadenitis virus

Swollen, Reddened Joints
*Corynebacterium kutscheri*
*Mycoplasma arthritidis*
*Streptobacillus moniliformis*

Tremors
Theiler's virus

Wasting Syndrome
- Mouse hepatitis virus [athymic (*nu/nu*) mice]
- Polyoma virus [athymic (*nu/nu*) mice]

Weight Loss
- *Chlamydia trachomatis*
- *Citrobacter freundii* (Biotype 4280)
- *Corynebacterium kutscheri*
- *Haemobartonella muris*
- *Hymenolepis nana*
- Kilham rat virus
- *Mycoplasma pulmonis*
- *Salmonella enteritidis*
- Sialodacryoadenitis virus
- *Streptococcus pneumoniae*

# Pathology

Abscesses
- Cervical lymph nodes
  - *Klebsiella pneumoniae*
  - *Pasteurella pneumotropica*
  - *Streptococcus pyogenes*
- Face, orbits, and tail
  - *Staphylococcus aureus*
- Kidney
  - *Corynebacterium kutscheri*
  - *Klebsiella pneumoniae*
- Liver
  - *Bacillus piliformis*
  - *Corynebacterium kutscheri*
  - *Klebsiella pneumoniae*
- Lung
  - Cilia-associated respiratory bacillus
  - *Mycoplasma pulmonis*
- Mesenteric lymph nodes
  - *Klebsiella pneumoniae*
- Preputial glands
  - *Pasteurella pneumotropica*
  - *Staphylococcus aureus*

Age-Dependent Polioencephalomyelitis
- Lactic dehydrogenase-elevating virus

Alopecia (see Dermatitis and Alopecia)

Amputations, Necrotic, of Limbs or Tails
- *Corynebacterium kutscheri*
- Ectromelia virus
- *Mycoplasma arthritidis*
- Poxvirus(es) in rats
- Ringtail
- *Streptobacillus moniliformis*

Amyloidosis
- *Myobia musculi*

Anemia
- *Haemobartonella muris*
- Murine leukemia viruses
- *Streptobacillus moniliformis*

Ankylosis
- *Streptobacillus moniliformis*

Arthritis
- *Corynebacterium kutscheri*
- *Mycoplasma arthritidis*

*Mycoplasma pulmonis* [athymic (*nu*/*nu*) mice]
*Streptobacillus moniliformis*

Ascites
- *Encephalitozoon cuniculi*
- Lymphocytic choriomeningitis virus

Atelectasis (Lung)
- Cilia-associated respiratory bacillus
- K virus (experimental)
- *Mycoplasma pulmonis*
- Sendai virus

Blood parasites
- *Eperythrozoon coccoides*
- *Haemobartonella muris*

Brain
- Cerebellar hypoplasia
  - Kilham rat virus
- Choroiditis
  - Lymphocytic choriomeningitis virus
- Ependymitis
  - Lymphocytic choriomeningitis virus
- Glial nodules
  - *Encephalitozoon cuniculi*
- Hemorrhage
  - Kilham rat virus
- Intranuclear inclusions
  - Kilham rat virus
- Leptomeningitis
  - *Encephalitozoon cuniculi*
  - Lymphocytic choriomeningitis virus
  - *Streptococcus pneumoniae*
- Syncytial giant cells
  - Mouse hepatitis virus

Bronchiectasis and Bronchiolectasis
- Cilia-associated respiratory bacillus
- *Mycoplasma pulmonis*

Bronchiolar Scarring
- Cilia-associated respiratory bacillus
- Sendai virus

Bronchiolitis Obliterans
- Cilia-associated respiratory bacillus

Cell Fragment Thrombi
- *Salmonella enteritidis*

Cerebellar Hypoplasia
- Kilham rat virus

Colon and Cecum
- Cecocolitis
  - *Bacillus piliformis*
- Colonic hyperplasia
  - *Citrobacter freundii* (Biotype 4280)
- Goblet cell hyperplasia
  - *Citrobacter freundii* (Biotype 4280)
- Helminth parasites
  - *Aspicularis tetraptera*
  - *Syphacia* sp.
- Hyperplastic typhlocolitis
  - Hepatitis virus, mouse [athymic (*nu*/*nu*) mice]
- Protozoan parasites
  - *Entamoeba muris*
  - *Tritrichomonas muris*

Cutaneous Papules, Erosions or Encrustations
- Ectromelia virus
- Mouse papule virus

Demyelination and Remyelination
- Theiler's virus

Dermatitis and Alopecia (see Clinical Signs above)

Ear
- Otitis interna
  - *Mycoplasma pulmonis*
  - *Pseudomonas aeruginosa*
  - *Streptobacillus moniliformis*
- Otitis media
  - Cilia-associated respiratory bacillus

Hypersensitivity, Cutaneous
- *Myobia musculi*
- *Myocoptes musculinus*
- *Staphylococcus aureus*

Immune Complex
- Glomerulonephritis
- Lactic dehydrogenase-elevating virus
- Lymphocytic choriomeningitis virus

Inclusions
- Intracytoplasmic (skin)
  - Ectromelia virus
  - Mouse papule virus
  - Poxvirus(es) in rats
- Intracytoplasmic and intranuclear (bronchi, ureters, and renal pelvis)
  - Polyoma virus [athymic (*nu/nu*) mice]
- Intranuclear
  - Harderian gland
    - Sialodacryoadenitis virus
  - Intestinal mucosa
    - Adenovirus, mouse (MAd-2)
  - Lung endothelium
    - K virus
  - Salivary gland
    - Mouse cytomegalovirus
    - Rat cytomegalovirus
  - Thymus
    - Mouse thymic virus

Infarcts
- Central nervous system, epididymis, and testes
  - Kilham rat virus
- Spleen and testes
  - *Streptococcus pneumoniae*

Intestine, Small
- Blunting of villi
  - *Bacillus piliformis*
  - Mouse hepatitis virus
  - Mouse rotavirus
  - Rat rotavirus-like agent
- Enteritis
  - *Bacillus piliformis*
  - *Giardia muris*
  - *Hymenolepis nana*
  - Mouse adenovirus (MAd-2)
  - Mouse hepatitis virus
  - Rat rotavirus-like agent
  - Reovirus-3 (evidence uncertain)
  - *Salmonella enteritidis*
  - *Spironucleus muris*
- Enteritis with ulceration
  - Mouse hepatitis virus
- Enteritis with ulceration and hemorrhage
  - *Bacillus piliformis*
  - *Citrobacter freundii* (Biotype 4280)
  - Ectromelia virus
- Helminth parasite
  - *Hymenolepis nana*
- Ileocecocolitis
  - *Bacillus piliformis*
  - *Citrobacter freundii*
  - *Salmonella enteritidis* (Biotype 4280)
- Protozoan parasites
  - *Giardia muris*
  - *Spironucleus muris*
- Syncytial epithelial giant cells
  - Mouse hepatitis virus
  - Rat rotavirus-like agent

Keratitis
- Sialoacryoadenitis virus

Kidney
- Cortical pitting and scarring
  - *Encephalitozoon cuniculi*
- Nephritis
  - *Corynebacterium kutscheri*
  - *Encephalitozoon cuniculi*
  - *Klebsiella pneumoniae*
- Protozoan parasite
  - *Encephalitozoon cuniculi*

Lacrimal Glands (dacryoadenitis, intranuclear inclusions, necrosis, squamous metaplasia)
- Sialodacryoadenitis virus

- Necrosis, Multifocal
  - Ectromelia virus
  - *Salmonella enteritidis*
  - *Streptobacillus moniliformis*
- Teratogenic effects
  - Kilham rat virus
- Thrombi
  - *Salmonella enteritidis*
  - *Streptococcus pneumoniae*

Splenitis
- Acute bacterial
  - *Streptococcus pneumoniae*
- Granulomatous
  - *Mycobacterium avium-intracellulare*
- Pyogranulomatous
  - *Salmonella enteritidis*

Splenomegaly
- *Corynebacterium kutscheri*
- Ectromelia virus
- *Eperythrozoon coccoides*
- *Haemobartonella muris*
- Lymphocytic choriomeningitis virus
- Mouse hepatitis virus
- *Myobia musculi*
- *Myocoptes musculinus*
- *Salmonella enteritidis*
- *Streptobacillus moniliformis*
- *Streptococcus pneumoniae*

Synctial Giant Cells
- Brain
  - Mouse hepatitis virus
- Bronchial epithelium
  - *Mycoplasma pulmonis* (mouse)
  - Sendai virus
- Intestinal epithelium
  - Mouse hepatitis virus
  - Rat rotavirus-like agent
- Multiple organs
  - Hepatitis virus, mouse [athymic (*nu*/*nu*) mice]
- Nasal epithelium
  - *Mycoplasma pulmonis* (mouse)

Teratogenic Effects
- Kilham rat virus

Testes
- Hemorrhage
  - Kilham rat virus
- Infarction
  - Kilham rat virus
  - *Streptococcus pneumoniae*

Thrombocytopenia
- Mouse cytomegalovirus

Thrombosis
- Central nervous system, epididymis, and testes
  - Kilham rat virus
- Liver and spleen
  - *Salmonella enteritidis*
- Spleen and testes
  - *Streptococcus pneumoniae*

Thymus
- Enlargement
  - Murine leukemia viruses
- Necrosis
  - Ectromelia virus
  - Lactic dehydrogenase-elevating virus
  - Mouse thymic virus
  - Sialodacryoadenitis virus

Tracheitis
- Cilia-associated respiratory bacillus
- *Corynebacterium kutscheri*
- *Mycoplasma pulmonis*
- Sendai virus
- Sialodacryoadenitis virus
- *Streptococcus pneumoniae*

Typhlocolitis
- Mouse hepatitis virus [athymic (*nu*/*nu*) mice]

Ulcerative Cecitis in Rats
*Salmonella enteritidis*

Ulcerative Dermatitis
*Myobia musculi*
*Myocoptes musculinus*
*Staphylococcus aureus*

Uterus
Endometritis
*Mycoplasma pulmonis*
Fetal resorption
Kilham rat virus
Sendai virus
*Streptobacillus piliformis*
Pyometra
*Mycoplasma pulmonis*

# Research Complications

Altered Immune Response
- Ectromelia virus
- *Encephalitozoon cuniculi*
- *Eperythrozoon coccoides*
- *Giardia muris*
- *Haemobartonella muris*
- Kilham rat virus
- Lactic dehydrogenase-elevating virus
- Lymphocytic choriomeningitis virus
- Minute virus of mice
- Mouse cytomegalovirus
- Mouse hepatitis virus
- Mouse thymic virus
- *Mycoplasma pulmonis*
- *Myobia musculi*
- *Myocoptes musculinus*
- *Salmonella enteritidis*
- Sendai virus
- *Spironucleus muris*
- *Syphacia* sp.

Altered Physiologic, Pharmacologic, or Toxicologic Response
- *Bacillus piliformis*
- *Haemobartonella muris*
- Kilham rat virus
- Lactic dehydrogenase-elevating virus
- Mouse hepatitis virus
- *Mycoplasma pulmonis*
- *Salmonella enteritidis*
- *Streptococcus pneumoniae*

Altered Susceptibility to Other Infections
- *Encephalitozoon cuniculi*
- *Eperythrozoon coccoides*
- *Haemobartonella muris*
- K virus (experimental)
- Lactic dehydrogenase-elevating virus
- Lymphocytic choriomeningitis virus
- Mouse cytomegalovirus
- Mouse hepatitis virus
- Mouse rotavirus
- *Mycoplasma pulmonis*
- *Salmonella enteritidis*
- Sendai virus
- Sialodacryoadenitis virus

Carcinogenesis or Spontaneous Neoplasia
- *Citrobacter freundii* (Biotype 4280)
- H-1 virus
- Lactic dehydrogenase-elevating virus
- Lymphocytic choriomeningitis virus
- Mouse mammary tumor virus
- *Mycoplasma pulmonis*
- Polyoma virus
- Sendai virus

Contamination of Cell Cultures
- Kilham rat virus
- Lymphocytic choriomeningitis virus
- Minute virus of mice
- *Mycoplasma arthritidis*
- *Mycoplasma pulmonis*
- Polyoma virus
- Reovirus-3

Contamination of Transplantable Tumors and Altered Host Response
- *Encephalitozoon cuniculi*
- *Haemobartonella muris*
- H-1 virus
- Kilham rat virus
- Lactic dehydrogenase-elevating virus
- Lymphocytic choriomeningitis virus
- Minute virus of mice
- *Mycoplasma arthritidis*
- *Mycoplasma neurolyticum*
- *Mycoplasma pulmonis*
- Polyoma virus
- Reovirus-3
- Sendai virus

Inapparent Infection Exacerbated by Experimental Immunosuppression
- *Bacillus piliformis*
- *Corynebacterium kutscheri*
- Ectromelia virus
- *Eperythrozoon coccoides*
- *Giardia muris*
- *Haemobartonella muris*
- Kilham rat virus
- Mouse hepatitis virus
- *Mycoplasma pulmonis*
- *Pneumocystis carinii*
- *Pseudomonas aeruginosa*
- *Salmonella enteritidis*
- *Spironucleus muris*

Zoonotic Agents (Infectious for Humans)
- Dermatophytes (fungi)
- Hantaviruses
- *Hymenolepis nana*
- *Leptospira interrogans* serovar *ballum*
- Lymphocytic choriomeningitis virus
- Poxvirus(es) in rats
- Rat rotavirus-like agent
- *Salmonella enteritidis*
- *Streptobacillus moniliformis*
- *Streptococcus pneumoniae*

# References


AALAS (American Association of Laboratory Animal Science). 1981. Ectromelia (mousepox) in the United States. Proceedings of a seminar presented at the 31st annual meeting of AALAS held in Indianapolis, Indiana, October 8, 1980. Lab. Anim. Sci. 31:549-631.

Abrams, G. D., H. Schneider, S. B. Formal, and H. Sprinz. 1963. Cellular renewal and mucosal morphology in experimental enteritis. Infection with *Salmonella typhimurium* in the mouse. Lab. Invest. 12:1241-1248.

Ackerman, J. I., and J. G. Fox. 1981. Isolation of *Pasteurella ureae* from reproductive tracts of congenic mice. J. Clin. Microbiol. 13:1049-1053.

Ackerman, J. I., J. G. Fox, and J. C. Murphy. 1984. An enzyme linked immunosorbent assay for detection of antibodies to *Corynebacterium kutscheri*. Lab. Anim. Sci. 34:38-43.

Ackermann, R. 1973. Epidemiologic aspects of lymphocytic choriomeningitis in man. Pp. 233-237 in Lymphocytic Choriomeningitis Virus and Other Adenoviruses, F. Lehmann-Grube, ed. New York: Springer-Verlag.

Adams, W. R., and L. M. Kraft. 1963. Epizootic diarrhea of infant mice. Identification of the etiologic agent. Science 141:359-360.

Adams, W. R., and L. M. Kraft. 1967. Electron-microscopic study of the intestinal epithelium of mice infected with agent of epizootic diarrhea of infant mice (EDIM virus). Am. J. Pathol. 51:39-60.

Adlam, C., and C. S. F. Easmon. 1983. Immunity and hypersensitivity to staphylococcal infection. Pp. 275-323 in Staphylococci and Staphylococcal Infections, vol. 1, C. S. F. Easmon and C. Adlam, eds. New York: Academic Press.

Afzelius, B. A. 1979. The immotile-cilia syndrome and other ciliary diseases. Internat. Rev. Exp. Pathol. 19:1-43.

Aguila, H. N., W. C. Lai, Y. S. Lu, and S. P. Pakes. 1988. Experimental *Mycoplasma pulmonis* infection of rats suppresses humoral but not cellular immune response. Lab. Anim. Sci. 38:138-142.

Akimaru, K., G. M. Stuhlmiller, and H. F. Siegler. 1981. Influence of mouse hepatitis virus on the growth of human melanoma in the peritoneal cavity of the athymic nude mouse. J. Surg. Oncol. 17:327-339.

Alexander, A. D. 1984. Leptospirosis in laboratory mice. Science 224:1158 (letter).

Alexander, A. D. 1985. Leptospira. Pp. 473-478 in Manual of Clinical Microbiology, 4th ed., E. H. Lennette, A. Balows, W. J. Hausler, Jr., and H. J. Shadomy, eds. Washington, D.C.: American Society for Microbiology.

Allan, J. E., G. R. Shellam, and J. R. Grundy. 1982. Effect of murine cytomegalovirus infection on mitogen responses in genetically resistant and susceptible mice. Infect. Immun. 36:235-242.

Allen, A. M., J. R. Ganaway, T. D. Moore, and R. F. Kinard. 1965. Tyzzer's disease syndrome in laboratory rabbits. Am. J. Pathol. 46:859-882.

Allen, A. M., G. L. Clarke, J. R. Ganaway, A. Lock, and R. M. Werner. 1981. Pathology and diagnosis of mousepox. Lab. Anim. Sci. 31:599-608.

Allen, A. M., M. J. Collins, Jr., and F. Fenner. 1986. Ectromelia. Pp. I.A.1-I.A.3 in Manual of Microbiologic Monitoring of Laboratory Animals, A. M. Allen and T. Nomura, eds. NIH Pub. No. 86-2498. Washington, D.C.: U.S. Department of Health and Human Services.

Aleu, F., and L. Thomas. 1966. Studies of PPLO infection. III. Electron microscopic study of brain lesions caused by *Mycoplasma neurolyticum* toxin. J. Exp. Med. 124:1083-1088.

Allison, A. C. 1980. Immune responses to polyoma virus and polyoma virus-induced tumors. Pp. 481-487 in Viral Oncology, G. Klein, ed. New York: Raven Press.

Amor, B., A. Kahan, and F. Delbane. 1964. La polyarthrite du rat a *Mycoplasma arthritidis*. III. Caracteristiques; roles des "peri pneumonia like organisms." C.R. Soc. Biol. 158:1244-1246.

Anderson, M. J., J. R. Pattison, R. J. R. Cureton, S. Argent, and R. B. Heath, 1980. The role of host responses in the recovery of mice from Sendai virus infection. J. Gen. Virol. 46:373-379.

Anderson, C. A., J. C. Murphy, and J. G. Fox. 1983. Evaluation of murine cytomegalovirus antibody detection by serological techniques. J. Clin. Microbiol. 18:753-758.

Anderson, C. A., J. C. Murphy, and J. G. Fox. 1986. Surveillance of mice for antibodies to murine cytomegalovirus. J. Clin. Microbiol. 23:1152-1154.

Anderson, L. C., S. L. Leary, and P. J. Manning. 1983. Rat-bite fever in animal research laboratory personnel. Lab. Anim. Sci. 33:292-294.

Andrews, J. S., J. J. Ellner, and D. P. Stevens. 1980. Identification of anti-*Giardia* antibodies in murine breast milk. Clin. Res. 27:340A.

Ansari, K. A., C. F. Neilson, and P. G. Stansly. 1963. Pathogenesis of infectious splenic enlargement in mice. Exp. Mol. Pathol. 2:61-68.

Ansbacher, L., M. F. Nichols, and A. W. Hahn. 1988. The influence of *Encephalitozoon cuniculi* on nerual tissue responses to implanted biomaterials in the rabbit. Lab. Anim. Sci. 38:689-695.

Antopol, W. 1950. Anatomic changes in mice treated with excessive doses of cortisone. Proc. Soc. Exp. Biol. Med. 73:262-265.

Antopol, W., S. Glaubach, H. Quittner, and I. Saphra. 1951. Experimental observations with massive doses of cortisone. Rheumatism 7:187-197.

Antopol, W., H. Quittner, and I. Saphra. 1953. "Spontaneous" infections after the administration of cortisone and ACTH. Am. J. Pathol. 29:599-600.

Appell, L. H., R. M. Kovatch, J. M. Reddecliff, and P. J. Gerone. 1971. Pathogenesis of Sendai virus infection in mice. Am. J. Vet. Res. 32:1835-1841.

Argyris, T. S. 1963. Hair growth cycles and skin neoplasia. Pp. 33-43 in Conference on Biology of Cutaneous Cancer. NCI Monograph 10. Washington, D.C.: U.S. Department of Health, Eduation, and Welfare. 140 pp.

Arison, R. N., J. A. Cassaro, and C. E. Shonk. 1963. Factors which affect plasma lactic dehydrogenase in tumor bearing mice. Proc. Soc. Exp. Biol. Med. 113:497-501.

Arison, R. N., J. A. Cassaro, and M. P. Pruss. 1966. Studies on murine ascites-producing agent and its effect on tumor development. Cancer Res. 26:1915-1920.

Ash, G. W. 1971. An epidemic of chronic skin ulceration in rats. Lab. Anim. 5:112-115.

Ashley, M. P., S. H. Neoh, I. Kotlarski, and D. Hardy. 1976. Local and systemic effects in the non-specific tumour resistance induced by attenuated *Salmonella enteritidis* llRX in mice. Aust. J. Exp. Biol. Med. Sci. 54:157-168.

Astell, C. R., M. Thomson, M. Merchlinsky, and D. C. Ward. 1983. The complete DNA sequence of minute virus of mice, and autonomous parvovirus. Nucleic Acids Res. ll:999-1018.

Ata, F. A., E. H. Stephenson, and J. Storz. 1971. Inapparent respiratory infection of inbred Swiss mice with sulfadiazine-resistant, iodine-negative chlamydiae. Infect. Immun. 4:506-507.

Attwood, H. D., and R. D. Sutton. 1965. *Encephalitozoon* granulomata in rats. J. Pathol. Bacteriol. 89:735-738.

Baer, H. 1967. *Diplococcus pneumoniae* type 16 in laboratory rats. Can. J. Comp. Med. 31:216-218.

Baer, H., and A. Preiser. 1969. Type 3 *Diplococcus pneumoniae* in laboratory rats. Can. J. Comp. Med. 33:113-117.

Baer, P. N., and L. Kilham. 1962a. Rat virus and periodontal disease. I. The periodontium in the mongoloid hamster. Oral Surg., Oral Med. and Oral Pathol. 15:756-763.

Baer, P. N., and L. Kilham. 1962b. Rat virus and periodontal disease. II. Onset and effect of age at time of inoculation. Oral Surg., Oral Med. and Oral Pathol. 15:1302-1311.

Baer, P. N., and L. Kilham. 1964. Rat virus and periodontal disease. III. The histopathology of the early lesions in the first molar. Oral. Surg., Oral Med. and Oral Pathol. 17:116-124.

Baer, P. N., and L. Kilham. 1974. Dental defects in hamsters infected with minute virus of mice. Oral Surg. 37:385-389.

Baggs, R. B., and S. A. Miller. 1974. Defect in resistance to *Salmonella typhimurium* in iron deficient rats. J. Infect. Dis. 130:409-411.

Bailey, J. M., J. Clough, and A. Lohaus. 1965a. Influence of LDH viruses on growth of Erhlich ascites tumor in mice. Proc. Soc. Exp. Biol. Med. 119:1200-1204.

Bailey, J. M., J. Clough, A. Lohaus, and D. Wright. 1965b. A comparative study of LDH viruses from different tumors. Fed. Proc. 24:597-602.

Bailey, O. T., A. M. Pappenheimer, F. S. Cheever, and J. B. Daniels. 1949. A murine virus (JHM) causing disseminated encephalomyelitis with extensive destruction of myelin. II. Pathology. J. Exp. Med. 90:195-212.

Baker, E. W., T. M. Evans, D. J. Gould, W. B. Hull, and H. L. Keegan. 1956. A Manual of Parasitic Mites of Medical or Economic Importance. New York: National Pest Control Association. 170 pp.

Baker, H. J., G. H. Cassell, and J. R. Lindsey. 1971. Research complications due to *Haemobartonella* and *Eperythrozoon* infections in experimental animals. Am. J. Pathol. 64:625-635.

Baker, H. J., J. R. Lindsey, and S. H. Weisbroth. 1979. Housing to control research variables. Pp. 169-172 in The Laboratory Rat. Vol. I: Biology and Diseases, H. J. Baker, J. R. Lindsey, and S. H. Weisbroth, eds. New York: Academic Press.

Bakken, K., and T. M. Vogelsang. 1950. The pathogenesis of *Salmonella typhimurium* infection in mice. Acta Pathol. Microbiol. 27:41-50.

Balk, M. W. 1983. Overview of the state of the art in health monitoring. Pp. 3-23 in The Importance of Laboratory Animal Genetics, Health, and the Environment in Biomedical Research, E. C. Melby, Jr. and M. W. Balk, eds. Orlando, Fla.: Academic Press.

Balsari, A., C. Bianchi, A. Cocilova, I. Dragoni, G. Poli, and W. Ponti. 1981. Dermatophytes in clinically healthy laboratory animals. Lab. Anim. 15:75-77.

Baltimore, D. 1970. RNA-dependent DNA polymerase in virions of RNA tumor viruses. Nature 226:1209-1211.

Banfield, W. G., G. Kasnic, and J. H. Blakwell. 1968. Further observations on the virus of epizootic diarrhea of infant mice. An electron microscopic study. Virology 36:411-422.

Bang, F. B., and A. Warwick. 1960. Mouse macrophages as host cells for the mouse hepatitis virus and the genetic basis of their susceptibility. Proc. Natl. Acad. Sci. USA 46:1065-1075.

Bangaru, B., R. Morecki, J. H. Glaser, L. M. Gartner, and M. S. Horowitz. 1980. Comparative studies of biliary atresia in the human newborn and reovirus-induced cholangitis in weanling mice. Lab. Invest. 43:456-462.

Baquiche, M. 1959. Le dimorphisme sexuel de la glande de Loewenthal chez le rat albinos. Acta Anat. 36:247-280.

Barden, J. A., and J. G. Tully. 1969. Experimental arthritis in mice with *M. pulmonis*. J. Bacteriol. 100:5-10.

Barile, M. F. 1973. Mycoplasmal contamination of cell cultures: *Mycoplasma*, virus-cell interactions. Pp. 131-172 in Contamination in Tissue Culture. New York: Academic Press.

Baringer, J. R., and N. Nathanson. 1972. Parvovirus hemorrhagic encephalopathy of rats. Electron microscopic observations of the vascular lesions. Lab. Invest. 27:514-522.

Barkin, R. M., J. C. Guckian, and J. W. Glosser. 1974. Infection by *Leptospira ballum*: A laboratory associated case. South. Med. J. 67:155-176.

Barlow, J. L. 1964. Hyperreactivity to endotoxin in mice infected with lymphocytic choriomeningitis virus. Pp. 448-454 in Bacterial Endotoxins, M. Landy and W. Braun, eds. Rahway, N.J.: Quinn and Boden.

Barthold, S. W. 1980. The microbiology of transmissible murine colonic hyperplasia. Lab. Anim. Sci. 30:167-173.

Barthold, S. W. 1986a. Research complications and state of knowledge of rodent coronaviruses. Pp. 53-89 in Complications of Viral and Mycoplasma Infections in Rodents to Toxicology Research and Testing, T. E. Hamm, Jr., ed. Washington, D.C.: Hemisphere Press.

Barthold, S. W. 1986b. Mouse hepatitis virus biology and epizootiology. Pp. 571-601 in Viral and Mycoplasmal Infections of Laboratory Rodents: Effects on Biomedical Research. P. N. Bhatt, R. O. Jacoby, H. C. Morse III, and A. E. New, eds. Orlando, FL: Academic Press.

Barthold, S. W. 1987. Host age and genotype effects on enterotropic mouse hepatitis virus infection. Lab. Anim. Sci. 37:36-40.

Barthold, S. W., and D. S. Beck. 1987. Intranasal challenge immunity of mice to antigenically homologous and heterologous strains of mouse hepatitis virus. Adv. Exp. Med. Biol. 218:449-450.

Barthold, S. W., and D. G. Brownstein. 1988. The effect of selected viruses on *Corynebacterium kutscheri* infection in rats. Lab. Anim. Sci. 38:580-583.

Barthold, S. W., and A. M. Jonas. 1977. Morphogenesis of early 1,2-dimethylhydrazine-induced lesions and latent period reduction of colon carcinogenesis in mice by a variant of *Citrobacter freundii*. Cancer Res. 37:4352-4360.

Barthold, S. W., and C. Olson. 1974. Papovavirus-induced neoplasia. Pp. 70-75 in Handbook of Laboratory Animal Science, vol. II, E. C. Melby and N. H. Altman, eds. Cleveland: CRC Press.

Barthold, S. W., and A. L. Smith. 1983. Mouse hepatitis virus S in weanling Swiss mice following intranasal inoculation. Lab. Anim. Sci. 33:355-360.

Barthold, S. W., and A. L. Smith. 1984. Mouse hepatitis virus strain-related patterns of tissue tropism in suckling mice. Arch. Virol. 81:103-112.

Barthold, S. W., G. L. Coleman, P. N. Bhatt, G. W. Osbaldiston, and A. M. Jonas. 1976. The etiology of transmissible murine colonic hyperplasia. Lab. Anim. Sci. 26:889-894.

Barthold, S. W., G. W. Osbaldiston, and A. M. Jonas. 1977. Dietary, bacterial and host genetic interactions in the pathogenesis of transmissible murine colonic hyperplasia. Lab. Anim. Sci. 27:938-945.

Barthold, S. W., G. L. Coleman, R. O. Jacoby, E. M. Livstone, and A. M. Jonas. 1978. Transmissible murine colonic hyperplasia. Vet. Pathol. 15:223-236.

Barthold, S. W., A. L. Smith, P. F. S. Lord, P. N. Bhatt, R. O. Jacoby, and A. J. Main. 1982. Epizootic coronaviral typhlocolitis in suckling mice. Lab. Anim. Sci. 32:376-383.

Barthold, S. W., A. L. Smith, and M. L. Povar. 1985. Enterotropic mouse hepatitis virus infection in nude mice. Lab. Anim. Sci. 35:613-618.

Bartlett, M. S., P. A. Verbanc, and J. W. Smith. 1979. Growth of *Pneumocystis carinii* with WI-38 cells. J. Clin. Microbiol. 10:796-799.

Bartlett, M. S., M. M. Durkin, M. A. Jay, S. F. Queener, and J. W. Smith. 1987a. Sources of rats free of latent *Pneumocystis carinii*. J. Clin. Microbiol. 25:1794-1795.

Bartlett, M. S., S. F. Queener, M. A. Jay, M. M. Durkin, and J. W. Smith. 1987b. Improved rat model for studying *Pneumocystis carinii* pneumonia. J. Clin. Microbiol. 25:480-484.

Barton, E. G., Jr., and W. G. Campbell, Jr. 1967. Further observations on the ultrastructure of *Pneumocytis*. Arch. Pathol. 83:527-534.

Barton, E. G., Jr., and W. G. Campbell, Jr. 1969. *Pneumocystis carinii* in lungs of rats treated with cortisone acetate. Ultrastructural observations relating to the life cycle. Am. J. Pathol. 54:209-236.

Baskar, J. F., S. C. Stanat, K. K. Sulik, and E. S. Huang. 1983. Murine cytomegalovirus-induced congenital defects and fetal maldevelopment. J. Infect. Dis. 148:836-843.

Baskar, J. F., J. Peacock, K. K. Sulik, and E. S. Huang. 1987. Early-stage developmental abnormalities induced by murine cytomegalovirus. J. Infect. Dis. 155:661-666.

Bass, R., and F. M. Hetrick. 1978. Persistent infection of a human lymphocyte cell line (Molt-4) with the Kilham rat virus. J. Infect. Dis. 137:210-212.

Baum, S. G., A. M. Lewis, Jr., W. P. Rowe, and R. J. Huebner. 1966. Epidemic nonmeningitic lymphocytic-choriomeningitis-virus infection. An outbreak in a population of laboratory personnel. N. Engl. J. Med. 274:934-936.

Beall, J. R., F. E. Tornung, and R. S. Runkle. 1971. A laminar flow system for animal maintenance. Lab. Anim. Sci. 21:206-212.

Beaver, D. L., L. L. Ashburn, E. G. McDaniel, and N. D. Brown. 1963. Lipid deposits in the lungs of germ free animals. Arch. Pathol. 76:108-114.

Beck, R. W. 1963. A study in the control of *Pseudomonas aeruginosa* in a mouse breeding colony by the use of chlorine in the drinking water. Lab. Anim. Care 13:41-46.

Beckwith, C., N. Peterson, J. J. Liu, and J. A. Shadduck. 1988. Dot enzyme-linked immunosorbent assay (dot ELISA) for antibodies to *Encephalitozoon cuniculi*. Lab. Anim. Sci. 38:573-576.

Belosevic, M., and G. M. Faubert. 1983. *Giardia muris*: Correlation between oral dosage, course of infection and trophozoite distribution in the mouse small intestine. Exp. Parasitol. 56:93-100.

Belosevic, M., G. M. Faubert, E. Skamene, and J. D. MacLean. 1984. Susceptibility and resistance of inbred mice to *Giardia muris*. Infect. Immun. 44:282-286.

Belosevic, M., G. M. Faubert, and J. D. MacLean. 1985. Suppression of primary antibody response to sheep erythrocytes in susceptible and resistant mice infected with *Giardia muris*. Infect. Immun. 47:21-25.

Bender, L. 1925. Spontaneous central nervous system lesions in the laboratory rabbit. Am. J. Pathol. 1:653-656.

Benedettini, G., G. DeLibero, L. Mori, and M. Campa. 1984. *Staphylococcus aureus* inhibits contact sensitivity to oxazolone by activating suppressor B cells in mice. Int. Arch. Allergy Appl. Immunol. 73:269-273.

Bennette, J. G. 1960. Isolation of a non-pathogenic tumour-destroying virus from mouse ascites. Nature 187:72-73.

Bennette, J. G., P. V. Bush, and R. D. Steele. 1967. Characteristics of a newborn runt disease induced by neonatal infection with an oncolytic strain of reovirus type 3 (reo3MH). I. Pathological investigations in rats and mice. Br. J. Exp. Pathol. 48:251-266.

Bentley, D. M., S. R. Watson, and R. E. Morris. 1983. Age-related loss of Lyt-1,2 cells in C58 mice results in susceptibility to lactic dehydrogenase virus-induced polioencephalomyelitis. Infect. Immun. 41:1389-1390.

Bentvelzen, P., and J. Brinkhof. 1980. Ubiquity of natural antibodies to the mammary tumour virus in mice. Arch. Ges. Wulstforsch. 50:193-203.

Bentvelzen, P., and J. Hilgers. 1980. Murine mammary tumor virus. Pp. 311-355 in Viral Oncology, G. Klein, ed. New York: Raven Press.

Berendt, R. F., G. G. Long, R. B. Abeles, P. G. Canonico, M. R. Elwell, and M. C. Powanda. 1977. Pathogenesis of respiratory *Klebsiella pneumoniae* infection in rats: Bacteriological and histological findings and metabolic alterations. Infect. Immun. 15:586-593.

Berger, H., and W. H. Linkenheimer. 1962. Activation of *Bartonella muris* infection in x-irradiated rats. Proc. Soc. Exp. Biol. Med. 109:271-273.

Bergs, V. V. 1969. Rat virus-mediated suppression of leukemia induction by Maloney virus in rats. Cancer Res. 28:1669-1672.

Bergs, V. V., and R. M. Scotti. 1967. Virus-induced peliosis hepatitis in rats. Science 158:377-378.

Berkenkamp, S. D., and R. B. Wescott. 1988. Arthropod transmission of *Eperythrozoon coccoides* in mice. Lab. Anim. Sci. 38:398-401.

Bernard, C. 1865. An Introduction to the Study of Experimental Medicine (English translation by H. C. Greene, 1927). New York: MacMillan. 226 pp.

Bernhard, W. 1958. Electron microscopy of tumor cells and tumor viruses. A review. Cancer Res. 18:494-509.

Bertram, M. A., C. B. Inderlied, S. Yadegar, P. Kolanoski, J. K. Yamada, and L. S. Young. 1986. Confirmation of the beige mouse model for study of disseminated infection with *Mycobacterium avium* complex. J. Infect. Dis. 154:194-195.

Bhatt, P. N., and R. O. Jacoby. 1977. Experimental infection of adult axenic rats with Parker's rat coronavirus. Arch. Virol. 54:345-352.

Bhatt, P. N., and R. O. Jacoby. 1986. Mousepox: Pathogenesis, diagnosis and rederivation. Chapt. 24, pp. 557-570 in Viral and Mycoplasmal Infections of Laboratory Rodents: Effects on Biomedical Research. P. N. Bhatt, R. O. Jacoby, H. C. Morse III, and A. E. New, eds. Orlando, Fla.: Academic Press.

Bhatt, P. N., and R. O. Jacoby. 1987a. Mousepox in inbred mice innately resistant or susceptible to lethal infection with ectromelia virus. I. Clinical responses. Lab. Anim. Sci. 37:11-15.

Bhatt, P. N., and R. O. Jacoby. 1987b. Mousepox in inbred mice innately resistant or susceptible to lethal infection with ectromelia virus. III. Experimental transmission of infection and derivation of virus-free progeny from previously infected dams. Lab. Anim. Sci. 37:23-28.

Bhatt, P. N., and R. O. Jacoby. 1987c. Stability of ectromelia virus strain NIH-79 under various laboratory conditions. Lab. Anim. Sci. 37:33-35.

Bhatt, P. N., and R. O. Jacoby. 1987d. Effect of vaccination on the clinical response, pathogenesis and transmission of mousepox. Lab. Anim. Sci. 37:610-614.

Bhatt, P. N., and A. M. Jonas. 1974. An epizootic of Sendai virus infection with mortality in a barrier-maintained mouse colony. Am. J. Epidemiol. 100:222-229.

Bhatt, P. N., D. H. Percy, and A. M. Jonas. 1972. Characterization of the virus of sialodacryoadenitis of rats: A member of the coronavirus group. J. Infect. Dis. 126:123-130.

Bhatt, P. N., R. O. Jacoby, and A. M. Jonas. 1977. Respiratory infection in mice with sialodacryoadenitis virus, a coronavirus of rats. Infect. Immun. 18:823-827.

Bhatt, P. N., W. G. Downs, S. M. Buckley, J. Casals, R. E. Shope, and A. M. Jonas. 1981. Mousepox epizootic in an experimental and barrier mouse colony at Yale University. Lab. Anim. Sci. 31:560-564.

Bhatt, P. N., R. O. Jacoby, and S. W. Barthold. 1986. Contamination of transplantable murine tumors with lymphocytic choriomeningitis virus. Lab. Anim. Sci. 36:136-139.

Bhatt, P. N., R. O. Jacoby, and L. Gras. 1988. Mousepox in inbred mice innately resistant or susceptible to lethal infection with ectromelia virus. IV. Studies with the Moscow strain. Arch. Virol. 100:221-230.

Bieniek, V. H., and B. Tober-Meyer. 1976. Zur Atiologie der Colitis und des Prolapsus recti bei der Maus. Z. Versuchstierkd. 18:337-348.

Biggar, W. D., D. Bogart, B. Holmes, and R. A. Good. 1972. Impaired phagocytosis of *Pneumococcus* type 3 in splenectomized rats. Proc. Soc. Exp. Biol. Med. 139:903-908.

Biggar, R. J., R. Deibel, and J. P. Woodall. 1976. Implications, monitoring, and control of accidental transmission of lymphocytic choriomeningitis virus within hamster tumor cell lines. Cancer Res. 36:537-553.

Biggers, D. C., L. M. Kraft, and H. Sprinz. 1964. Lethal intestinal virus infection of mice (LIVIM). An important new model for study of the response of the intestinal mucosa to injury. Am. J. Pathol. 75:413-422.

Bishop, J. M., and H. E. Varmus. 1975. The molecular biology of RNA tumor viruses. Pp. 1-48 in Cancer: A Comprehensive Treatise, vol. 2., F. F. Becker, ed. New York: Plenum.

Bismanis, J. E. 1970. Detection of latent murine nosematosis and growth of *Nosema cuniculi* in cell culture. Can. J. Microbiol. 16:237-242.

Bittner, J. J. 1936. Some possible effects of nursing on the mammary gland tumor incidence in mice. Science 84:162.

Blackmore, D. K., and S. Casillo. 1972. Experimental investigation of uterine infections of mice due to *Pasteurella pneumotropica*. J. Comp. Pathol. 82:471-475.

Blackmore, D. K., and R. A. Francis. 1970. The apparent transmission of staphylococci of human origin to laboratory animals. J. Comp. Pathol. 80:645-651.

Blackwell, J. H., R. W. Tennant, and T. G. Ward. 1966. Serological studies with an agent of epizootic diarrhea of infant mice. Pp. 63-67 in Viruses of Laboratory Rodents, R. Holdenried, ed. National Cancer Institute Monograph 20. Washington, D.C.: U.S. Department of Health, Education, and Welfare.

Blailock, Z. R., E. R. Rabin, and J. L. Melnick. 1967. Adenovirus endocarditis in mice. Science 157:69-70.

Blailock, Z. R., E. R. Rabin, and J. L. Melnick. 1968. Adenovirus myocarditis in mice. An electron microscopic study. Exp. Mol. Pathol. 9:84-96.

Blanden, R. V., and C. A Mims. 1973. Macrophage activation in mice infected with ectromelia or lymphocytic choriomeningitis viruses. Aust. J. Exp. Biol. Med. Sci. 51:393-398.

Blanden, R. V., G. B. Mackaness, and F. M. Collins. 1966. Mechanisms of acquired resistance in mouse typhoid. J. Exp. Med. 124:585-600.

Blandford, G. 1975. Studies on the immune response and pathogenesis of Sendai virus infection of mice. III. The effects of cyclophosphamide. Immunology 28:871-883.

Blandford, G., and R. B. Heath. 1972. Studies on the immune response and pathogenesis of Sendai virus infection in mice. I. The fate of viral antigens. Immunology 22:637-649.

Blank, F. 1957. Favus of mice. Can. J. Microbiol. 3:885-896.

Boak, R. A., W. D. Linscott, and R. E. Bodfish. 1960. A case of *Leptospirosis ballum* in California. Calif. Med. 93:163-165.

Bogart, D., W. D. Biggar, and R. A. Good. 1972. Impaired intravascular clearance of *Pneumococcus* type 3 following splenectomy. J. Reticuloendothel. Soc. 11:77-87.

Bohme, D. H., H. A. Schneider, and J. M. Lee. 1959. Some physiopathological parameters of natural resistance to infection in murine salmonellosis. J. Exp. Med. 110:9-25.

Bohnhoff, M., and C. P. Miller. 1962. Enhanced susceptibility to *Salmonella* infection in streptomycin-treated mice. J. Infect. Dis. 111:117-127.

Bohnhoff, M., B. L. Drake, and C. P. Miller. 1954. Effect of streptomycin on susceptibility of intestinal tract to experimental *Salmonella* infection. Proc. Soc. Exp. Biol. Med. 86:132-137.

Bonath, K., ed. 1983. Schwerpunkte der Infektionsuberwachung in Versuchstierbestanden. Berlin: Paul Parey, Verlag. 79 pp.

Bond, S. B., P. M. Howley, and K. K. Takemoto. 1978. Characterization of K virus and its comparison with polyoma virus. J. Virol. 28:337-343.

Bonnard, B. D., E. K. Manders, D. A. Campbell, R. B. Herbermann, and M. J. Collins. 1976. Immunosuppressive activity of a subline of the mouse El-4 lymphoma. Evidence for minute virus of mice causing the inhibition. J. Exp. Med. 143:187-205.

Bonventre, P. F., H. C. Hubel, J. G. Michael, and A. D. Nickol. 1980. Impaired resistance to bacterial infection after tumor implant is traced to lactic dehydrogenase virus. Infect. Immun. 30:316-319.

Boorman, G. A., P. H. C. Lina, C. Zurcher, and H. T. M. Nieuwerkerk. 1973a. *Hexamita* and *Giardia* as a cause of mortality in congenitally thymus-less (nude) mice. Clin. Exp. Immunol. 15:623-627.

Boorman, G. A., J. I. M. Van Hooft, D. Van Der Waaij, and M. J. van Noord. 1973b. Synergistic role of intestinal flagellates and normal intestinal bacteria in post weaning mortality seen in mice. Lab. Anim. Sci. 23:187-193.

Boorman, G. A., M. I. Luster, J. H. Dean, M. L. Campbell, L. A. Lauer, F. A. Talley, R. E. Wilson, and M. J. Collins. 1982. Peritoneal macrophage alterations caused by naturally occurring mouse hepatitis virus. Am. J. Pathol. 106:110-117.

Booss, J., and E. F. Wheelock. 1977a. Role of viremia in the suppression of T-cell function during murine cytomegalovirus infection. Infect. Immun. 17:378-381.

Booss, J., and E. F. Wheelock. 1977b. Progressive inhibition of T-cell function preceding clinical signs of cytomegalovirus infection in mice. J. Infect. Dis. 135:478-481.

Booth, B. H. 1952. Mouse ringworm. Arch. Dermatol. Syphilol. 66:65-69.

Borum, K. 1954. Hair pattern and hair succession in the albino mouse. Acta Pathol. Microbiol. Scand. 34:521-541.

Boschert, K. R., T. R. Schoeb, D. B. Chandler, and D. L. Dillehay. 1988. Inhibition of phagocytosis and interleukin-1 production in pulmonary macrophages from rats with sialodacryoadenitis virus infection. J. Leukocyte Biol. 44:87-92.

Bowen, G. S., C. H. Calisher, W. G. Winkler, A. L. Kraus, E. H. Fowler, R. H. Garman, D. W. Fraser, and A. R. Hinman. 1975. Laboratory studies of a lymphocytic choriomeningitis virus outbreak in man and laboratory animals. Am. J. Epidemiol. 102:233-240.

Boyle, J. F., D. G. Weismiller, and K. V. Holmes. 1987. Genetic resistance to mouse hepatitis virus correlates with absence of virus-binding activity on target tissues. J. Virol. 61:185-189.

Brahic, M., W. G. Stroop, and J. R. Brainger. 1981. Theiler's virus persists in glial cells during demyelinating disease. Cell 26:123-128.

Braunsteiner, H., and C. Friend. 1954. Viral hepatitis associated with transplantable mouse leukemias. I. Acute hepatic manifestations following treatment with urethane or methylformamide. J. Exp. Med. 100:665-677.

Brautigam, A. R., and M. B. A. Oldstone. 1980. Replication of murine cytomegalovirus in reproductive tissues. Am. J. Pathol. 98:213-223.

Brennan, P. C., R. J. Flynn, and T. E. Fritz. 1965a. The isolation of *Salmonella cerro* from a closed colony of CF1 mice. Lab. Anim. Care 15:260-261.

Brennan, P. C., T. E. Fritz, and R. J. Flynn. 1965b. *Pasteurella pneumotropica:* Cultural and biochemical characteristics, and its association with disease in laboratory animals. Lab. Anim. Care 15:307-313.

Brennan, P. C., T. E. Fritz, R. J. Flynn, and C. M. Poole. 1965c. *Citrobacter freundii* associated with diarrhea in laboratory mice. Lab. Anim. Care 15:266-275.

Brennan, P. C., T. E. Fritz, and R. J. Flynn. 1969a. Murine pneumonia: A review of the etiologic agents. Lab. Anim. Care 19:360-371.

Brennan, P. C., T. E. Fritz, and R. J. Flynn. 1969b. Role of *Pasteurella pneumotropica* and *Mycoplasma pulmonis* in murine pneumonia. J. Bacteriol. 97:337-349.

Brett, S. J. 1983. Immunodepression in *Giardia muris* and *Spironucleus muris* infections in mice. Parasitology 87:507-515.

Brett, S. J., and F. E. G. Cox. 1982a. Immunological aspects of *Giardia muris* and *Spironucleus muris* infections in inbred and outbred strains of laboratory mice: A comparative study. Parasitology 85:85-99.

Brett, S. J., and F. E. G. Cox. 1982b. Interactions between the intestinal flagellates *Giardia muris* and *Spironucleus muris* and the blood parasites *Babesia microti, Plasmodium yoelii* and *Plasmodium berghei* in mice. Parasitology 85:101-110.

Brick, J. O., R. F. Newell, and D. G. Doherty. 1969. A barrier system for a breeding and experimental rodent colony: Description and operation. Lab. Anim. Care 19:92-97.

Briles, D. E., W. H. Benjamin, Jr., C. A. Williams, and J. M. Davie. 1981. A genetic locus responsible for *Salmonella* susceptibility in BSVS mice is not responsible for the limited T-dependent immune responsiveness of BSVS mice. J. Immunol. 127:906-911.

Brinton, M. A. 1982. Lactate dehydrogenase-elevating virus. Pp. 193-208 in The Mouse in Biomedical Research. Vol. II: Diseases, H. L. Foster, J. D. Small, and J. G. Fox, eds. New York: Academic Press.

Brinton, M. A., and I. Brand. 1977. Delayed foreign-body tumorigenesis in mice infected with lactate dehydrogenase-elevating virus: Brief communication. J. Natl. Cancer Inst. 59:1027-1029.

Briody, B. A. 1955. Mousepox (ectromelia) in the United States. Proc. Anim. Care Panel 6:1-8.

Briody, B. A. 1959. Response of mice to ectromelia and vaccinia viruses. Bacteriol. Rev. 23:61-95.

Briody, B. A. 1966. The natural history of mousepox. Pp. 105-116 in Viruses of Laboratory Rodents, R. Holdenried. ed. National Cancer Institute Monograph 20. Washington, D.C.: U.S. Department of Health, Education, and Welfare.

Briody, B. A., T. S. Hauschka, and E. A. Mirand. 1956. The role of genotype in resistance to an epizootic of mousepox (ectromelia). Am. J. Hyg. 63:59-68.

Bro-Jorgensen, K., and M. Volkert. 1972. Haemopoietic defects in mice infected with lymphocytic choriomeningitis virus. I. The enhanced x-ray sensitivity of the virus infected mice. Acta Pathol. Microbiol. Scand. 80:845-852.

Bro-Jorgensen, K., and M. Volkert. 1974. Defects in the immune system of mice infected with lymphocytic choriomeningitis virus. Infect. Immun. 9:605-614.

Bro-Jorgensen, K., F. Guttler, P. N. Jorgensen, and M. Volkert. 1975. T lymphocyte function as the principal target of lymphocytic choriomeningitis virus-induced immunosuppression. Infect. Immun. 11:622-629.

Broderson, J. R., J. R. Lindsey, and J. Crawford. 1976a. Role of environmental ammonia in respiratory mycoplasmosis of the rat. Am. J. Pathol. 85:115-130.

Broderson, J. R., F. A. Murphy, and J. C. Hierholzer. 1976b. Lethal enteritis in infant mice caused by mouse hepatitis virus. Lab. Anim. Sci. 26:824.

Brody, A. R., and J. E. Craighead. 1974. Pathogenesis of pulmonary cytomegalovirus infection in immunosuppressed mice. J. Infect. Dis. 129:677-689.

Brown, G. W., and I. I. Suter. 1969. Human infections with mouse favus in a rural area of South Australia. Med. J. Aust. 2:541-543.

Brownstein, D. G. 1978. Pathogenesis of *Pseudomonas aeruginosa* bacteremia in cyclophosphamide treated mice and potentiation of endogenous streptococcal virulence. J. Infect. Dis. 137:795-801.

Brownstein, D. G. 1983. Genetics of natural resistance to Sendai virus infection in mice. Infect. Immun. 41:308-312.

Brownstein, D. G. 1986. Sendai virus. Pp. 37-61. In Viral and Mycoplasmal Infections of Laboratory Rodents: Effects on Biomedical Research. P. N. Bhatt, R. O. Jacoby, H. C. Morse III, and A. E. New, eds. Orlando, Fla.: Academic Press.

Brownstein, D. G. 1987a. Tacheal mucociliary transport in laboratory mice: Evidence for genetic polymorphism. Exp. Lung Res. 13: 185-191.

Brownstein, D. G. 1987b. Resistance/susceptibility to lethal Sendai virus infection genetically linked to a mucocilary transport polymorphism. J. Virol. 61:1670-1671.

Brownstein, D. G., and S. W. Barthold. 1982. Mouse hepatitis virus immunofluorescence in formalin- or Bouin's-fixed tissue using trypsin digestion. Lab. Anim. Sci. 32:37-39.

Brownstein, D. G., and E. C. Weir. 1987. Immunostimulation in mice infected with Sendai virus. Am. J. Vet. Res. 12:1692-1696.

Brownstein, D. G., and S. Winkler. 1986. Genetic resistance to lethal Sendai virus pneumonia: virus replication and interferon production in C57BL/6J and DBA/2J mice. Lab. Anim. Sci. 36:126-129.

Brownstein, D. G., and S. Winkler. 1987. Genetic determinants of lung virus titers and resistance to lethal Sendai virus pneumonia. Arch. Virol. 96:201-214.

Brownstein, D. G., A. L. Smith, and E. A. Johnson. 1981. Sendai virus infection in genetically resistant and susceptible mice. Am. J. Pathol. 105:156-163.

Brownstein, D. G., S. W. Barthold, R. L. Adams, G. A. Terwilliger, and J. G. Aftosmis. 1985. Experimental *Corynebacterium kutscheri* infection in rats: bacteriology and serology. Lab. Anim. Sci. 36:135-138.

Brugerolle, G., I. Kunstyr, J. Senaud, and K. T. Friedhoff. 1980. Fine structure of trophozoites and cysts of the pathogenic diplomonad *Spironucleus muris*. Z. Parasitenkd. 62:47-61.

Bruggeman, C. A., H. Meijer, P. H. J. Dormans, W. M. H. Debie, G. E. L. M. Grauls, and C. P. A. van Boven. 1982. Isolation of a cytomegalovirus-like agent from wild rats. Arch. Virol. 73:231-241.

Bruggeman, C. A., W. M. H. Debie, G. Grauls, G. Majoors, and C. P. A. van Boven. 1983a. Infection of laboratory rats with a new cytomegalo-like virus. Arch. Virol. 76:189-199.

Bruggeman, C. A., H. Schellekens, G. Grauls, W. M. H. Debie, and C. P. A. van Boven. 1983b. Rat cytomegalovirus: Induction of and sensitivity to interferon. Antiviral Res. 3:315-324.

Bruggeman, C. A., H. Meijer. F. Bosman, and C. P. A. van Boven. 1985. Biology of rat cytomegalovirus infection. Intervirol 24:1- 9.

Bruggeman, C. A., J. H. Bruning, G. Grauls, A. E. J. M. van den Bogaard, and F. Bosman. 1987. Presence of cytomegalovirus in brown rat. Study in a rat model. Intervirol. 27:32-37.

Bruning, J. H., C. A. Bruggeman, C. P. A. van Boven, and P. J. C. van Breda Vriesman. 1986. Passive transfer of cytomegalovirus by cardiac and renal organ transplants in a rat model. Transplantation 41:695-698.

Brynjolfsson, G., and L. S. Lombard. 1969. Colitis cystica in mice. Cancer 23:225-229. (Note: This paper describes an entity that is very similar to *C. freundii* disease in mice. The etiology was not determined.)

Buchbinder, L., L. Hall, S. L. Wilens, and C. A. Slanetz. 1935. Observations on enzootic paratyphoid infection in a rat colony. Am. J. Hyg. 22:199-213.

Buchmeier, M. J., and M. B. A. Oldstone. 1978. Virus-induced immune complex disease: Identification of specific viral antigens and antibodies deposited in complexes during chronic lymphocytic choriomeningitis infection. J. Immunol. 120:1297-1304.

Budillon, G., M. Carrella, and M. Coltorti. 1972. Phenobarbital liver microsomal induction in MHV-3 viral hepatitis of the mouse. Experientia 28:1011-1012.

Budillon, G., M. Carrella, F. DeMarco, and G. Mazzacca. 1973. Effect of phenobarbital on MHV-3 viral hepatitis of the mouse. Pathol. Microbiol. 39:461-466.

Buhles, W. C., Jr., and M. Shifrine. 1977. Adjuvant protection against bacterial infection in granulocytopenic mice. J. Infect. Dis. 136:90-95.

Bukowski, J. F., B. A. Woda, S. Habu, K. Okumura, and R. M. Welsh. 1983. Natural killer cell depletion enhances virus synthesis and virus-induced hepatitis in vivo. J. Immunol. 131:1531-1538.

Bukowski, J. F., B. A. Woda, and R. M. Welsh. 1984. Pathogenesis of murine cytomegalovirus infection in natural killer cell-depleted mice. J. Virol. 52:119-128.

Buller, R. M. L., P. N. Bhatt, and G. D. Wallace. 1983. Evaluation of an enzyme-linked immunosorbent assay for the detection of ectromelia (mousepox) antibody. J. Clin. Microbiol. 18:1220-1225.

Buller, R. M. L., M. Potter, and G. D. Wallace. 1986. Variable resistance to ectromelia (mousepox) virus among genera of *Mus*. Curr. Top. Microbiol. Immunol. 127:319-322.

Buller, R. M. L., K. L. Holmes, A. Hugin, T. N. Frederickson, and H. C. Morse III. 1987a. Induction of cytotoxic T-cell responses in vivo in the absence of CD4 helper cells. Nature 328:77-79.

Buller, R. M. L., A. C. Weinblatt, A. W. Hamburger, and G. D. Wallace. 1987b. Observations on the replication of ectromelia virus in mouse-derived cell lines: Implications for epidemiology of mousepox. Lab. Anim. Sci. 37:28-32.

Buller, R. M. L., R. A. Yetter, T. N. Frederickson, and H. C. Morse III. 1987c. Abrogation of resistance to severe mousepox in C57BL/6 mice infected with LP-BM5 murine leukemia virus. J. Virol. 61:383-387.

Burek, J. D., G. C. Jersey, C. K. Whitehair, and G. R. Carter. 1972. The pathology and pathogenesis of *Bordetella bronchiseptica* and *Pasteurella pneumotropica* in conventional and germfree rats. Lab. Anim. Sci. 22:844-849.

Burek, J. D., C. Zurcher, M. C. J. van Nunen, and C. F. Hollander. 1977. A naturally occurring epizootic caused by Sendai virus in breeding and aging rodent colonies. II. Infection in the rat. Lab. Anim. Sci. 27:963-971.

Burnett, F. M., and D. Lush. 1936. Inapparent (Subclinical) infection of the rat with the virus of infectious ectromelia of mice. J. Pathol. Bacteriol. 43:469-476.

Buxton, A., and G. Fraser. 1977a. Reoviruses (and other diplornaviruses). Pp. 625-637 in Animal Microbiology, vol. 2. Oxford: Blackwell Scientific.

Buxton, A., and G. Fraser. 1977b. Adenoviruses. Pp. 725-735 in Animal Microbiology, vol. 2, Rickettsias and Viruses. Oxford: Blackwell.

Buxton, A., and G. Fraser. 1977c. Herpesviruses. Pp. 737-773 in Animal Microbiology, vol. 2: Rickettsias and Viruses. Oxford: Blackwell.

Buxton, I. K., S. P. K. Chan, and P. G. W. Plagemann. 1988. The Ia antigen is not the major receptor for lactate dehydrogenase-elevating virus on macrophages from CBA and BALB/c mice. Virus Res. 9:205-219.

Bywater, J. E., and B. S. Kellett. 1978. *Encephalitozoon cuniculi* antibodies in a specific-pathogen-free rabbit unit. Infect. Immun. 21:360-364.

Cacciatore, L., and S. Antoniello. 1971. Arginase activity of mouse serum and liver tissue in some conditions of experimental liver damage. Enzymologia 41:112-120.

Cafruny, W. A., and P. G. W. Plagemann. 1982. Immune response to lactate dehydrogenase-elevating virus: Serologically specific rabbit neutralizing antibody to the virus. Infect. Immun. 37:1007-1012.

Campa, M., C. Garizelli, and G. Falcone. 1975. Depression of contact sensitivity and enhancement of antibody response in *Pseudomonas aeruginosa* infected mice. Infect. Immun. 12:1252-1257.

Campa, M., C. Garizelli, E. Ferrannini, and G. Falcone. 1976. Evidence for suppressor cell activity associated with depression of contact sensitivity in *Pseudomonas aeruginosa* infected mice. Clin. Exp. Immunol. 26:355-362.

Campa, M., E. Ferrannini, V. Colizzi, and G. Garzelli. 1977. Distribution of 51Cr-labeled lymph node cells in *Pseudomonas aeruginosa*-infected mice. J. Nucl. Med. Allied Sci. 21:37-42.

Campbell, D. A., E. K. Manders, J. R. Oehle, G. D. Bonnard, R. K. Oldham, and R. B. Herbermann. 1977a. Inhibition of in vitro lymphoproliferative responses by in vivo passaged rat 13762 mammary adenocarcinoma cells. I. Characteristics of inhibition and evidence for an infectious agent. Cell. Immunol. 33:364-377.

Campbell, D. A., S. P. Staal, E. K. Manders, G. D. Bonnard, R. K. Oldman, L. A. Salzman, and R. B. Herbermann. 1977b. Inhibition of in vitro lymphoproliferative responses by in vivo passaged rat 13762 mammary adenocarcinoma cells. II. Evidence that Kilham rat virus is responsible for the inhibitory effect. Cell. Immunol. 33:378-391.

Campbell, W. G., Jr. 1972. Ultrastructure of *Pneumocystis carinii* in human lung. Arch. Pathol. 93:312-324.

Canonico, P. G., J. D. White, and M. C. Powanda. 1975. Peroxisome depletion in rat liver during pneumococcal sepsis. Lab. Invest. 33:147-150.

Carrano, V. A., S. W. Barthold, D. S. Beck, and A. L. Smith. 1984. Alteration of viral respiratory infections of mice by prior infection with mouse hepatitis virus. Lab. Anim. Sci. 34:573-576.

Carter, E. A., J. R. Wands, and K. J. Isselbacher. 1977. Effect of active murine hepatitis (MHV-1-59) on ethanol oxidation in vivo. Gastroenterology 73:321-326.

Carter, G. R. 1984. Genus 1. *Pasteurella*. Pp. 552-558 in Bergey's Manual of Systematic Bacteriology, vol. I, N. R. Krieg and J. G. Holt, eds. Baltimore: Williams & Wilkins.

Carter, P. B., and F. M. Collins. 1974. The role of enteric infection in normal mice. J. Exp. Med. 139:1189-1203.

Carter, P. B., J. B. Woolcock, and F. M. Collins. 1975. Involvement of the upper respiratory tract in orally induced salmonellosis in mice. J. Infect. Dis. 131:570-574.

Carthew, P. 1977a. Lethal intestinal virus of infant mice in mouse hepatitis virus. Vet. Rec. 101:465.

Carthew, P. 1977b. A method for the serological diagnosis of epizootic diarrhea in infant mice. Vet. Rec. 101:386.

Carthew, P. 1981. Inhibition of the mitotic response in regenerating mouse liver during viral hepatitis. Infect. Immun. 33:641-642.

Carthew, P., and R. P. Slinger. 1981. Diagnosis of sialodacryoadenitis virus infection of rats in a virulent enzootic outbreak. Lab. Anim. 15:339-342.

Carthew, P., and S. Sparrow. 1980a. A comparison in germ-free mice of the pathogenesis of Sendai virus and mouse pneumonia virus infections. J. Pathol. 130:153-158.

Carthew, P., and S. Sparrow. 1980b. Persistence of pneumonia virus of mice and Sendai virus in germ-free (*nu/nu*) mice. Br. J. Exp. Pathol. 61:172-175.

Carthew, P., and S. Sparrow. 1980c. Sendai virus in nude and germ-free rats. Res. Vet. Sci. 29:289-292.

Carthew, P., and A. Verstraete. 1978. A serological survey of accredited breeding colonies in the United Kingdom for common rodent viruses. Lab. Anim. 12:29-32.

Carthew, P., M. J. Wood, C. Kirby. 1983. Elimination of Sendai (parainfluenza type I) virus infection from mice by embryo transfer. J. Reprod. Fertil. 69:253-257.

Casebolt, D. B., and T. R. Schoeb. 1988. An outbreak in mice of salmonellosis caused by *Salmonella enteritidis* serotype enteritidis. Lab. Anim. Sci. 38:190-192.

Casebolt, D. B., D. M. Spalding, T. R. Schoeb, and J. R. Lindsey. 1987. Suppression of immune response induction in Peyer's patch lymphoid cells from mice infected with mouse hepatitis virus. Cell. Immunol. 109:97-103.

Casebolt, D. B., J. R. Lindsey, and G. H. Cassell. 1988. Prevalence rates of infectious agents among commercial breeding populations of rats and mice. Lab. Anim. Sci. 38:327-329.

Casillo, S., and D. K. Blackmore. 1972. Uterine infections caused by bacteria and mycoplasma in mice and rats. J. Comp. Pathol. 82:477-482.

Cassell, G. H. 1982. The pathogenic potential of mycoplasmas: *Mycoplasma pulmonis* as a model. Rev. Infect. Dis. 4:S18-S34.

Cassell, G. H., and M. B. Brown. 1983. Enzyme-linked immunosorbent assay (ELISA) for detection of anti-mycoplasmal antibody. Pp. 457-469 in Methods in Mycoplasmology, vol. I, S. Razin and J. G. Tully, eds. New York: Academic Press.

Cassell, G. H., and A. Hill. 1979. Murine and other small animal mycoplasmas. Pp. 235-273 in The Mycoplasmas, vol. 2, J. G. Tully and R. F. Whitcomb, eds. New York: Academic Press.

Cassell, G. H., J. R. Lindsey, H. J. Baker, and J. K. Davis. 1979. Mycoplasmal and rickettsial diseases. Pp. 243-269 in The Laboratory Rat. Vol. I, H. J. Baker, J. R. Lindsey, and S. H. Weisbroth, eds. New York: Academic Press.

Cassell, G. H., J. R. Lindsey, J. K. Davis, M. K. Davidson, M. B. Brown, and J. G. Mayo. 1981. Detection of natural *Mycoplasma pulmonis* infection in rats and mice by an enzyme-linked immunosorbent assay. Lab. Anim. Sci. 31:676-682.

Cassell, G. H., M. K. Davidson, J. K. Davis, and J. R. Lindsey. 1983a. Recovery and identification of murine mycoplasmas. Pp. 129-142 in Methods in Mycoplasmology. Vol. II, J. G. Tully and S. Razin, eds. New York: Academic Press.

Cassell, G. H., J. K. Davis, J. R. Lindsey, M. K. Davidson, M. B. Brown, and H. J. Baker. 1983b. Detection of *Mycoplasma pulmonis* infections by ELISA. Lab. Anim. 12:27-38.

Cassell, G. H., N. R. Cox, J. K. Davis, M. B. Brown, F. C. Minion, and J. R. Lindsey. 1986. State-of-the-art detection methods for rodent mycoplasmas. Pp. 143-160 in Complications of Viral and Mycoplasmal Infections in Rodents to Toxicology Research and Testing. T. E. Hamm, Jr., ed. Washington, D.C.: Hemisphere Press.

Castleman, W. L. 1983. Respiratory tract lesions in weanling outbred rats infected with Sendai virus. Am. J. Vet. Res. 44:1024-1031.

Castleman, W. L. 1984. Alterations in pulmonary ultrastructure and morphometric parameters induced by parainfluenza (Sendai) virus in rats during postnatal growth. Am. J. Pathol. 114:322-335.

Castleman, W. L., L. J. Brundage-Anguish, L. Kreitzer, and S. B. Neuenschwander. 1987. Pathogenesis of bronchiolitis and pneumonia induced in neonatal and weanling rats by parainfluenza (Sendai) virus. Am. J. Pathol. 129:277-286.

Cavallero, C. 1967. Relative effectiveness of various steroids in an androgen assay using the exorbital lacrimal gland of the castrated rat. Acta Endocrinol. 55:119-130.

Cetin, E. T., M. Tashinoglu, and S. Volkan. 1965. Epizootic of *Trichophyton mentagrophytes* in white mice. Pathol. Microbiol. 28:839-846.

Chalmer, J. E., J. S. Mackenzie, and N. F. Stanley. 1977. Resistance to murine cytomegalovirus linked to the major histocompatibility complex in the mouse. J. Gen. Virol. 37:107-114.

Chalupsky, J., J. Vavra, and P. Bedmik. 1973. Detection of antibodies to *Encephalitozoon cuniculi* in rabbits by the indirect immunofluorescent antibody test. Folia Parasitol. 20:281-284.

Chantler, J. K., V. Misra, and J. B. Hudson. 1979. Vertical transmission of murine cytomegalovirus. J. Gen. Virol. 42:621-625.

Chapman, J. S. 1982. The atypical mycobacteria. Am. Rev. Resp. Dis. 125:119-124.

Charlton, D., and G. Blandford. 1977. Immunoglobulin class-specific antibody response in serum, spleen, lungs, and bronchoalveolar washings after primary and secondary Sendai virus infection of germfree mice. Infect. Immun. 17:521-527.

Chase, H. B. 1954. Growth of the hair. Physiol. Rev. 34:113-126.

Chase, H. B., and G. J. Eaton. 1959. The growth of hair follicles in waves. Ann. N.Y. Acad. Sci. 83:365-368.

Cheever, F. S. 1956. Diarrheal disease of suckling mice. Ann. N.Y. Acad. Sci. 66:196-203.

Cheever, F. S., and J. H. Mueller. 1947. Epidemic diarrheal disease of suckling mice. I. Manifestations, epidemiology, and attempts to transmit the disease. J. Exp. Med. 85:405-416.

Cheever, F. S., and J. H. Mueller. 1948. Epidemic diarrheal disease of suckling mice. III. The effect of strain, litter, and season upon the incidence of the disease. J. Exp. Med. 88:309-316.

Cheever, F. S., J. B. Daniels, O. T. Bailey, and A. M. Pappenheimer. 1949. A murine virus (JHM) causing disseminated encephalomyelitis with extensive destruction of myelin. I. Isolation and biological properties of the virus. J. Exp. Med. 90:181-194.

Childs, J. E., G. W. Korch, G. A. Smith, A. D. Terry, and J. W. LeDuc. 1985. Geographical distribution and age related prevalence of antibody to Hantaan-like virus in rat populations of Baltimore, Maryland, U.S.A. Am. J. Trop. Med. Hyg. 34:385-387.

Childs, J. E., G. E. Glass, G. W. Korch, J. W. LeDuc. 1987a. Prospective seroepidemiology of hantaviruses and population dynamics of small mammal communities of Baltimore, Maryland. Am. J. Trop. Med. Hyg. 37:648-662.

Childs, J. E., G. W. Korch, G. E. Glass, J. W. LeDuc, and K. V. Shah. 1987b. Epizootiology of *Hantavirus* infections in Baltimore: Isolation of a virus from Norway rats, and characteristics of infected rat populations. Am. J. Epidemiol. 126:55-68.

Childs, J. E., G. E. Glass, G. W. Korch, R. R. Arthur, K. V. Shah, D. Glasser, C. Rossi, and J. W. LeDuc. 1988. Evidence of human infection with a rat-associated hantavirus in Baltimore, Maryland. Am. J. Epidemiol. 127:875-878.

Christensen, L. R., S. H. Weisbroth, and B. Matanic. 1966. Detection of ectromelia virus and ectromelia antibodies by immunofluorescence. Lab. Anim. Care 16:129-141.

Christoffersen, P. J., and K. Bro-Jorgensen. 1977. Erythropoietic activity and interferon production in LCM virus infected nude mice. Acta Pathol. Microbiol. Scand. 85:435-439.

Christoffersen, P. J., M. Volkert, and J. Rygaard. 1976. Immunological unresponsiveness of nude mice to LCM virus infection. Acta Pathol. Microbiol. Scand. 84:520-523.

Chumakov, M. P., I. N. Gavrilovskaya, V. A. Boiko, M. A. Zakharova, Y. A. Myasnikov, T. A. Bashkirov, N. S. Apekina, R. S. Safiullin, and V. S. Potapov. 1981. Detection of hemorrhagic fever with renal syndrome (HFRS) virus in the lungs of bank voles *Clethrionomys glareolus* and red backed voles *Clethrionomys rutilus* trapped in HFRS foci in the European part of U.S.S.R., and serodiagnosis of this infection in man. Arch. Virol. 69:295-300.

Clark, E. A., P. H. Russell, M. Egghart, and M. A. Horton. 1979. Characteristics and genetic control of NK-cell-mediated cytotoxicity activated by naturally acquired infection in the mouse. Int. J. Cancer 24:688-699.

Clark, S. L. 1959. The ingestion of proteins and colloidal materials by columnar absorptive cells of the small intestines in suckling rats and mice. J. Biophy. Biochem. Cytol. 5:41-50.

Clarke, M. C., R. J. Taylor, G. A. Hall, and P. W. Jones. 1978. The occurrence of facial and mandibular abscesses associated with *Staphylococcus aureus*. Lab. Anim. (London) 12:121-123.

Classen, D. C., J. M. Moringstar, and J. D. Shanley. 1987. Detection of antibody to murine cytomegalovirus by enzyme-linked immunosorbent and indirect immunofluorescence assays. J. Clin. Microbiol. 25:600-604.

Clatch, R. J., R. W. Melvold, S. D. Miller, and H. L. Lipton. 1985. Theiler's murine encephalomyelitis virus (TMEV)-induced demyelinating disease in mice is influenced by the H-2D region: Correlation with TMEV specific delayed-type hypersensitivity. J. Immunol. 135:1408-1414.

Cohen, B. J., and F. G. de Groot. 1976. Adenovirus infection in athymic (*nu/nu*) mice. Lab. Anim. Sci. 26:955-956.

Cohen, J. C., and H. E. Varmus. 1979. Endogenous mammary tumor virus DNA varies among wild mice and segregates during inbreeding. Nature 278:418-422.

Cohen, P. L., S. S . Cross, and D. E. Mosier. 1975. Immunologic effects of neonatal infection with mouse thymic virus. J. Immunol. 115:706-710.

Cohn, D. A., and G. Schiffman. 1987. Immunoregulatory role of the spleen in antibody responses to pneumococcal polysaccharide antigens. Infect. Immun. 55:1375-1380.

Coid, C. R., and G. Wardman. 1971. The effect of parainfluenza type 1 (Sendai) virus infection on early pregnancy in the rat. J. Reprod. Fertil. 24:39-43.

Coid, C. R., and G. Wardman. 1972. The effect of maternal respiratory disease induced by parainfluenza type 1 (Sendai) virus on fetal development and neonatal mortality in the rat. Med. Microbiol. Immunol. 157:181-185.

Cole, A. G., N. Nathanson, and H. Rivet. 1970. Viral hemorrhagic encephalopathy of rats. II. Pathogenesis of central nervous system lesions. Am. J. Epidemiol. 91:339-350.

Cole, B. C., and G. H. Cassell. 1979. *Mycoplasma* infections as models of chronic joint inflammation. Arth. Rheum. 22:1375-1381.

Cole, B. C., and J. R. Ward. 1979. Mycoplasmas as arthritogenic agents. Pp. 367-398 in The Mycoplasmas, vol. II, J. G. Tully and R. F. Whitcomb, eds. New York: Academic Press.

Cole, B. C., M. L. Miller, and J. R. Ward. 1967. A comparative study on the virulence of *Mycoplasma arthritidis* and "*Mycoplasma hominis*" type 2 strains in rats. Proc. Soc. Exp. Biol. Med. 124:103-107.

Cole, B. C., M. L. Miller, and J. R. Ward. 1969. The role of *Mycoplasma* in rat arthritis induced by 6-sulfanilamidoindazole (6-SAI). Proc. Soc. Exp. Biol. Med. 130:994-1000.

Cole, B. C., L. Golightly-Rowland, and J. R. Ward. 1975. Arthritis in mice induced by *Mycoplasma pulmonis*: Humoral antibody and lymphocyte responses of CBA mice. Infect. Immun. 12:1083-1092.

Cole, B. C., L. Golightly-Rowland, and J. R. Ward. 1976a. Arthritis of mice induced by *Mycoplasma arthritidis*: Humoral antibody and lymphocyte responses of CBA mice. Ann. Rheum. Dis. 35:14-22.

Cole, B. C., J. C. Overall, Jr., P. S. Lombardi, and L. A. Glasgow. 1976b. Induction of interferon in ovine and human lymphocyte cultures by mycoplasmas. Infect. Immun. 14:88-92.

Cole, B. C., K. E. Aldridge, and J. R. Ward. 1977. *Mycoplasma*-dependent activation of normal lymphocytes: Mitogenic potential of mycoplasmas for mouse lymphocytes. Infect. Immun. 18:383-399.

Cole, B. C., R. A. Daynes, and J. R. Ward. 1981. Stimulation of mouse lymphocytes by a mitogen derived from *Mycoplasma arthritidis*. I. Transformation is associated with an H-2-linked gene that maps to the 1-E/1-C subregion. J. Immunol. 127:1931-1936.

Cole, B. C., G. J. Sullivan, R. A. Daynes, I. A. Sayed, and J. R. Ward. 1982. Stimulation of mouse lymphocytes by a mitogen derived from *Mycoplasma arthritidis*. II. Cellular requirements for T-cell transformation mediated by a soluble mycoplasma mitogen. J. Immunol. 128:2013-2018.

Coleman, G. L., R. O. Jacoby, P. N. Bhatt, A. L. Smith, and A. M. Jonas. 1983. Naturally occurring lethal parvovirus infection in juvenile and young adult rats. Vet. Pathol. 20:44-45.

Collier, W. A. 1939. Infectious polyarthritis of rats. J. Pathol. Bacteriol. 48:579-589.

Collins, D. N., H. Weigand, and J. Hotchin. 1961. The effects of pretreatment with x-rays on the pathogenesis of lymphocytic choriomeningitis in mice. J. Immunol. 87:682-687.

Collins, F. M. 1972. Salmonellosis in orally infected specific pathogen-free C57BL mice. Infect. Immun. 5:191-198.

Collins, F. M., and P. B. Carter. 1978. Growth of salmonellae in orally infected germfree mice. Infect. Immun. 21:41-47.

Collins, J., W. G. Starkey, T. S. Walls, G. J. Clarke, K. K. Worton, A. J. Spencer, S. J. Haddon, M. P. Osborne, D. C. A. Candy, and J. Stephen. 1988. Intestinal enzyme profiles in normal and rotavirus-infected mice. J. Pediat. Gastroenterol. Nutr. 7:264-272.

Collins, M. J., Jr., and J. C. Parker. 1972. Murine virus contaminants of leukemia viruses and transplantable tumors. J. Natl. Cancer Inst. 49:1139-1143.

Collins, M. J., R. L. Peters, and J. C. Parker. 1981. Serological detection of ectromelia virus antibody. Lab. Anim. Sci. 31:595-598.

Colwell, D. E., S. M. Michalek, D. E. Briles, E. Jirillo, and J. R. McGhee. 1984. Monoclonal antibodies to *Salmonella* lipopolysaccharide: Anti-O-polysaccharide antibodies protect C3H mice against challenge with virulent *Salmonella typhimurium*. J. Immunol. 133:950-957.

Contag, C. H., S. P. K. Chan, S. W. Wietgrefe, and P. G. W. Plagemann. 1986. Correlation between presence of lactate dehydrogenase-elevating virus RNA and antigens in motor neurons and paralysis in infected C58 mice. Virus Res. 6:195-209.

Cook, I. 1963. Reovirus type 3 infection in laboratory mice. 1963. Aust. J. Exp. Biol. Med. Sci. 41:651-660.

Cooney, D. R., J. C. Dearth, S. E. Swanson, M. K. Dewanjee, and R. L. Telander. 1979a. Relative merits of partial splenectomy, splenic reimplantation, and immunization in preventing postsplenectomy infection. Surgery 86:561-569.

Cooney, D. R., S. E. Swanson, J. C. Dearth, M. K. Dewanjee, and R. L. Telander. 1979b. Heterotopic splenic auto-transplantation in prevention of overwhelming postsplenectomy infection. J. Pediat. Surg. 14:336-342.

Coonrod, J. D. 1981. Pulmonary opsonins in *Klebsiella pneumoniae* pneumonia in rats. Infect. Immun. 33:533-539.

Coonrod, J. D., and K. Yoneda. 1982. Comparative role of complement in pneumococcal and staphylococcal pneumonia. Infect. Immun. 37:1270-1277.

Coonrod, J. D., S. R. Rehm, and K. Yoneda. 1983. Pneumococcal killing in the alveolus. Evidence for a nonphagocytic defense mechanism for early clearance. Chest 83:89S-90S.

Cordier, R., and E. de Haven. 1960. Les inclusions nucleaires de la glande de Loewenthal du rat male en microscopie electronique. C. R. Acad. Sci. 250:398-400.

Coriell, L. L., and G. J. McGarrity. 1973. Biomedical applications of laminar airflow. Pp. 43-47 in Germfree Research: Biological Effect of Gnotobiotic Environments, J. B. Heneghan, ed. New York: Academic Press.

Cotmore, S. F., and P. Tattersall. 1986. Organization of nonstructural genes of the autonomous parvovirus minute virus of mice. J. Virol. 58:724-732.

Cotmore, S. F., L. J. Sturzenbecker, and P. Tattersall. 1983. The autonomous parvovirus MVM encodes two nonstructural proteins in addition to its capsid polypeptides. Virology 129:333-343.

Coutelier, J.-P., E. V. Roost, P. Lambotte, and J. Van Snick. 1986. The murine antibody response to lactate dehydrogenase-elevating virus. J. Gen. Virol. 67:1099-1108.

Cox, H. W., and G. Calaf-Iturri. 1976. Autoimmune factors associated with anemia in acute *Haemobartonella* and *Eperythrozoon* infections of rodents. Ann. Trop. Med. Parasitol. 70:73-79.

Cox, J. C. 1977. Altered immune responsiveness associated with *Encephalitozoon cuniculi* infection in rabbits. Infect. Immun. 15:392-395.

Cox, J. C., and H. A. Gallichio. 1978. Serological and histological studies on adult rabbits with recent, naturally acquired encephalitozoonosis. Res. Vet. Sci. 24:260-261.

Cox, J. C., and D. Pye. 1975. Serodiagnosis of nosematosis by immunofluorescence using cell-culture-grown organisms. Lab. Anim. 9:297-304.

Cox, J. C., A. G. Heather, D. Pye, and N. B. Walden. 1977. Application of immunofluorescence to the establishment of an *Encephalitozoon cuniculi*-free rabbit colony. Lab. Anim. Sci. 27:204-209.

Cox, J. C., R. C. Hamilton, and H. D. Attwood. 1979. An investigation of the route and progression of *Encephalitozoon cuniculi* infection in adult rabbits. J. Protozool. 26:260-265.

Cox, J. C., R. Horsburgh, and D. Pye. 1981. Simple diagnostic test for antibodies to *Encephalitozoon cuniculi* based on enzyme immunoassay. Lab. Anim. 15:41-43.

Cox, N. R., J. R. Lindsey, and J. G. Mayo. 1977. Tail lesions in weanling mice. Program of the 114th Annual Meeting of the American Veterinary Medical Association, held July 11-14, 1977, in Atlanta, Ga. Abstract no. 170.

Cox, N. R., M. K. Davidson, J. K. Davis, J. R. Lindsey, and G. H. Cassell. 1988. Natural mycoplasmal infections in isolator-maintained LEW/Tru rats. Lab. Anim. Sci. 38:381-388.

Coyle, M. B., D. G. Hollis, and N. B. Groman. 1985. *Corynebacterium* spp. and other coryneform organisms. Pp. 193-204 in Manual of Clinical Microbiology, 4th ed. E. H. Lennette, A. Balows, W. J. Hausler, Jr., and H. J. Shadomy, eds. Washington, D.C.: American Society for Microbiology.

Craigie, J. 1966a. *Bacillus piliformis* (Tyzzer) and Tyzzer's disease of the laboratory mouse. I. Propagation of the organism in embryonated eggs. Proc. R. Soc. London 165:35-61.

Craigie, J. 1966b. *Bacillus piliformis* (Tyzzer) and Tyzzer's disease of the laboratory mouse. II. Mouse pathogenicity of *B. piliformis* grown in embryonated eggs. Proc. R. Soc. London 165:61-78.

Crawford, L. V. 1966. A minute virus of mice. Virology 29:605-612.

Crawford, L. V., E. A. C. Hullett, M. G. Burdon, and D. J. McGeoch. 1969. The DNA of a minute virus of mice. J. Gen. Virol. 4:37-46.

Crispens, C. G. 1964. On the epizootiology of the lactic dehydrogenase agent. J. Natl. Cancer Inst. 35:975-979.

Crispens, C. G. 1971. Studies on the response of SJL/J mice to infection with the lactate dehydrogenase virus. Arch. Ges. Virusforsch. 35:177-182.

Crispens, C. G. 1972. Genetic control of the response of SJL/J mice to LDH virus infection. Arch. Ges. Virusforsch. 38:225-227.

Cross, S. S. 1973. Development of Bioassays and Studies on the Biology of Mouse Thymic Virus. Ph.D. Dissertation. Washington, D.C.: George Washington University.

Cross, S. S., and J. C. Parker. 1972. Some antigenic relationships of the murine parvoviruses: Minute virus of mice, rat virus and H-1 virus. Proc. Soc. Exp. Biol. Med. 139:105-108.

Cross, S. S., H. C. Morse III, and R. Asofsky. 1976. Neonatal infection with mouse thymic virus. Differential effects on T cells mediating the graft-versus-host reaction. J. Immunol. 117:635-638.

Cross, S. S., J. C. Parker, W. P. Rowe, and M. L. Robbins. 1979. Biology of mouse thymic virus, a herpesvirus of mice, and the antigenic relationship to mouse cytomegalovirus. Infect. Immun. 26:1186-1195.

Crystal, M. M. 1958. The mechanism of transmission of *Haemobartonella muris* (Mayer) of rats by the spined rat louse, *Polyplax spinulosa* (Burmeister). J. Parasitol. 44:603-606.

Crystal, M. M. 1959a. Extrinsic incubation period of *Haemobartonella muris* in the spined rat louse, *Polyplax spinulosa*. J. Bacteriol. 77:511.

Crystal, M. M. 1959b. The infective index of the spine rat louse, *Polyplax spinulosa* (Burmeister), in the transmission of *Haemobartonella muris* (Mayer) of rats. J. Econ. Entomol. 52:543-544.

Cryz, S. J. , Jr., E. Furer, and R. Germanier. 1984. Protection against *Pseudomonas aeruginosa* infection in a murine burn wound sepsis model by passive transfer of antitoxin A, antielastase and anti-polysaccharide. Infect. Immun. 39:1072-1079.

Csiza, C. K., and M. K. Abelseth. 1973. An epizootic of protozoan enteritis in a closed mouse colony. Lab. Anim. Sci. 23:858-861.

Csiza, C. K., and D. N. McMartin. 1976. Apparent acaridal dermatitis in a C57BL/6Nya mouse colony. Lab. Anim. Sci. 26:781-787.

Cukor, G., M. K. Berry, and N. R. Blacklow. 1978. Simplified radioimmunoassay for detection of human rotavirus in stools. J. Infect. Dis. 138:906-910.

Cumming, C. N. W., and C. Elias. 1957. The establishment by a commercial company of a colony of rats free from certain pathogens. Proc. Anim. Care Panel 7:41-49.

Cushion, M. T., and P. D. Walzer. 1984a. Growth and serial passage of *Pneumocystis carinii* in the A549 cell line. Infect. Immun. 44:245-251.

Cushion, M. T., and P. D. Walzer. 1984b. Cultivation of *Pneumocystis carinii* in lung-derived cell lines. J. Infect. Dis. 149:644.

Cushion, M. T., J. J. Ruffolo, M. J. Linke, and P. D. Walzer. 1985. *Pneumocystis carinii*: Growth variables and estimates in the A549 and WI-38 VA 13 human cell lines. Exp. Parasitol. 60:43-54.

Dal Canto, M. C., and R. L. Barbano. 1984. Remyelination during remission in Theiler's virus infection. Am. J. Pathol. 116:30-45.

Dal Canto, M. C., and H. L. Lipton. 1975. Primary demyelination in Theiler's virus infection. An ultrastructural study. Lab. Invest. 33:626-627.

Dal Canto, M. C., and H. L. Lipton. 1979. Recurrent demyelination in chronic central nervous system infection produced by Theiler's murine encephalomyelitis virus. J. Neurol. Sci. 42:391-405.

Dal Canto, M. C., and H. L. Lipton. 1980. Schwann cell remyelination and recurrent demyelination in the central nervous system of mice infected with attenuated Theiler's virus. Am. J. Pathol. 98:101-122.

Dal Canto, M. C., and H. L. Lipton. 1982. Ultrastructural immunohistochemical localization of virus in acute and chronic demyelinating Theiler's virus infection. Am. J. Pathol. 106:20-29.

Dalldorf, G. 1939. The simultaneous occurrence of the viruses of canine distemper and lymphocytic choriomeningitis. J. Exp. Med. 70:19-27.

Dalton, A. J., L. Kilham, and R. F. Zeigel. 1963. A comparison of polyoma, "K" and Kilham rat viruses with the electron microscope. Virology 20:391-398.

Darrigrand, A. A., S. B. Singh, and C. M. Lang. 1984. Effects of Kilham rat virus on natural killer cell-mediated cytotoxicity in Brown Norway and Wistar Furth rats. Am. J. Vet. Res. 45:200-202.

Davidson, M. K., J. R. Lindsey, M. B. Brown, T. R. Schoeb, and G. H. Cassell. 1981. Comparison of methods for detection of *Mycoplasma pulmonis* in experimentally and naturally infected rats. J. Clin. Microbiol. 14:644-646.

Davidson, M. K., J. R. Lindsey, M. B. Brown, G. H. Cassell, and G. H. Boorman. 1983. Natural infection of *Mycoplasma arthritidis* in mice. Curr. Microbiol. 8:205-208.

Davidson, M. K., J. R. Lindsey, R. F. Parker, J. G. Tully, and G. H. Cassell. 1988a. Differences in virulence for mice among strains of *Mycoplasma pulmonis*. Infect. Immun. 56:2156-2162.

Davidson, M. K., S. E. Ross, J. R. Lindsey, and G. H. Cassell. 1988b. Colony opacity, hemadsorption, hemolysis, and mitogenicity are not associated with virulence of *Mycoplasma pulmonis*. Infect. Immun. 56:2169-2173.

Davies, R. R., and J. Shewell. 1965. Ringworm carriage and its control in mice. J. Hyg. 63:507-515.

Davis, B. D., R. Dulbeco, H. N. Eisen, and H. S. Ginsburg. 1980. Reoviruses and epidemic acute gastroenteritis virus. Pp. 1203-1216 in Microbiology, 3rd ed. Hagerstown, Md.: Harper and Row.

Davis, G. L., and M. M. Hawrisiak. 1977. Experimental cytomegalovirus infection and the developing mouse inner ear. Lab. Invest. 37:20-29.

Davis, G. L., K. W. Krawczyk, and M. M. Hawrisiak. 1979. Age-related eurocytotropism of mouse cytomegalovirus in explanted trigeminal ganglia. Am. J. Pathol. 97:261-275.

Davis, J. K., and G. H. Cassell. 1982. Murine respiratory mycoplasmosis in LEW and F344 rats: Strain differences in lesion severity. Vet. Pathol. 19:280-293.

Davis, J. K., R. B. Thorp, P. A. Maddox, M. B. Brown, and G. H. Cassell. 1982. Murine respiratory mycoplasmosis in F344 and LEW rats: Evolution of lesions and lung lymphoid cell populations. Infect. Immun. 36:720-729.

Davis, J. K., R. F. Parker, H. White, D. Dziedzic, G. Taylor, M. K. Davidson, N. R. Cox, and G. H. Cassell. 1985. Strain differences in susceptibility to murine respiratory mycoplasmosis in C57BL/6N and C3H/HeN mice. Infect. Immun. 50:647-654.

Davis, J. K., G. H. Cassell, G. Gambill, N. Cox, H. Watson, and M. Davidson. 1987. Diagnosis of murine mycoplasmal infections by enzyme-linked immunosorbent assay (ELISA). Isr. J. Med. Sci. 23:717-722.

Dawe, C. J., L. Kilham, and W. D. Morgan. 1961. Intranuclear inclusions in tissue cultures infected with rat virus. J. Natl. Cancer Inst. 27:221-238.

de Souza, M., and Smith, A. L. 1989. Comparison of isolation in cell culture with conventional and modified mouse antibody production tests for detection of murine viruses. J. Clin. Microbiol. 27:185-187.

Dean, D. J. 1951. Mouse encephalomyelitis: Immunologic studies of a non-infected colony. J. Immunol. 66:347-359.

DeBurgh, P., A. V. Jackson, and A. E. Williams. 1945. Spontaneous infection of laboratory mice with a psittacosis-like organism. Aust. J. Exp. Biol. Med. Sci. 23:107-110.

DeBuryn, W. M. 1949. A lymphopenia-causing agent, probably a virus, found in mice after injection with tumor tissue and with cell-free filtrates of lymphosarcoma T 86157(MB). Cancer Res. 9:395-397.

Degre, M., and L. A. Glasgow. 1968. Synergistic effect in viral bacterial infection. I. Combined infection of the respiratory tract in mice with parainfluenza virus and *Hemophilus* influenza. J. Infect. Dis. 118:449-462.

Degre, M., and T. Midtvedt. 1971. Respiratory infection with parainfluenza 1, Sendai virus in gnotobiotic and conventional mice. Acta Pathol. Microbiol. Scand. 79:123-124.

Degre, M., and L. A. Solberg. 1971. Synergistic effect in viral bacteria infection. III. Histopathologic changes in the trachea of mice following viral and bacterial infection. Acta Pathol. Microbiol. Scand. 79:129-136.

Deibel, R. H., and H. W. Seeley, Jr. 1974. Streptoccaceae. Pp. 490-517 in Bergey's Manual of Determinative Bacteriology, 8th ed., R. E. Buchanan and N. E. Gibbons, eds. Baltimore: Williams & Wilkins.

DeLellis, R. A., and H. J. Wolfe. 1987. New techniques in gene product analysis. Arch. Pathol. Lab. Med. 111:620-627.

Della Porta, G., L. Chieco-Bianchi, and N. Pennelli. 1979. Tumours of the haemopoietic system. Pp. 527-576 in Pathology of Tumours of the Mouse. V, S. Turusov, ed. Lyon: International Agency for Research on Cancer.

DeOme, K. B., L. J. Faulkin, Jr., H. A. Bern, and P. B. Blair. 1959. Development of mammary tumors from hyperplastic alveolar nodules transplanted into gland-free mammary fat pads of female C3H mice. Cancer Res. 19:515-520.

DeRubertis, F. R., and K. A. Woeber. 1972. The effect of acute infection with *Diplococcus pneumoniae* on hepatic mitochondrial alpha-glycerophosphate dehydrogenase activity. Endocrinology 90:1384-1387.

Descoteaux, J.-P., and P. Payment. 1981. Comparison of hemagglutination inhibition serum neutralization and ELISA-PVM tests for the detection of antibodies to pneumonia virus of mice in rat sera. J. Virol. Meth. 3:83-87.

Descoteaux, J.-P., D. Grignon-Archambault, and G. Lussier. 1977. Serologic study on the prevalence of murine viruses in five Canadian mouse colonies. Lab. Anim. Sci. 27:621-626.

Descoteaux, J.-P., P. Payment, and M. Trudel. 1980. Comparison of the hemagglutination inhibition procedure and an enzyme-linked immunosorbent assay for detection of specific antibodies to pneumonia virus of mice in experimentally infected laboratory rats. J. Clin. Microbiol. 11:162-166.

Desmyter, J., K. M. Johnson, C. Deckers, J. W. LeDuc, F. Brasseur, and C. van Ypersele de Strihou. 1983. Laboratory rat associated outbreak of hemorrhagic fever with renal syndrome due to Hantaan-like virus in Belgium. Lancet ii:1445-1448.

Didier, E. S., and J. A. Shadduck. 1988. Modulated immune responsiveness associated with experimental *Encephalitozoon cuniculi* infection in BALB/c mice. Lab. Anim. Sci. 38:680-684.

Dietz, J. N., and B. C. Cole. 1982. Direct activation of the J774.1 murine macrophage cell line by *Mycoplasma arthritidis*. Infect. Immun. 37:811-819.

DiGiacomo, R. F., and T. D. Koepsell. 1986. Sampling for detection of infection or disease in animal populations. J. Am. Vet. Med. Assoc. 189:22-23.

Dillberger, J. E., P. Monroy, and N. H. Altman. 1987a. The effect of three bleeding techniques on lactic dehydrogenase levels in mice: Implications for lactic dehydrogenase virus assay. Lab. Anim. Sci. 37:356-359.

Dillberger, J. E., P. Monroy, and N. H. Altman. 1987b. Delayed increase in plasma lactic dehydrogenase activity in mouse hepatitis virus-infected mice subsequently infected with lactic dehydrogenase virus. Lab. Anim. Sci. 37:792-794.

Doherty, P. C., R. M. Zinkernagel, and I. A. Ramshaw. 1974. Specificity and development of cytotoxic thymus-derived lymphocytes in lymphocytic choriomeningitis. J. Immunol. 112:1548-1552.

Doi, K., A. Yasoshima, A. Kojima, H. Okawa, S. Kurabe, and A. Okaniwa. 1980. Pathological observations on natural cases of sialodacryoadenitis of rats. Exp. Anim. 29:419-426.

Dolan, M. M., and A. J. Fendrick. 1959. Incidence of *Trichophyton mentagrophytes* in laboratory rats. Proc. Anim. Care Panel 9:161-164.

Dolan, M. M., A. M. Kligman, P. G. Kobylinski, and M. A. Motsavage. 1958. Ringworm epizootics in laboratory mice and rats: Experimental and accidental transmission of infection. J. Invest. Dermatol. 30:23-35.

Domenico, P., W. G. Johanson, Jr., and D. C. Straus. 1982. Lobar pneumonia in rats produced by clinical isolates of *Klebsiella pneumoniae*. Infect. Immun. 37:327-335.

Dournon, E., B. Moriniere, S. Matheron, P. M. Girard, J.-P. Gonzalez, F. Hirsch, and J. B. McCormick. 1984. HFRS after a wild rodent bite in the Haute-Savoie and risk of exposure to Hantaan-like virus in a Paris laboratory. Lancet i:676-677.

Dowling, J. N., B. C. Wu, J. A. Armstrong, and M. Ho. 1977. Enhancement of murine cytomegalovirus infection during graft-vs.-host reaction. J. Infect. Dis. 135:990-994.

Downs, W. G. 1982. Mouse encephalomyelitis virus. Pp. 341-352 in The Mouse in Biomedical Research, vol. II, H. L. Foster, J. D. Small, and J. G. Fox, eds. New York: Academic Press.

Dubensky, T. W., F. A. Murphy, and L. P. Villarreal. 1984. Detection of DNA and RNA virus genomes in organ systems of whole mice: Patterns of mouse organ infection by polyomavirus. J. Virol. 50:779-783.

Dubos, R. J., R. W. Schaedler, R. Costello, and P. Hoet. 1965. Indigenous, normal and autochthonous flora of the gastrointestinal tract. J. Exp. Med. 122:67-82.

DuBuy, H., S. Baron, C. Uhlendorf, and M. L. Johnson. 1973. Role of interferon in murine lactic dehydrogenase virus infection in vivo and in vitro. Infect. Immun. 8:977-984.

Duffey, P. S., D. Martinez, G. D. Abrams, and W. H. Murphy. 1976. Pathogenetic mechanisms in immune polioencephalomyelitis: Induction of disease in immunosuppressed mice. J. Immunol. 116:475-481.

DuMoulin, G. C., and K. D. Stottmeier. 1978. Use of cetylpyridinium chloride in the decontamination of water for culture of mycobacteria. Appl. Environ. Microbiol. 36:771-773.

Duncan, D. W., and W. E. Razzell. 1972. *Klebsiella* biotypes among coliforms isolated from forest environments and farm produce. Appl. Microbiol. 24:933-938.

Dunn, T. B. 1954. Normal and pathologic anatomy of reticular tissue in laboratory mice with classification and discussion of neoplasms. J. Natl. Cancer Inst. 14:1281-1433.

Dunn, T. B. 1959. Morphology of mammary tumors in mice. Pp. 38-84 in The Pathophysiology of Cancer, F. Homburger, ed. New York: Hoeber.

Dupuy, J., E. Levy-Leblond, and C. LePrevost. 1975. Immunopathology of mouse hepatitis type 3 infection. II. Effect of immunosuppression in resistant mice. J. Immunol. 114:226-230.

Dvorak, S., and M. Otechenasek. 1964. Geophilic zoophilic and anthropophilic dermatophytes: A review. Mycopathol. Mycol. Appl. 23:294-296.

Dyrberg, T., P. L. Schwimmbeck, and M.B.A. Oldstone. 1988. Inhibition of diabetes in BB rats by virus infection. J. Clin. Invest. 81:928-931.

Eamons, G. J. 1984. Bacterial and mycoplasmal flora of the middle ear of laboratory rats with otitis media. Lab. Anim. Sci. 34:480-483.

Earle, D. P. 1954. Analysis of sequential physiologic derangements in epidemic hemorrhagic fever, with a commentary on management. Am. J. Med. 16:690-709.

Easmon, C. S. F., and A. A. Glynn. 1975. Cell mediated immune response in *Staphylococcus aureus* infections in mice. Immunology 29:75-85.

Easmon, C. S. F., and A. A. Glynn. 1977. Effect of cyclophosphamide on delayed hypersensitivity to *Staphylococcus aureus* in mice. Immunology 33:767-776.

Easmon, C. S. F., and A. A. Glynn. 1979. The cellular control of delayed hypersensitivity to *Staphylococcus aureus* in mice. Immunology 38:103-108.

East, J., D. M. V. Parrot, F. C. Chesterman, and A. Pomerance. 1963. The appearance of hepatotrophic virus in mice thymectomized at birth. J. Exp. Med. 118:1069-1082.

Eaton, G. J., A. Lerro, R. P. Custer, and A. R. Crane. 1982. Eradication of Sendai pneumonitis from a conventional mouse colony. Lab. Anim. Sci. 32:384-386.

Eckner, R. J., T. Han, and V. Kumar. 1974. Enhancement of murine leukemia by mycoplasmas. Suppression of cell-mediated immunity but not humoral immunity. Fed. Proc. 33:769 (abstr.)

Edberg, S. C. 1986. Nucleic acid hybridization analysis to elucidate microbial pathogens. Lab. Med. 17:735-738.

Eddy, B. E. 1982. Polyomavirus. Pp. 293-311 in The Mouse in Biomedical Research. Vol. II: Diseases, H. L. Foster, J. D. Small, and J. G. Fox, eds. New York: Academic Press.

Eddy, B. E., S. E. Stewart, R. Young, and G. B. Mider. 1958. Neoplasms in hamsters induced by a mouse tumor agent passed in tissue culture. J. Natl. Cancer Inst. 29:747-761.

Ediger, R. D., M. M. Rabstein, and L. D. Olson. 1971. Circling in mice caused by *Pseudomonas aeruginosa*. Lab. Anim. Sci. 21:845-848.

Ediger, R. D., R. M. Kovatch, and M. M. Rabstein. 1974. Colitis in mice with a high incidence of rectal prolapse. Lab. Anim. Sci. 24:488-494.

Edwards, P. R., and M. A. Fife. 1952. Capsule types of *Klebsiella*. J. Infect. Dis. 91:92-104.

Edwards, P. R., D. W. Bruner, and A. B. Moran. 1948. Further studies on the occurrence and distribution of salmonella types in the United States. J. Infect. Dis. 83:220-231.

Ehresmann, D. W., and R. N. Hogan. 1986. Acceleration of scrapie disease in mice by an adenovirus. Intervirol. 25:103-110.

Eiden, J., S. Vonderfecht, and R. H. Yolken. 1985. Evidence that a novel rotavirus-like agent of rats can cause gastroenteritis in man. Lancet ii:8-11.

Eiden, J., H. M. Lederman, S. Vonderfecht, and R. Yolken. 1986a. T-cell-deficient mice display normal recovery from experimental rotavirus infection. J. Virol. 57:706-708.

Eiden, J., S. Vonderfecht, K. Theil, A. Torres-Medina, and R.H. Yolken. 1986b. Genetic and antigenic relatedness of human and animal strains of antigenically distinct rotavirus. J. Infect. Dis. 154:972-982.

Eisenbrandt, D. L., and R. J. Russell. 1979. Scanning electron microscopy of *Spironucleus* (*Hexamita*) *muris* infection in mice. Scanning Electron Microsc. 3:23-27.

Eisenbrandt, D. L., G. B. Hubbard, and R. E. Schimdt. 1982. A subclinical epizootic of sialodacryoadenitis in rats. Lab. Anim. Sci. 32:655-659.

Eisenstein, T. K., and B. M. Sultzer. 1983. Immunity to *Salmonella* infection. Adv. Exp. Med. Biol. 162:261-296.

El Dadah, A. H., N. Nathanson, K. O. Smith, R. A. Squire, G. W. Santos, and E. C. Melby. 1967. Viral hemorrhagic encephalopathy of rats. Science 156:392-394.

Elko, E. E., and W. Cantrell. 1968. Phagocytosis and anemia in rats infected with *Haemobartonella muris*. J. Infect. Dis. 118:324-332.

Elwell, M. R., M. L. Sammons, C. T. Liu, and W. R. Beisel. 1975. Changes in blood pH in rats after infection with *Streptococcus pneumoniae*. Infect. Immun. 11:724-726.

Emmons, C. W., H. Chapman, J. P. Binford, and K. J. Kwon-Chung. 1977. Medical Mycology, 3rd ed. Philadelphia: Lea and Febiger. 592 pp.

Engers, H. D., J. A. Louis, R. H. Zubler, and B. Hirt. 1981. Inhibition of T cell mediated functions by MVM(i), a parvovirus closely related to minute virus of mice. J. Immunol. 127:2280-2285.

Ertl, H. C. J., and R. W. Finberg. 1984a. Characteristics and functions of Sendai virus-specific T-cell clones. J. Virol. 50:425-443.

Ertl, H. C. J., and R. W. Finberg. 1984b. Sendai virus-specific T-cell clones: Induction of cytolytic T cells by an anti-idiotypic antibody directed against a helper T-cell clone. Proc. Natl. Acad. Sci. USA 81:2850-2854.

Ertl, H. C. J., W. Gerlich, and U. Koszinowski. 1979. Detection of antibodies to Sendai virus by enzyme-linked immunosorbent assay (ELISA). J. Immunol. Meth. 28:163-176.

Evans, R., and V. Riley. 1968. Circulating interferon in mice infected with lactic dehydrogenase-elevating virus (LDV virus). J. Gen. Virol. 3:449-452.

Ewing, W. H. 1972. The nomenclature of *Salmonella*, its usage, and definitions for the three species. Can. J. Microbiol. 18:1629-1637.

Exon, J. H., N. M. Patton, and L. D. Koller. 1975. Hexamitiasis in cadmium-exposed mice. Arch. Environ. Health 31:463-464.

Eydelloth, R. S., S. L. Vonderfecht, J. F. Sheridan, L. D. Enders, and R. H. Yolken. 1984. Kinetics of viral replication and local and systemic immune responses in experimental rotavirus infection. J. Virol. 50:947-950.

Facklam, R. R., and R. B. Carey. 1985. Streptococci and aerococci. Pp. 154-175 in Manual of Clinical Microbiology, 4th ed., E. H. Lennette, A. Balows, W. J. Hausler, Jr., and H. J. Shadomy, eds. Washington, D.C.: American Society for Microbiology.

Fallon, M. T., M. K. Reinhard, B. M. Gray, T. W. Davis, and J. R. Lindsey. 1988. Inapparent Streptococcus pneumoniae type 35 infections in commercial rats and mice. Lab. Anim. Sci. 38:129-132.

Famulari, N. G. 1983. Murine leukemia viruses with recombinant *env* genes: A discussion of their role in leukemogenesis. Curr. Top. Microbiol. Immunol. 103:75-108.

Farmer, J. J., III, B. R. Davis, F. W. Hickman-Brenner, A. McWhorter, G. P. Huntley-Carter, M. A. Asbury, C. Riddle, H. G. Wathen-Grady, C. Elias, G. R. Fanning, A. G. Steigerwalt, C. M. O'Hara, G. K. Morris, P. B. Smith, and D. J. Brenner. 1985. Biochemical identification of new species and biogroups of Enterobacteriaceae isolated from clinical specimens. J. Clin. Microbiol. 21:46-76.

Fastier, L. B. 1950. Studies on haemagglutination with the GDVII strain of murine encephalomyelitis. J. Immunol. 65:323-330.

Fastier, L. B. 1951. Factors involved in haemagglutination by the GDVII strain of murine encephalomyelitis virus. J. Immunol. 66:365-378.

Fauve, R. M., C. H. Pierce-Chase, and R. Dubos. 1964. Corynebacterial pseudotuberculosis in mice. II. Activation of natural and experimental latent infections. J. Exp. Med. 120:283-304.

Feigin, R. D., and D. C. Anderson. 1975. Human leptospirosis. Crit. Rev. Clin. Lab. Sci. 5:413-467.

Feigin, R. D., V. H. San Joaquin, M. W. Haymond, and R. G. Wyatt. 1969. Daily periodicity of susceptibility of mice to pneumococcal infection. Nature 224:379-380.

Fenner, F. 1948a. The clinical features and pathogenesis of mousepox (infectious ectromelia of mice). J. Pathol. Bacteriol. 60:529-552.

Fenner, F. 1948b. The epizootic behavior of mousepox (infectious ectromelia). Br. J. Exp. Pathol. 29:69-91.

Fenner, F. 1948c. The epizootic behavior of mousepox (infectious ectromelia of mice). II. The course of events in long-continued epidemics. J. Hyg. 46:383-393.

Fenner, F. 1949. Mousepox (infectious ectromelia of mice): A review. J. Immunol. 63:341-373.

Fenner, F. 1981. Mousepox (infectious ectromelia): Past, present, and future. Lab. Anim. Sci. 31:553-559.

Fenner, F. 1982. Mousepox. Pp. 209-230 in The Mouse in Biomedical Research. Vol. II: Diseases, H. L. Foster, J. D. Small, and J. G. Fox, eds. New York: Academic Press.

Fenner, F., B. R. McAuslan, C. A. Mims, J. Sambrook, and D. O. White. 1974. Reoviruses. Pp. 139-145 in The Biology of Animal Viruses, 2nd ed. New York: Academic Press.

Ferm, V. H., and L. Kilham. 1964. Congenital anomalies induced in hamster embryos with H-1 virus. Science 145:510-511.

Ferm, V. H., and L. Kilham. 1965. Histopathologic basis of the teratogenic effects of H-1 virus on hamster embryos. J. Embryol. Exp. Morphol. 13:151-158.

Ferner, W. T., R. L. Miskuff, R. H. Yolken, and S. L. Vonderfecht. 1987. Comparison of methods for detection of serum antibody to murine rotavirus. J. Clin. Microbiol. 25:1364-1369.

Feuerman, E., I. Alteras, E. Honig, and N. Lehrer. 1975. Saprophytic occurrence of *Trichophyton mentagrophytes* and *Microsporum gypseum* in the coats of healthy laboratory animals. Mycopathologia 55:13-16.

Fidler, I. J. 1977. Depression of macrophages in mice drinking hyperchlorinated water. Nature 270:735-736.

Field, E. J., and D. H. Adams. 1968. Riley virus in wild mice. Lancet i:868.

Finberg, R., H. Cantor, B. Benacerraf, and S. Burakoff. 1980. The origins of alloreactivity: Differentiation of prekiller cells to virus infection results in alloreactive cytolytic T lymphocytes. J. Immunol. 124:1858-1860.

Finch, S. C., and A. M. Jonas. 1973. Ethyl palmitate-induced bartonellosis as an index of functional splenic ablation. J. Reticuloendothel. Soc. 13:20-26.

Findlay, G. M., N. S. Alcock, and R. O. Stern. 1936. The virus aetiology of one form of lymphocytic meningitis. Lancet 1:650-654.

Findlay, G., E. Klieneberger, F. O. MacCallum, and R. D. MacKenzie. 1938. Rolling disease: New syndrome in mice associated with a pleuropneumonia-like organism. Lancet 235:1511-1513.

Findlay, G. M., R. D. Mackenzie, F. O. MacCallum, and E. Klieneberger. 1939. The aetiology of polyarthritis in the rat. Lancet 237:7-10.

Fisher, E. R., and L. Kilham. 1953. Pathology of a pneumotropic virus recovered from C3H mice carrying the Bittner milk agent. Arch. Pathol. 55:14-19.

Fishman, O., Z. P. DeCamargo, and M. Grinblat. 1976. *Trichophyton mentagrophytes* infection in laboratory white mice. Mycopathologia 59:113-115.

Fitzmaurice, M. A., V. Riley, and G.A. Santisteban. 1974. Biological synergism between the LDH-virus and *Eperythrozoon coccoides:* Studies on the mechanism. Pathol. Biol. 20:743-750.

Flamm, H. 1957. *Klebsiella*-Enzootic in einer Mausezucht. Schweiz. Z. Pathol. Bakteriol. 20:23-27.

Flatt, R. E., and S. J. Jackson. 1970. Renal nosematosis in young rabbits. Pathol. Vet. 7:492-497.

Flatt, R. E., J. A. Halvorsen, and R. L. Kemp. 1978. Hexamitiasis in a laboratory mouse colony. Lab. Anim. Sci. 28:62-64.

Flewett, T. H., and G. N. Woode. 1978. The rotavirus: A brief review. Arch. Virol. 57:1-23.

Flodh, H., G. Magnusson, and O. Magnusson. 1974. Pulmonary foam cells in rats at different ages. Z. Versuchstierkd. 16:299-312.

Flynn, R. J. 1955. Ectoparasites in mice. Proc. Anim. Care Panel 6:75-91.

Flynn, R. J. 1959. Studies on the etiology of ringtail of rats. Proc. Anim. Care Panel 9:155-160.

Flynn, R. J. 1963a. *Pseudomonas aeruginosa* infection and its effects on biological and medical research. Lab. Anim. Care 13:1-6.

Flynn, R. J. 1963b. The diagnosis of *Pseudomonas aeruginosa* infection in mice. Lab. Anim. Care 13:126-130.

Flynn, R. J. 1963c. *Pseudomonas aeruginosa* infection and radio-biological research at the Argonne National Laboratory: Effects, diagnosis, epizootiology, and control. Lab. Anim. Care 13:25-35.

Flynn, R. J. 1963d. The diagnosis and control of ectromelia infection in mice. Lab. Anim. Care 13:130-137.

Flynn, R. J. 1963e. The diagnosis of some forms of ectoparasitism of mice. Proc. Anim. Care Panel 13:111-115.

Flynn, R. J. 1973a. Parasites of Laboratory Animals. Ames, Iowa: Iowa State University Press. 884 pp.

Flynn, R. J. 1973b. Cestodes. Pp. 155-202 in Parasites of Laboratory Animals. Ames, Iowa: Iowa State University Press.

Flynn, R. J. 1973c. Nematodes. Pp. 203-320 in Parasites of Laboratory Animals. Ames, Iowa: Iowa State University Press.

Ford, T. M. 1965. An outbreak of pneumonia in laboratory rats associated with *Diplococcus pneumoniae*. Lab. Anim. Care 15:448-451.

Ford, T. M., and G. N. Joiner. 1968. Pneumonia in a rat associated with *Corynebacterium pseudotuberculosis*, a case report and literature survey. Lab. Anim. Care 18:220-223.

Forsberg, C. M., and J. J. Buyllen. 1972. Effects of passage and iron on virulence of *Pseudomonas aeruginosa*. J. Clin. Pathol. 45:65-68.

Forster, U., and G. Wachendorfer. 1973. Inapparent infection of Syrian hamsters with the virus of lymphocytic choriomeningitis. Pp. 113-127 in Lymphocytic Choriomeningitis Virus and Other Arenaviruses, F. Lehmann-Grube, ed. New York: Springer-Verlag.

Foster, H. L. 1958. Large scale production of rats free of commonly occurring pathogens and parasites. Proc. Anim. Care Panel 8:92-100.

Foster, H. L., S. J. Foster, and E. S. Pfau. 1963. The large scale production of cesarean-originated barrier-sustained mice. Lab. Anim. Care 13:711-718.

Fox, J. G., and C. M. Beaucage. 1979. The incidence of *Salmonella* in random-source cats purchased for use in research. J. Infect. Dis. 139:362-365.

Fox, J. G., and J. B. Brayton. 1982. Mycoses. Pp. 411-413 in The Mouse in Biomedical Research. Vol. II: Diseases, H. L. Foster, J. D. Small, and J. G. Fox, eds. New York: Academic Press.

Fox, J. G., J. C. Murphy, and V. E. Igras. 1977a. Adverse effects of mouse hepatitis virus on ascites myeloma passage in the BALB/cJ mouse. Lab. Anim. Sci. 27:173-179.

Fox, J. G., S. M. Niemi, J. C. Murphy, and F. W. Quimby. 1977b. Ulcerative dermatitis in the rat. Lab. Anim. Sci. 27:671-678.

Fox, J. G., S. M. Niemi, J. Ackerman, and J. C. Murphy. 1987. Comparison of methods to diagnose an epizootic of *Corynebacterium kutscheri* pneumonia in rats. Lab. Anim. Sci. 37:72-75.

Francis, S. J., P. J. Southern, A. Valsamakis, and M. B. A. Oldstone. 1987. State of viral genome and proteins during persistent lymphocytic choriomeningitis virus infection. Curr. Top. Microbiol. Immunol. 133:67-88.

Franklin, J., and C. B. Richter. 1968. The isolation of *Salmonella poona* and a nonmotile variant from laboratory mice. Lab. Anim. Care 18:92-93.

Fraser, L. R., and D. Taylor-Robinson. 1977. The effect of *Mycoplasma pulmonis* on fertilization and preimplantation development in vitro of mouse eggs. Fertil. Steril. 28:488-498.

Fredericson, E., and E. A. Birnbaum. 1954. Competitive fighting between mice with different hereditary backgrounds. J. Gen. Psychol. 85:271-280.

French, G. R., R. S. Foulke, O. A. Brand, G. A. Eddy, H. W. Lee, and P. W. Lee. 1981. Korean hemorrhagic fever: Propagation of the etiologic agent in a cell line of human origin. Science 211:1046-1048.

Frenkel, J. K. 1956. Pathogenesis of toxoplasmosis and of infection with organisms resembling toxoplasma. Ann. N.Y. Acad. Sci. 64:215-251.

Frenkel, J. K., J. T. Good, and J. A. Schultz. 1966. Latent *Pneumocystis* infection of rats, relapse and chemotherapy. Lab. Invest. 15:1559-1577.

Freundt, E. A. 1956. *Streptobacillus moniliformis* infection in mice. Acta Pathol. Microbiol. Scand. 38:231-245.

Freundt, E. A. 1959. Arthritis caused by *Streptobacillus moniliformis* and pleuropneumonia-like organisms in small rodents. Lab. Invest. 8:1358-1366.

Friedman, S., and S. H. Weisbroth. 1975. The parasitic ecology of the rodent mite, *Myobia musculi*. II. Genetic factors. Lab. Anim. Sci. 25:440-445.

Friedman, S., and S. H. Weisbroth. 1977. The parasitic ecology of the rodent mite, *Myobia musculi*. IV. Life cycle. Lab. Anim. Sci. 27:34-37.

Friedmann, C. T., E. L. Spiegel, E. Aaron, and R. McIntyre. 1973. Leptospirosis contracted from pet mice. Calif. Med. 118:51-52.

Friend, C. 1957. Cell-free transmission in adult Swiss mice of a disease having the character of a leukemia. J. Exp. Med. 105:307-318.

Fries, A. S. 1977a. Studies on Tyzzer's disease: Application of immunofluorescence for detection of *Bacillus piliformis* and for demonstration and determination of antibodies to it in sera from mice and rats. Lab. Anim. 11:69-73.

Fries, A. S. 1977b. Studies on Tyzzer's disease: Isolation and propagation of *Bacillus piliformis*. Lab. Anim. 11:75-78.

Fries, A. S. 1979. Studies on Tyzzer's disease: A long-term study of the humoral antibody response in mice, rats and rabbits. Lab. Anim. 13:37-41.

Fries, A. S. 1980. Antibodies to *Bacillus piliformis* (Tyzzer's disease) in sera from man and other species. Pp. 249-250 in Animal Quality and Models in Research, A. Spiegel, S. Erichsen, and H. A. Solleveld, eds. Stuttgart: Gustav Fischer Verlag.

Fries, A. S., and O. Ladefoged. 1979. The influence of *Bacillus piliformis* (Tyzzer) infections on the reliability of pharmacokinetic experiments in mice. Lab. Anim. 13:257-261.

Fries, A. S., and O. Svendsen. 1978. Studies on Tyzzer's disease in rats. Lab. Anim. 12:1-4.

Fujiwara, K. 1967. Complement fixation reaction and agar-gel double diffusion test in Tyzzer's disease of mice. Jpn. J. Microbiol. 11:103-117.

Fujiwara, K. 1971. Problems in checking inapparent infections in laboratory mouse colonies, an attempt at serological checking by anamnestic response. Pp. 77-92 in Defining the Laboratory Animal. Washington, D.C.: National Academy of Sciences.

Fujiwara, K. 1980. Microbiological control of laboratory animals, possibilities and limitations with the emphasis on bacteriological aspects. Pp. 173-179 in Animal Quality and Models in Biomedical Research, A. Spiegel, S. Erichsen, and H. A. Solleveld, eds. Stuttgart: Gustav Fischer Verlag.

Fujiwara, K., Y. Takagaki, K. Maejima, K. Kato, M. Naiki, and Y. Tajima. 1963. Tyzzer's disease in mice: Pathologic studies on experimentally infected animals. Jpn. J. Exp. Med. 33:183-202.

Fujiwara, K., R. Takahashi, H. Kurashina, and N. Matsunuma. 1969. Protective serum antibodies in Tyzzer's disease of mice. Jpn. J. Exp. Med. 39:491-504.

Fujiwara, K., N. Hirano, S. Takenaka, and K. Sato. 1973. Peroral infection in Tyzzer's disease of mice. Jpn. J. Exp. Med. 43:33-42.

Fujiwara, K., S. Takenaka, and S. Shumiya. 1976. Carrier state of antibody and viruses in a mouse breeding colony persistently infected with Sendai and mouse hepatitis viruses. Lab. Anim. Sci. 26:153-159.

Fujiwara, K., T. Tamura, F. Taguchi, N. Hirano, and K. Ueda. 1977. Wasting disease in nude mice with faculatively virulent mouse hepatitis virus. Pp. 53-60 in Proceedings of the Second International Workshop on Nude Mice. Stuttgart: Gustav Fischer Verlag.

Fujiwara, K., Y. Tanishima, and M. Tanaka. 1979. Seromonitoring of laboratory mouse and rat colonies for common murine pathogens. Exp. Anim. 28:297-306.

Fujiwara, K., M. Nakayama, and K. Takahashi. 1981. Serologic detection of inapparent Tyzzer's disease in rats. Jpn. J. Exp. Med. 51:197-200.

Fukumi, H., and Y. Takeuchi. 1975. Vaccination against parainfluenza 1 virus (typhus muris) infection in order to eradicate this virus in colonies of laboratory animals. Dev. Biol. Stand. 28:477-481.

Fukumi, H., H. Mizutani, Y. Takeuchi, Y. Tajima, K. Imaizumi, T. Tanaka, and J. I. Kaneko. 1962. Studies of Sendai virus infection in laboratory mice. Jpn. J. Med. Sci. Biol. 15:153-163.

Furmanski, P., and M. A. Rich. 1982. Neoplasms of the hematopoietic system. Pp. 352-371 in The Mouse in Biomedical Research. Vol. IV: Experimental Biology and Oncology, H. L. Foster, J. D. Small, and J. G. Fox, eds. New York: Academic Press.

Furth, J. 1946. Prolongation of life with prevention of leukemia by thymectomy in mice. J. Gerontol. 1:46-52.

Furth, J., H. R. Seibold, and R. R. Rathbone. 1933. Experimental studies on lymphomatosis of mice. Am. J. Cancer 19:521-604.

Furuta, T., Y. Goto, T. Tamura, C. Kai, and K. Ueda. 1979. Pulmonary vascular lesions in nude mice persistently infected with mouse hepatitis virus. Jpn. J. Exp. Med. 49:423-428.

Furuta, T., K. Ueda, K. Fujiwara, and K. Yamanouchi. 1985. Cellular and humoral immune responses of mice subclinically infected with *P. carinii*. Infect. Immun. 47:544-548.

Gaertner, D. J., J. R. Lindsey, and J. O. Stevens. 1988. Cytomegalovirus-like lesions in lacrimal glands of laboratory rats. Lab. Anim. Sci. 38:79-82.

Gajdusek, D. C. 1962. Virus hemorrhagic fevers: special reference to hemorrhagic fever with renal syndrome (epidemic hemorrhagic fever). J. Pediatr. 60:841-857.

Gallily, R., A. Warwick, and G. Barry. 1964. Effect of cortisone on genetic resistance to mouse hepatitis virus in vivo and in vitro. Proc. Natl. Acad. Sci. USA 51:1158-1164.

Galton, M. 1963. Myobic mange in the mouse leading to skin ulceration and amyloidosis. Am. J. Pathol. 43:855-865.

Ganaway, J. R. 1980. Effect of heat and selected chemical disinfectants upon infectivity of spores of *Bacillus piliformis* (Tyzzer's disease). Lab. Anim. Sci. 30:192-196.

Ganaway, J. R. 1982. Bacterial and mycotic diseases of the digestive system. Pp. 1-20 in The Mouse in Biomedical Research. Vol. II: Diseases, H. L. Foster, J. D. Small, and J. G. Fox, eds. New York: Academic Press.

Ganaway, J. R., A. M. Allen, and T. D. Moore. 1971. Tyzzer's disease. Am. J. Pathol. 64:717-732.

Ganaway, J. R., A. M. Allen, T. D. Moore, and H. J. Bohner. 1973. Natural infection of germfree rats with *Mycoplasma pulmonis*. J. Infect. Dis. 127:529-537.

Ganaway, J. R., R. S. McReynolds, and A. M. Allen. 1976. Tyzzer's disease in free-living cottontail rabbits (*Sylvilagus floridanus*) in Maryland. J. Wildlife Dis. 12:545-549.

Ganaway, J. R., T. H. Spencer, T. D. Moore, and A. M. Allen. 1985. Isolation, propagation, and characterization of a newly recognized pathogen, cilia-associated respiratory (CAR) bacillus of rats, an etiological agent of chronic respiratory disease. Infect. Immun. 47:472-479.

Gang, D. L., L. V. Barrett, E. J. Wilson, R. H. Rubin, and D. N. Medearis. 1986. Myopericarditis and enhanced dystrophic cardiac calcification in murine cytomegalovirus infection. Am. J. Pathol. 124:207-215.

Gangadharam, P. R. J., P. F. Pratt, and P. T. Davidson. 1981. Experimental infections with *Mycobacterium avium-intracellulare*. Rev. Infect. Dis. 3:973-978.

Gangadharam, P. R. J., C. K. Edwards III, P. S. Murthy, and P. F. Pratt. 1983. An acute infection model for *Mycobacterium avium-intracellulare* disease using beige mice: Preliminary results. Am. Rev. Resp. Dis. 127:648-649.

Gannon, J. 1978. The immunoperoxidase test for diagnosis of *Encephalitozoon cuniculi* in rabbits. Lab. Anim. 12:125-127.

Gannon, J. 1980a. A survey of *Encephalitozoon cuniculi* in laboratory animal colonies in the United Kingdom. Lab. Anim. 14:91-94.

Gannon, J. 1980b. The course of infection of *Encephalitozoon cuniculi* in immunodeficient and immunocompetent mice. Lab. Anim. 14:189-192.

Gannon, J., and P. Carthew. 1980. Prevalence of indigenous viruses in laboratory animal colonies in the United Kingdom 1978-1979. Lab. Anim. 14:309-311.

Gard, S. 1943. Purification of poliomyelitis viruses. Acta Med. Scand. 143:1-173.

Gard, S. 1944. *Bacillus piliformis* infection in mice, and its prevention. Acta Pathol. Microbiol. Scand. 54:123-134.

Gardiner, E. M., and P. Tattersall. 1988a. Evidence that developmentally regulated control of gene expression by a parvoviral allotropic determinant is particle mediated. J. Virol. 62:1713-1722.

Gardiner, E. M., and P. Tattersall. 1988b. Mapping of the fibrotropic and lymphotropic host range determinants of the parvovirus minute virus of mice. J. Virol. 62:2605-2613.

Gardner, M. B., J. E. Officer, J. Parker, J. D. Estes, and R. W. Rongey. 1974. Induction of disseminated virulent cytomegalovirus infection by immunosuppression of naturally chronically infected wild mice. Infect. Immun. 10:966-969.

Garlinghouse, L. E., Jr., and A. L. Smith. 1985. Responses of mice susceptible or resistant to lethal infection with mouse hepatitis virus, strain JHM, after exposure by a natural route. Lab. Anim. Sci. 35:469-472.

Garlinghouse, L. E., and G. L. Van Hoosier. 1978. Studies on adjuvant-induced arthritis, tumor transplantability and serologic response to bovine serum albumin in Sendai virus infected rats. Am. J. Vet. Res. 39:297-300.

Garlinghouse, L. E., Jr., A. L. Smith, and T. Holford. 1984. The biological relationship of mouse hepatitis virus (MHV) strains and interferon: In vitro induction and sensitivities. Arch. Virol. 82:19-29.

Garlinghouse, L. E., Jr., G. L. Van Hoosier, Jr., and W. E. Giddens, Jr. 1987. Experimental Sendai virus infection in laboratory rats. I. Virus replication and immune response. Lab. Anim. Sci. 37:437-441.

Gay, W. I., ed. Undated. Health Benefits of Animal Research. Washington, D.C.: Foundation for Biomedical Research. 82 pp.

Genest, P. 1959. Transmission congenitale do la psittacose experimentale chex la Souris Blanche. Bull. Acad. Vet. France 32:75-80.

Georg, L. K. 1960. Animal Ringworm in Public Health. PHS Publ. No. 727. Washington, D.C.: U.S. Department of Health, Education, and Welfare. 61 pp.

Georgii, A., and I. Kirschenhofer. 1965. Uber die Isolierung von Lactate-Hydrogenase-Erhohendem Virus aus wilden Mausen. Z. Naturforsch. 20:3-10.

Gerber, M. A., K. V. Shah, S. N. Thung, and G. M. ZuRhein. 1980. Immunohistochemical demonstration of common antigen of polyomaviruses in routine histologic tissue sections of animals and man. Am. J. Clin. Pathol. 73:794-797.

Gerloff, R. K., and R. O. Watson. 1970. A *Chlamydia* from the peritoneal cavity of mice. Infect. Immun. 1:64-68.

Ghose, L. H., R. D. Schnagl, and I. H. Holmes. 1978. Comparison of an enzyme-linked immunosorbent assay for quantitation of rotavirus antibodies with complement fixation in an epidemiological survey. J. Clin. Microbiol. 8:268-276.

Gibson, S. V., K. S. Waggie, J. E. Wagner, and J. R. Ganaway. 1987. Diagnosis of subclinical *Bacillus piliformis* infection in a barrier-maintained mouse production colony. Lab. Anim. Sci. 37:786-788.

Giddens, W. E., K. K. Keahey, G. R. Carter, and C. K. Whitehair. 1968. Pneumonia in rats due to infection with *Corynebacterium kutscheri*. Pathol. Vet. 5:227-237.

Giddens, W. E., Jr., G. L. Van Hoosier, Jr., and L. E. Garlinghouse, Jr. 1987. Experimental Sendai virus infection in laboratory rats. II. Pathology and immunohistochemistry. Lab. Anim. Sci. 37:442-448.

Gigliotti, F., and W. T. Hughes. 1988. Passive immunoprophylaxis with specific monoclonal antibody confers partial protection against *Pneumocystis carinii* pneumonitis in animal models. J. Clin. Invest. 81:1666-1668.

Gilardi, G. L. 1985. *Pseudomonas*. Pp. 350-356 in Manual of Clinical Microbiology, 4th ed., E. H. Lennette, A. Balows, W. J. Hausler, Jr., and H. J. Shadomy, eds. Washington, D.C.: American Society for Microbiology.

Giles, R. B., J. A. Sheedy, C. N. Ekman, H. F. Froeb, C. C. Conley, J. L. Stockard, D. W. Cugell, J. W. Vester, R. K. Kiyasu, G. Entwisle, and R. H. Yoe. 1954. The sequelae of epidemic hemorrhagic fever, with a note on causes of death. Am. J. Med. 16:629-638.

Ginder, D. R. 1964. Increased susceptibility of mice infected with mouse adenoviruses to *Escherichia coli*-induced pyelonephritis. J. Exp. Med. 120:1117-1128.

Ginsberg, H. S., and F. L. Horsfall, Jr. 1951. Therapy of infection with pneumonia virus of mice (PVM). Effect of a polysaccharide on the multiplication cycles of the virus and on the course of the viral pneumonia. J. Exp. Med. 93:161-171.

Glasgow, L. A., T. Odugbemi, P. Dwyer, and A. L. Ritterson. 1971. *Eperythrozoon coccoides*. I. Effect on the interferon response in mice. Infect. Immun. 4:425-430.

Glasgow, L. A., A. T. Murrer, and P. S. Lombardi. 1974. *Eperythrozoon coccoides*. II. Effect on interferon production and role of humoral anti-body in host resistance. Infect. Immun. 9:266-272.

Gledhill, A. W. 1961. Enhancement of the pathogenicity of mouse hepatitis virus (MHV-1) by prior infection of mice with certain leukemia agents. Br. J. Cancer 15:531-538.

Gledhill, A. W. 1962. Latent ectromelia. Nature 196:298.

Gledhill, A. W., and C. H. Andrewes. 1951. A hepatitis virus of mice. Br. J. Exp. Pathol. 32:559-568.

Gledhill, A. W., and G. W. A. Dick. 1955. The nature of mouse hepatitis virus infection in weanling mice. J. Pathol. Bacteriol. 69:311-320.

Gledhill, A. W., and J. S. F. Niven. 1955. Latent virus as exemplified by mouse hepatitis virus (MHV). Vet. Rev. Anat. 1:82-90.

Gledhill, A. W., and J. S. F. Niven. 1957. The toxicity of some bacterial filtrates for mice pre-infected with *Eperythrozoon coccoides*. Br. J. Exp. Pathol. 38:284-290.

Gledhill, A. W., G. W. A. Dick, and J. S. F. Niven. 1955. Mouse hepatitis virus and its pathogenic action. J. Pathol. Bacteriol. 69:299-309.

Gledhill, A. W., D. L. J. Bilbey, and J. S. F. Niven. 1965. Effect of certain murine pathogens on phagocytic activity. Br. J. Exp. Pathol. 46:433-442.

Gleiser, C. A., and F. C. Heck. 1972. The pathology of experimental K-virus infection in suckling mice. Lab. Anim. Sci. 22:865-869.

Goeth, H., and K. R. Appel. 1974. Experimentelle Untersuchungen uber die beeintrachtigung der fertilitat durch mycoplasmeninfektionen des genitaltraktes. Zentralbl. Bakteriol. (Hyg.) 228:282-289.

Goff, S. P. 1984. The genetics of murine leukemia viruses. Curr. Top. Microbiol. Immunol. 112:45-71.

Gogolak, F. M. 1953. The histopathology of murine pneumonitis infection and the growth of the virus in the mouse lung. J. Infect. Dis. 92:254-272.

Goldgaber, D., C. J. Gibbs, Jr., D. C. Gajdusek, and A. Svedmyr. 1985. Definition of three serotypes of hantaviruses by a double sandwich ELISA with biotin-avidin amplification system. J. Gen. Virol. 66:1733-1740.

Goldstein, E., and G. M. Green. 1967. Alteration of the pathogenicity of *Pasteurella pneumotropica* for the murine lung caused by changes in pulmonary antibacterial activity. J. Bacteriol. 93:1651-1656.

Gonnert, R. 1941. Die Bronchopneumonie, eine neue Viruskrankheit der Maus. Z. Bakteriol. 147:161-174.

Gonnert, R. 1942. Uber einige Eigenschaften des Bronchopneumonievirus der Maus. Z. Bakteriol. 148:331-337.

Goodman, D. G., and F. M. Garner. 1972. A comparison of methods for detecting *Nosema cuniculi* in rabbit urine. Lab. Anim. Sci. 22:568-572.

Gordon, F. B., G. Freeman, and J. M. Clampit. 1938. A pneumonia-producing filtrable agent from stock mice. Proc. Soc. Exp. Biol. Med. 39:450-453.

Gorrill, R. H. 1956. Spinning disease of mice. J. Pathol. Bacteriol. 71:353-358.

Goslee, S., and E. Wolinsky. 1976. Water as a source of potentially pathogenic mycobacteria. Am. Rev. Resp. Dis. 113:287-292.

Goto, H., and K. Shimizu. 1978. The role of maternal antibody in contact infection of mice with Sendai virus. Exp. Anim. 27:423-426.

Graffi, A. 1957. Chloroleukemia of mice. Ann. N.Y. Acad. Sci. 68:540-558.

Graham, W. R. 1963. Recovery of pleuropneumonia-like organisms (P.P.L.O.) from the genitalia of the female rat. Lab. Anim. Care 13:719-724.

Gray, D. G., and A. L. Campbell. 1953. The use of chloramphenicol and foster mothers in the control of natural pasteurellosis in experimental mice. Aust. J. Exp. Biol. 31:161-166.

Greenberg, H., V. McAuliffe, J. Valdesuso, R. Wyatt, J. Flores, A. Kalica, Y. Hoshino, and N. Singh. 1983. Serological analysis of the subgroup protein of rotavirus, using monoclonal antibodies. Infect. Immun. 39:91-99.

Greenberg, H. B., P. T. Vo, and R. Jones. 1986. Cultivation and characterization of three strains of murine rotavirus. J. Virol. 57:585-590.

Greenlee, J. E. 1979. Pathogenesis of K virus infection in newborn mice. Infect. Immun. 26:703-705.

Greenlee, J. E. 1981. Effect of host age on experimental K virus infection in mice. Infect. Immun. 33:297-303.

Greenlee, J. E., and W. K. Dodd. 1984. Reactivation of persistent papovavirus K infection in immunosuppressed mice. J. Virol. 51:425-429.

Greenlee, J. E., and M. F. Law. 1984. Persistent infection and transformation of mouse glial cultures by K virus, a mouse papovavirus. J. Gen. Virol. 65:1253-1258.

Greenlee, J. E., W. K. Dodd, and M. L. Oster-Granite. 1982. An in vitro assay for K-papovavirus of mice. J. Virol. Methods 4:139-146.

Gregg, M. B. 1975. Recent outbreaks of lymphocytic choriomeningitis in the United States. Bull. W.H.O. 52:549-553.

Griesemer, R. A. 1958. Bartonellosis. J. Natl. Cancer Inst. 20:949-955.

Griffith, J. W., W. J. White, P. J. Danneman, and C. M. Lang. 1988. Cilia associated respiratory bacillus infection of obese mice. Vet. Pathol. 25:72-76.

Griffiths, H. J. 1971. Some common parasites of small laboratory animals. Lab. Anim. 5:123-135.

Griffiths, P. D., and J. E. Grundy. 1987. Molecular biology and immunology of cytomegalovirus. Biochem. J. 241:313-324.

Grimwood, B. G. 1985. Viral contamination of a subline of *Toxoplasma gondii* RH. Infect. Immun. 50:917-918.

Grody, W. W., L. Cheng, and K. J. Lewin. 1987. Application of in situ DNA hybridization technology to diagnostic surgical pathology. Pathol. Annu. 22:151-175.

Gross, L. 1951a. "Spontaneous" leukemia developing in C3H mice following inoculation in infancy with AK leukemic extracts or AK embryos. Proc. Soc. Exp. Biol. Med. 76:27-32.

Gross, L. 1951b. Pathogenic properties and vertical transmission of the mouse leukemic agent. Proc. Soc. Exp. Biol. Med. 78:342-348.

Gross, L. 1953a. A filterable agent recovered from AK leukemic extracts, causing salivary gland carcinomas in C3H mice. Proc. Soc. Exp. Biol. Med. 83:414-421.

Gross, L. 1953b. Neck tumors, or leukemia, developing in adult C3H mice following inoculation, in early infancy, with filtered (Berkefeld, N.) or centrifuged (144,000 × g.) AK leukemic extracts. Cancer 6:948-957.

Gross, L. 1959. Serial cell-free passage of a radiation-activated mouse leukemia agent. Proc. Soc. Exp. Biol. Med. 100:102-105.

Gross, L. 1970. Oncogenic viruses. Oxford: Pergamon Press. 991 pp.

Gruber, H. E., and J. W. Osborne. 1979. Ultrastructural features of spironucleus (hexamitiasis) in x-irradiated rat small intestine. Lab. Anim. 13:199-202.

Guetta, E., Y. Graziani, and J. Tal. 1986. Suppression of Ehrlich ascites tumors in mice by minute virus of mice. J. Natl. Cancer Inst. 76:1177-1180.

Gustafsson, B. 1948. Germ-free rearing of rats. Acta Pathol. Microbiol. Scand. 73:1-130.

Guttler, F., K. Bro-Jorgensen, and P. N. Jorgensen. 1975. Transient impaired cell-mediated tumor immunity after acute infection with lymphocytic choriomeningitis virus. Scand. J. Immunol. 4:327-336.

Haas, V. H. 1960. Serial passage of a lymphocytic tumor and choriomeningitis virus in immune mice. J. Natl. Cancer Inst. 25:75-83.

Habermann, R. T., and F. P. Williams, Jr. 1958. Salmonellosis in laboratory animals. J. Natl. Cancer Inst. 20:933-947.

Halkett, J. A. E., A. J. Davis, and G. A. Natsios. 1968. The effect of cold stress and *Pseudomonas aeruginosa* gavage on the survival of three-week-old Swiss mice. Lab. Anim. Care 18:94-96.

Hall, W. C., and J. M. Ward. 1984. A comparison of the avidin-biotin-peroxidase complex (ABC) and peroxidase-anti-peroxidase (PAP) immunocytochemical techniques for demonstrating Sendai virus infection in fixed tissue specimena. Lab. Anim. Sci. 34:261-263.

Hall, W. C., R. A. Lubet, C. J. Henry, and M. J. Collins, Jr. 1985. Sendai virus ... disease processes and research complications. Chapter 3, pp. 25-52, In Complications of Viral and Mycoplasmal Infections in Rodents to Toxicology Research and Testing. T. E. Hamm, Jr., ed. Washington, DC:Hemisphere Press.

Hamelin, C., and G. Lussier. 1988. Genotypic differences between the mouse adenovirus strains FL and K87. Experientia 44:65-66.

Hamelin, C., C. Jacques, and G. Lussier. 1988. Genome typing of mouse adenoviruses. J. Clin. Microbiol. 26:31-33.

Hamilton, J. R., and J. C. Overall, Jr. 1978. Synergistic infection with murine cytomegalovirus and *Pseudomonas aeruginosa* in mice. J. Infect. Dis. 137:775-782.

Hamilton, J. R., J. C. Overall, and L. A. Glasgow. 1976. Synergistic effect on mortality in mice with murine cytomegalovirus and *Pseudomonas aeruginosa, Staphylococcus aureus,* or *Candida albicans* infections. Infect. Immun. 14:982-989.

Hamilton, J. R., J. C. Overall, and L. A. Glasgow. 1977. Synergistic infection with murine cytomegalovirus and *Candida albicans* in mice. J. Infect. Dis. 135:918-924.

Hamm, T. E., Jr. 1983. The effects of health and health monitoring on oncology studies. Pp. 45-60 in The Importance of Laboratory Animal Genetics, Health and the Environment in Biomedical Research, E. C. Melby, Jr., and M. W. Balk, eds. New York: Academic Press.

Hammond, C. W. 1963. *Pseudomonas aeruginosa* infection and its effects on radiobiological research. Lab. Anim. Care 13(1,Part 2):6-11.

Hammond, C. W., M. Tompkins, and C. P. Miller. 1954. Studies on the susceptibility to infection following ionizing radiation. I. The time of onset and duration of the endogenous bacteremias in mice. J. Exp. Med. 99:405-410.

Hammond, C. W., D. Ruml, D. B. Cooper, and C. P. Miller. 1955. Studies on susceptibility to infection following ionizing radiation. III. Susceptibility of the intestinal tract to oral inoculation with *Pseudomonas aeruginosa*. J. Exp. Med. 102:403-411.

Hanna, M. G., A. K. Szakal, and R. L. Tyndall. 1970a. Histoproliferative effect of Rauscher leukemia virus on lymphatic tissue: Histological and ultrastructural studies of germinal centers and their relation to leukemogenesis. Cancer Res. 30:1748 1763.

Hanna, M. G., H. E. Walburg, R. C. Tyndall, and M. J. Snodgrass. 1970b. Histoproliferative effect of Rauscher leukemia virus on lymphatic tissue. II. Antigen-stimulated germfree and conventional BALB/c mice. Proc. Soc. Exp. Biol. Med. 134:1132-1141.

Hanna, P. E., D. H. Percy, F. Paturzo, and P. N. Bhatt. 1984. Sialodacryoadenitis in rat: Effects of immunosuppression on the course of the disease. Am. J. Vet. Res. 45:2077-2083.

Harada, S., T. Ishibashi, Y. Kitahara, Y. Harada, M. Takamoto, and K. Sugiyama. 1979. Experimental *Pseudomonas* infection in mice: Effect of single cyclophosphamide administration on *Pseudomonas* infection. Jpn. J. Exp. Med 49:43-50.

Hard, G. C. 1966. Staphylococcal infections of the tail of the laboratory rat. Lab. Anim. Care 16:421-429.

Harding, B., F. Kenny, F. Given, B. Murphy, and S. Lavelle. 1987. Autotransplantation of splenic tissue after splenectomy in rats offers partial protection against intravenous pneumococcal challenge. Eur. Surg. Res. 19:135-139.

Harkness, J. E., and F. G. Ferguson. 1982. Bacterial, mycoplasmal, and mycotic disease of the lymphoreticular, musculoskeletal, cardiovascular, and endocrine systems. Pp. 83-97 in The Mouse in Biomedical Research. Vol. II: Diseases, H. L. Foster, J. D. Small, and J. G. Fox, eds. New York: Academic Press.

Harkness, J. E., and J. E. Wagner. 1975. Self-mutilation in mice associated with otitis media. Lab. Anim. Sci. 25:315-318.

Harper, J. S., III, C. J. Dawe, B. D. Trapp, P. E. McKeever, M. Collins, J. L. Woyclechowska, D. L. Madden, and J. L. Sever. 1983. Paralysis in nude mice caused by polyomavirus-induced vertebral tumors. Pp. 359-367 in Polyomaviruses and Human Neurological Diseases. New York: Alan R. Liss.

Hartley, J. W., and W. P. Rowe. 1960. A new mouse virus apparently related to the adenovirus group. Virology 11:645-647.

Hartley, J. W., W. P. Rowe, and R. J. Huebner. 1961. Recovery of reoviruses from wild and laboratory mice. Proc. Soc. Exp. Biol. Med. 108:390-395.

Hartley, J. W., N. K. Wolford, L. J. Old, and W. P. Rowe. 1977. A new class of murine leukemia virus associated with development of spontaneous lymphomas. Proc. Natl. Acad. Sci. USA 74:789-792.

Hartwich, J., and M. T. Shouman. 1965. Untersuchungen uber gehauft auftretende *Klebsiella*-Infectionen bei Versuchsratten. Z. Versuchstierkd. 6:141-146.

Harwell, J. F., and D. D. Boyd. 1968. Naturally occurring oxyuriasis in mice. J. Am. Vet. Med. Assoc. 153:950-953.

Hashimoto, K., and K. Umehara. 1977. Immunological study of experimental enteric adenovirus infection in nude mice. Pp. 71-75 in Proceedings of the Second International Workshop on Nude Mice. Stuttgart: Gustav Fischer Verlag.

Hashimoto, K., T. Sugiyama, and S. Sasaki. 1966. An adenovirus isolated from the feces of mice. I. Isolation and identification. Jpn. J. Microbiol. 10:115-125.

Hashimoto, K., T. Sugiyama, M. Yoshikawa, and S. Sasaki. 1970. Intestinal resistance in the experimental enteric infection of mice with a mouse adenovirus. I. Growth of the virus and appearance of a neutralizing substance in the intestinal tract. Jpn. J. Microbiol. 14:381-395.

Hashimoto, K., Y. Okada, T. Tajiri, H. Amano, N. Aoki, and S. Sasaki. 1973. Intestinal resistance in the experimental enteric infection of mice with mouse adenovirus. III. Suppressive effect of cyclophosphamide on the establishment and duration of the intestinal resistance. Jpn. J. Microbiol. 17:503-511.

Hathaway, S. C., D. K. Blackmore, and R. B. Marshall. 1983. Leptospirosis and the maintenance host: A laboratory mouse model. Res. Vet. Sci. 34:82-89.

Hauschka, T. S. 1952. Whisker-eating mice. J. Hered. 43:77-80.

Hazlett, L. D., D. D. Rosen, and R. S. Berk. 1977. *Pseudomonas* eye infections in cyclophosphamide-treated mice. Invest. Ophthalmol. Vis. Sci. 16:649-652.

Heck, F. C., W. G. Sheldon, and C. A. Gleiser. 1972. Pathogenesis of experimentally produced mouse adenovirus infection in mice. Am. J. Vet. Res. 33:841-846.

Hedrich, H. J. 1983. Overview of the state of the art in genetic monitoring. Pp. 75-100 in The Importance of Laboratory Animal Genetics, Health, and the Environment in Biomedical Research, E. C. Melby, Jr. and M. W. Balk, eds. Orlando, Fla.: Academic Press.

Heiniger, H. J., H. Meier, N. Kaliss, M. Cherry, H. W. Chen, and R. D. Stoner. 1974. Hereditary immunodeficiency and leukemogenesis in HRS/J mice. Cancer Res. 34:201-211.

Held, J. R. 1981. Summary—Ectromelia (mousepox) in the United States. Lab. Anim. Sci. 31:630-632.

Hemelt, I. E., D. L. Huxsoll, and A. R. Warner, Jr. 1974. Comparison of MHG virus with mouse encephalomyelitis viruses. Lab. Anim. Sci. 24:523-529.

Henderson, D. C., C. E. Tosta, and N. Wedderburn. 1978. Exacerbation of murine malaria by concurrent infection with lactic dehydrogenase-elevating virus. Clin. Exp. Immunol. 33:357-359.

Henderson, D. C., R. W. S. Chang, and J. L. Turk. 1979. Infection with LDH virus alters host response to tumours. Br. J. Cancer 39:453-456.

Hendrix, M. G. R., C. A. Bruggeman, and C. P.A. van Boven. 1986. Alterations of functional state of peritoneal macrophages during rat cytomegalovirus infection in vivo. Fed. Europ. Microbiol. Soc. Microbiol. Letters 33:111-115.

Herbermann, R. B., M. E. Nunn, H. T. Holden, S. Staal, and J. Y. Djeu. 1977. Augmentation of natural cytotoxic activity of mouse lymphoid cells against syngeneic and allogeneic target cells. Int. J. Cancer 19:555-564.

Hershberger, L. G., L. M. Hensen, and D. W. Calhoun. 1960. Immunization in experimental arthritis in rats. Arth. Rheum. 3:387-394.

Herweg, D., and I. Kunstyr. 1979. Effect of intestinal flagellate *Spironucleus (Hexamita) muris* and of dimetridazole on intestinal microflora in thymus-deficient (nude) mice. Z. Bakt. Hyg. 245:262-269.

Heston, W. E. 1975. Genetics: Animal tumors. Pp. 33-57 in Cancer: A Comprehensive Treatise, vol. I, F. F. Becker, ed. New York: Plenum Press.

Heston, W. E. 1974. Genetics of cancer. J. Hered. 65:262-272.

Heyl, J. G. 1963. A study of *Pasteurella* strains from animal sources. Antonie van Leeuwenhoek 29:79-83.

HFRS (Hemorrhagic Fever with Renal Syndrome Virus Guideline Committee). 1986. Guidelines for surveillance, prevention, and control of Hantaan virus infection in laboratory animal colonies. Pp. 209-216 in Viral and Mycoplasmal Infections of Laboratory Rodents: Effects on Biomedical Research, P. N. Bhatt, R. O. Jacoby, H. C. Morse III, and A. E. New, eds. Orlando, Fla.: Academic Press.

Hierholzer, J. D., J. R. Broderson, and F. A. Murphy. 1979. New strain of mouse hepatitis virus as a cause of lethal enteritis in infant mice. Infect. Immun. 24:508-522.

Hightower, D., H. S. Uhrig, and J. I. Davis. 1966. *Pseudomonas aeruginosa* infection in rats used in radiobiology research. Lab. Anim. Care 16:85-93.

Hill, A. 1972. Transmission of *Mycoplasma pulmonis* between rats. Lab. Anim. 6:331-336.

Hill, A. C. 1974a. Mycoplasmas of small animals. Pp. 311-316 in Mycoplasmas of Man, Animals, Plants and Insects, J. M. Bove and J. F. Duplan, eds. Paris: Institut National de la Sante et de la Recherche Medicale.

Hill, A. C. 1974b. Experimental and natural infection of the conjunctiva of rats. Lab. Anim. 8:305-310.

Hill, A. C. 1983. Mycoplasma collis, a new species from rats and mice. Int. J. Syst. Bacteriol. 33:847-851.

Hirano, N., S. Takenaka, and K. Fujiwara. 1975a. Pathogenicity of mouse hepatitis virus for mice depending upon host age and route of infection. Jpn. J. Exp. Med. 45:285-292.

Hirano, N., T. Tamura, F. Taguchi, K. Ueda, and K. Fujiwara. 1975b. Isolation of a low virulent mouse hepatitis virus from nude mice with wasting syndrome and hepatitis. Jpn. J. Exp. Med. 45:429-432.

Hirano, N., S. Hino, and K. Fujiwara. 1978. Physico-chemical properties of mouse hepatitis virus (MHV-2) grown on DBT cell culture. Microbiol. Immunol. 22:377-390.

Hirano, N., K. Ono, A. Inoue, T. Murakami, and H. Takamaru. 1985. Replication of rat coronavirus in a rat cell line, LBC. Arch. Virol. 75:301-304.

Hirano, N., H. Takamaru, K.Ono, T. Murakami, and K. Fujiwara. 1986. Replication of sialodacryoadenitis virus of rat in LBC cell culture. Arch. Virol. 88:121-125.

Hirsch, M. S., R. C. Moellering, Jr., H. G. Pope, and D. C. Poskanzer. 1974. Lymphocytic-choriomeningitis-virus infection traced to a pet hamster. N. Engl. J. Med. 291:610-612.

Hirst, R. G., and R. Campbell. 1977. Mechanisms of resistance to *Corynebacterium kutscheri* in mice. Infect. Immun. 17:319-324.

Hirst, R. G., and R. J. Olds. 1978a. *Corynebacterium kutscheri* and its alleged avirulent variant in mice. J. Hyg. 80:349-356.

Hirst, R. G., and R. J. Olds. 1978b. Serological and biochemical relationship between the alleged avirulent variant of *Corynebacterium kutscheri* and streptococci of group N. J. Hyg. 80:356-363.

Hirst, R. G., and M. E. Wallace. 1976. Inherited resistance to *Corynebacterium kutscheri* in mice. Infect. Immun. 14:475-482.

Ho, M. 1980. Role of specific cytotoxic lymphocytes in cellular immunity against murine cytomegalovirus. Infect. Immun. 27:767-776.

Hoag, W. G. 1961. Oxyuriasis in laboratory mouse colonies. Am. J. Vet. Res. 22:150-153.

Hoag, W. G. 1964. Animal health control for inbred mouse colonies of the Jackson Laboratory. Lab. Anim. Care 14:253-259.

Hoag, W. G., J. Strout, and H. Meier. 1964. Isolation of *Salmonella* spp. from laboratory mice and from diet supplements. J. Bacteriol. 88:534-536.

Hoag, W. G., J. Strout, and H. Meier. 1965. Epidemiological aspects of the control of *Pseudomonas* infection in mouse colonies. Lab. Anim. Care 15:217-225.

Hoag, W. G., P. W. Wetmore, J. Rogers, and H. Meier. 1962. A study of latent *Pasteurella* infection in a mouse colony. J. Infect. Dis. 11:135-140.

Hoenig, E., G. Margolis, and L. Kilham. 1974. Experimental adenovirus infection of the mouse adrenal gland. II. Electron microscopic observations. Am. J. Pathol. 75:375-394.

Holmes, K. V., J. F. Boyle, and M. F. Frana. 1986a. Mouse hepatitis virus: Molecular biology and implications for pathogenesis. Pp. 603-624 in Viral and Mycoplasmal Infections of Laboratory Rodents: Effects on Biomedical Research. P. N. Bhatt, R. O. Jacoby, H. C. Morse III, and A. E. New, eds. Orlando, Fla: Academic Press.

Holmes, K. V., R. M. Welsh, and M. V. Haspel. 1986b. Natural cytotoxicity against mouse hepatitis virus-infected target cells. I. Correlation of cytotoxicity with virus binding to leukocytes. J. Immunol. 136:1446-1453.

Holt, D. 1959. Presence of K-virus in wild mice in Australia. Aust. J. Exp. Biol. Med. Sci. 37:183-192.

Hong, C. C., and R. D. Ediger. 1978a. Preputial gland abscess in mice. Lab. Anim. Sci. 28:153-156.

Hong, C. C., and R. D. Ediger. 1978b. Self-mutilation of the penis in C57BL/6N mice. Lab. Anim. 12:55-57.

Hong, C. C., and R. D. Ediger. 1978c. Chronic necrotizing mastitis in rats caused by *Pasteurella pneumotropica*. Lab. Anim. Sci. 28:317-320.

Hook, W. E., R. R. Wagner, and R. C. Lancefield. 1960. An epizootic of Swiss mice caused by a group A streptococcus, newly designated type 50. Am. J. Hyg. 72:111-119.

Hooper, A., and A. Sebesteny. 1974. Variation in *Pasteurella pneumotropica*. J. Med. Microbiol. 7:137-140.

Horowitz, S. A., and G. H. Cassell. 1978. Enzyme-linked immunosorbent assay for detection of *Mycoplasma pulmonis* antibodies. Infect. Immun. 22:161-170.

Horowitz, J., J. E. Volanakis, and D. E. Briles. 1987. Blood clearance of *Streptococcus pneumoniae* by C-reactive protein. J. Immunol. 138:2598-2603.

Horsfall, F. L., Jr., and H. S. Ginsberg. 1951. The dependence of the pathological lesion upon the multiplication of pneumonia virus of mice (PVM). Kinetic relation between the degree of viral multiplication and the extent of pneumonia. J. Exp. Med. 93:139-150.

Horsfall, F. L., Jr., and R. G. Hahn. 1939. A pneumonia virus of Swiss mice. Proc. Soc. Exp. Biol. Med. 40:684-686.

Horsfall, F. L., Jr., and R. G. Hahn. 1940. A latent virus in normal mice capable of producing pneumonia in its natural host. J. Exp. Med. 71:391-408.

Horsfall, F. L., Jr., and M. McCarty. 1947. The modifying effects of certain substances of bacterial origin on the course of infection with pneumonia virus of mice (PVM). J. Exp. Med. 85:623-646.

Hotchin, J. 1962. The biology of lymphocytic choriomeningitis infection: Virus-induced immune disease. Cold Spring Harbor Symp. Quant. Biol. 27:479-499.

Hotchin, J. 1971a. Virus, cell surface, and self: Lymphocytic choriomeningitis of mice. Am. J. Clin. Pathol. 56:333-349.

Hotchin, J. 1971b. The contamination of laboratory animals with lymphocytic choriomeningitis virus. Am. J. Pathol. 64:747-769.

Hotchin, J., and L. Benson. 1963. The pathogenesis of lymphocytic choriomeningitis in mice: The effects of different inoculation routes and the footpad response. J. Immunol. 91:460-468.

Hotchin, J., and D. N. Collins. 1964. Glomerulonephritis and late onset disease following neonatal virus infection. Nature 203:1357-1359.

Hotchin, J., and E. Sikora. 1975. Laboratory diagnosis of lymphocytic choriomeningitis. Bull. W.H.O. 52:555-559.

Hottle, G. A., and D. N. Wright. 1966. Growth and survival of *Mycoplasma neurolyticum* in liquid media. J. Bacteriol. 91:1834-1839.

Howanitz, J. H. 1988. Immunoassaay. Arch. Pathol. Lab. Med. 112:771-779.

Hsu, C. K., A. E. New, and J. G. Mayo. 1980. Quality assurance of rodent models. Pp. 17-28 in Animal Quality and Models in Biomedical Research, A. Spiegel, S. Erichsen, and H. A. Solleveld, eds. Stuttgart: Gustav Fischer Verlag.

Howard, C. J., and G. Taylor. 1979. Variation in the virulence of strains of *Mycoplasma pulmonis* related to susceptibility to killing by macrophages in vivo. J. Gen. Microbiol. 114:289-294.

Howard, C. J., E. J. Stott, and G. Taylor. 1978. The effect of pneumonia induced in mice with *Mycoplasma pulmonis* on resistance to subsequent bacterial infection and the effect of a respiratory infection with Sendai virus on the resistance of mice to *Mycoplasma pulmonis*. J. Gen. Microbiol. 109:79-87.

Howard, R. J., and J. S. Najarian. 1974. Cytomegalovirus-induced immune suppression. I. Humoral immunity. Clin. Exp. Immunol. 18:109-118.

Howard, R. J., A. L. Notkins, and S. E. Mergenhagen. 1969. Inhibition of cellular immune reactions in mice infected with lactic dehydrogenase virus. Nature 221:873-874.

Howard, R. J., J. Miller, and J. S. Najarian. 1974. Cytomegalovirus-induced immune suppression. II. Cell-mediated immunity. Clin. Exp. Immunol. 18:119-126.

Howard, R. J., H. H. Balfour, Jr., M. V. Seidel, R. L. Simmons, and J. S. Najarian. 1977. Effect of murine cytomegalovirus on cell-mediated immunity. Transplant. Proc. 9:355-358.

Howard, R. J., D. M. Mattson, and H. H. Balfour, Jr. 1979. Effect of immunosuppression on humoral and cell-mediated immunity to murine cytomegalovirus. Proc. Soc. Exp. Biol. Med. 161:341-346.

Howell, E. V., and R. S. Jones. 1963. Factors influencing pathogenicity of *Mycoplasma arthritidis* (PPLO). Proc. Soc. Exp. Biol. Med. 112:69-75.

Howell, J. M., and N. Edington. 1968. The production of rabbits free from lesions associated with *Encephalitozoon cuniculi*. Lab. Anim. 2:143-148.

Hsu, C.-K. 1979. Parasitic diseases. Pp. 307-331 in The Laboratory Rat. Vol. I: Biology and Diseases, H. J. Baker, J. R. Lindsey, and S. H. Weisbroth, eds. New York: Academic Press.

Hsu, C.-K. 1982. Protozoa. Pp. 359-372 in The Mouse in Biomedical Research. Vol. II: Diseases, H. L. Foster, J. D. Small, and J. G. Fox, eds. New York: Academic Press.

Hsu, D. V. M., and Q. M. Geiman. 1952. Synergistic effect of *Haemobartonella muris* on *Plasmodium berghei* in white rats. Am. J. Trop. Med. Hyg. 1:747-760.

Huebner, R., and G. J. Todaro. 1969. Oncogenes of RNA tumor viruses as determinants of cancer. Proc. Natl. Acad. Sci. USA 64:1087-1094.

Hughes, W. T. 1979. Limited effect of trimethoprim-sulfamethoxazole prophylaxis on *Pneumocystis carinii*. Antimicrob. Agents Chemother. 16:333-335.

Hughes, W. T. 1988. Comparison of dosages, intervals, and drugs in the prevention of *Pneumocystis carinii* pneumonia. Antimicrob. Agents Chemother. 32:623-625.

Hung, T., S.-M. Xia, T.-X. Zhao, J.-Y. Zhou, G. Song, G. X. H. Liao, W. W. Ye, Y. L. Chu, and C. S. Hang. 1983. Morphological evidence for identifying the viruses of hemorrhagic fever with renal syndrome as candidate members of the Bunyaviridae family. Arch. Virol. 78:137-144.

Hung, T., G. Chen, C. Wang, H. Yao, Z. Fang, T. Chao, Z. Chou, W. Ye, X. Chang, S. Den, X. Liong, and W. Chang. 1984. Waterbourne outbreak of rotavirus diarrhea in adults in China caused by a novel rotavirus. Lancet i:1139-1142.

Hunstein, W., E. Perings, B. Eggeling, and N. Uhl. 1969. Panmyelophthisis and viral hepatitis. Experimental study with the MHV-3 mouse hepatitis virus. Acta Haematol. 42:336-346.

Hunt, R. D. 1963. Dacryoadenitis in the Sprague-Dawley rat. Am. J. Vet. Res. 24:638-641.

Hunt, R. D., N. W. King, and H. L. Foster. 1972. Encephalitozoonosis: Evidence for vertical transmission. J. Infect. Dis. 126:212-214.

Hunter, B. 1971. Eradication of Tyzzer's disease in a colony of barrier-maintained mice. Lab. Anim. 5:271-276.

Iftimovici, R., V. Iacobsecu, A. Mutiu, and D. Puca. 1976. Enzootic with ectromelia symptomatology in Sprague-Dawley rats. Rev. Roum. Med. Virol. 27:65-66.

Iida, T. 1972. Experimental study on the transmission of Sendai virus in specific pathogen free mice. J. Gen. Virol. 14:69-75.

Iida, T., M. Tajima, and Y. Murata. 1973. Transmission of maternal antibodies to Sendai virus in mice and its significance in enzootic infection. J. Gen. Virol. 18:247-254.

Ijaz, M. K., M. I. Sabara, P. J. Frenchick, and L. A. Babiuk. 1987. Assessment of intestinal damage in rotavirus infected neonatal mice by a D-xylose absorption test. J. Virol. Meth. 18:153-157.

ILAR (Institute of Laboratory Animal Resources). 1970. Gnotobiotes: Standards and Guidelines for the Breeding, Care, and Management of Laboratory Animals. A report of the Subcommittee on Standards for Gnotobiotes, Committee on Standards. Washington, D.C.: National Academy of Sciences. 52 pp.

ILAR (Institute of Laboratory Animal Resources). 1976a. Long-term holding of laboratory rodents. A report of the Committee on Long-Term Holding of Laboratory Rodents. ILAR News 19:L1-L25.

ILAR (Institute of Laboratory Animal Resources). 1976b. Guide for the Care and Use of the Nude (Thymus-Deficient) Mouse in Biomedical Research. A report of the Committee on Care and Use of the "Nude" Mouse. ILAR News 19(2):M1-M20.

ILAR (Institute of Laboratory Animal Resources). 1980. National Survey of Laboratory Animal Facilities and Resources, Fiscal Year 1978. A report of the Committee on Laboratory Animal Facilities and Resources. NIH Pub. No. 80-2091. Washington, D.C.: U.S. Department of Health and Human Services. 90 pp.

Inada, T., and C. A. Mims. 1984. Mouse Ia antigens are receptors for lactate dehydrogenase virus. Nature 309:59-61.

Inada, T., and C. A. Mims. 1985a. Pattern of infection and selective loss of Ia positive cells in suckling and adult mice inoculated with lactic dehydrogenase virus. Arch. Virol. 86:151-165.

Inada, T., and C. A. Mims. 1985b. Ia antigens and Fc receptors of mouse peritoneal macrophages as determinants of susceptibility to lactic dehydrogenase virus. J. Gen. Virol. 66:1469-1477.

Inada, T., and C. A. Mims. 1986. Infection of mice with lactic dehydrogenase virus prevents development of experimental allergic encephalomyelitis. J. Neuroimmunol. 11:53-56.

Inada, T., and C. A. Mims. 1987. Genetic basis for Ia positivity and susceptibility to lactic dehydrogenase virus in macrophages of SJL/J mice. Arch. Virol. 92:77-86.

Innes, J. R. M., and M. F. Stanton. 1961. Acute disease of the submaxillary and Harderian glands (sialodacryoadenitis) of rats with cytomegaly and no inclusion bodies, with comments on normal gross and microscopic structure of the exocrine glands in the head and neck of rats. Am. J. Pathol. 38:455-468.

Innes, J. R. M., W. Zeman, J. K. Frenkel, and G. Borner. 1962. Occult endemic encephalitozoonosis of the central nervous system of mice (Swiss-Bagg-O'Grady strain). J. Neuropathol. Exp. Neurol. 21:519-533.

Iralu, V., and K. D. Ganong. 1983. Agglutination of mouse erythrocytes by *Eperythrozoon coccoides*. Infect. Immun. 39:963-965.

Irvani, J., and A. van As. 1972. Mucus transport in the tracheobronchial tree of normal and bronchitic rats. J. Pathol. 106:81-93.

Isakov, N., M. Feldman, and S. Segal. 1981. Effect of lactic dehydrogenase virus infection on tumor induction and tumor growth. Cancer Res. 41:667-672.

Isakov, N., M. Feldman, and S. Segal. 1982a. Acute infection of mice with lactic dehydrogenase virus (LDV) impairs the antigen-presenting capacity of their macrophages. Cell. Immunol. 66:317-332.

Isakov, N., M. Feldman, and S. Segal. 1982b. Lactic dehydrogenase virus (LDV) impairs the antigen-presenting capacity of macrophages yet fails to affect their phagocytic activity. Immunobiology 162:15-27.

Isakov, N., M. Feldman, and S. Segal. 1982c. The mechanism of modulation of humoral immune responses after infection of mice with lactic dehydrogenase virus. J. Immunol. 128:969-975.

Ishida, T., and K. Fujiwara. 1979. Pathology of diarrhea due to mouse hepatitis virus in the infant mouse. Jpn. J. Exp. Med. 49:33-41.

Ishida, T., and K. Fujiwara. 1982. Maternally derived immune resistance to fatal diarrhea in infant mice due to mouse hepatitis virus. Jpn. J. Exp. Med. 52:231-235.

Ishida, T., T. Tamura, K. Ueda, and K. Fujiwara. 1978. Hepatosplenic myelosis in the nude mouse naturally infected with mouse hepatitis virus. Jpn. J. Vet. Sci. 40:739-743.

Ito, S., K. Imaizumi, Y. Tajima, M. Endo, and R. Koyama. 1957. A disease of rats caused by a pleuropneumonia-like organism (PPLO). Jpn. J. Exp. Med. 27:243-248.

Ito, Y. 1980. Organization and expression of the genome of polyoma virus. Pp. 447-480 in Viral Oncology, G. Klien, ed. New York: Raven Press.

Ito, Y., and Y. Hosaka. 1983. Component(s) of Sendai virus that can induce interferon in mouse spleen. Infect. Immun. 39:1019-1023.

Itoh, T. N. Kagiyama, H. Iwai, O. Okada, S. Takashina, and H. Goto. 1978. Sendai virus infection in a small mouse breeding colony. Jpn. J. Vet. Sci. 40:615-618.

Ivanov, A. P., V. N. Bashkirtsev, and E. A. Tkachenko. 1981. Enzyme-linked immunosorbent assay for detection of arenaviruses. Arch. Virol. 67:71-74.

Iwai, H., T. Itoh, and S. Shumiya. 1977. Persistence of Sendai virus in a mouse breeder colony and possibility to re-establish the virus free colonies. Exp. Anim. 26:205-212.

Iwai, H., Y. Goto, and K. Ueda. 1979. Response of athymic nude mice to Sendai virus. Jpn. J. Exp. Med. 49:123-130.

Iwai, H., T. Itoh, N. Nagiyama, and T. Nomura. 1980. Monitoring of murine infections in facilities for animal experimentation. Pp. 219-222 in Animal Quality and Models in Biomedical Research, A. Spiegel, S. Erichsen, and H. A. Solleveld, eds. Stuttgart: Gustav Fischer Verlag.

Iwai, H., R. Yamaguchi, Y. Otsuka, K. Ueda, and M. Saito. 1984. Immunoglobulin classes of anti-Sendai virus antibody detected by ELISA in infected nude mouse serum. Microbiol. Immunol. 28:481-491.

Iwai, H., K. Machii, Y. Otsuka, and K. Ueda. 1988. T cell subsets responsible for clearance of Sendai virus from infected mouse lungs. Microbiol. Immunol. 32:305-315.

Iwasaki, Y. 1978. Experimental virus infection in nude mice. Pp. 457-475 in The Nude Mouse in Experimental and Clinical Research. J. Fogh and B. C. Giovanella, eds. New York: Academic Press.

Jackson, G. G., and R. L. Muldoon. 1973. Viruses causing common respiratory infection in man. Reoviruses and adenoviruses. J. Infect. Dis. 128:811-866.

Jackson, N. N., H. G. Wall, C. A. Miller, and M. Rogul. 1980. Naturally acquired infections of *Klebsiella pneumoniae* in Wistar rats. Lab. Anim. 14:357-361.

Jackson, S., R. F. Solorzano, and C. Middleton. 1973. Indirect fluorescent antibody test for *Nosema cuniculi* (*Encephalitozoon*) in rabbits. Proc. U.S. Anim. Health Assoc. 77:478-483.

Jacobson, R. H., and N. D. Reed. 1974. The thymus dependency of resistance to pinworm infection in mice. J. Parasitol. 60:976-979.

Jacobson, S., R. M. Friedman, and C. J. Pfau. 1981. Interferon induction by lymphocytic choriomeningitis viruses correlates with maximum virulence. J. Gen. Virol. 57:275-283.

Jacoby, R. O. 1986. Rat coronavirus. Pp. 625-638 in Viral and Mycoplasmal Infections of Laboratory Rodents: Effects on Biomedical Research. P. N. Bhatt, R. O. Jacoby, H. C. Morse III, and A. E. New, eds. Orlando, FL; Academic Press.

Jacoby, R. O., and S. W. Barthold. 1981. Quality assurance for rodents used in toxicological research and testing. Pp. 27-55 in Scientific Considerations in

Monitoring and Evaluating Toxicological Research, E. J. Gralla, ed. Washington, D.C.: Hemisphere Press.

Jacoby, R. O., P. N. Bhatt, and A. M. Jonas. 1975. Pathogenesis of sialodacryoadenitis in gnotobiotic rats. Vet. Pathol. 12:196-209.

Jacoby, R. O., P. N. Bhatt, and A. M. Jonas. 1979. Viral diseases. Pp. 271-306 in The Laboratory Rat. Vol. I: Biology and Diseases, H. J. Baker, J. R. Lindsey, and S. H. Weisbroth, eds. New York: Academic Press.

Jacoby, R. O., P. N. Bhatt, D. J. Gaertner, A. L. Smith, and E. A. Johnson. 1987. The pathogenesis of rat virus infection in infant and juvenile rats after oronasal inoculation. Arch. Virol. 95:251-270.

Jacoby, R. O., D. J. Gaertner, P. N. Bhatt, F. X. Paturzo, and A. L. Smith. 1988. Transmission of experimentally-induced rat virus infection. Lab. Anim. Sci. 38:11-14.

Jakab, G. J. 1974. Effect of sequential inoculation of Sendai virus and *Pasteurella pneumotropica* in mice. J. Am. Vet. Med. Assoc. 164:723-728.

Jakab, G. J. 1981. Interactions between Sendai virus and bacterial pathogens in the murine lung: A review. Lab. Anim. Sci. 31:170-177.

Jakab, G. J., and G. A. Warr. 1981. Immune enhanced phagocytic dysfunction in pulmonary macrophages infected with parainfluenza 1 (Sendai) virus. Am. Rev. Resp. Dis. 124:575-581.

Jasmin, G. 1957. Experimental polyarthritis in rats injected with tumor exudate. Ann. Rheum. Dis. 16:365-370.

Jawetz, E. 1948. A latent pneumotropic *Pasteurella* of laboratory animals. Proc. Soc. Exp. Biol. Med. 68:46-48.

Jawetz, E. 1950. A pneumotropic *Pasteurella* of laboratory animals. I. Bacteriological and serologic characteristics of the organism. J. Infect. Dis. 86:172-183.

Jawetz, E., and W. H. Baker. 1950. A pneumotropic *Pasteurella* of laboratory animals. II. Pathological and immunological studies with the organism. J. Infect. Dis. 86:184-196.

Jenkin, C. R., D. Rowley, and I. Auzins. 1964. The basis of immunity to mouse typhoid. I. The carrier state. Aust. J. Exp. Biol. Med. Sci. 42:215-228.

Jennings, L. F., and R. M. Rumpf. 1965. Control of epizootic diarrhea in infant mice. Lab. Anim. Care 15:386-392.

Jenson, A. B., E. R. Rabin, C. A. Phillips, and J. L. Melnick. 1965. Reovirus encephalitis in newborn mice. Am. J. Pathol. 47:223-239.

Jersey, G., C. K. Whitehair, and G. R. Carter. 1973. *Mycoplasma pulmonis* as the primary cause of chronic respiratory disease in rats. J. Am. Vet. Med. Assoc. 163:599-604.

Johanson, W. G., Jr., S. J. Jay, and A. K. Pierce. 1974. Bacterial growth in vivo. An important determinant of the pulmonary clearance of *Diplococcus pneumoniae* in rats. J. Clin. Invest. 53:1320-1325.

Johnson, E., and S. W. Barthold. 1979. The ultrastructure of transmissible murine colonic hyperplasia. Am. J. Pathol. 97:291-313.

Johnson, J. E., III, L. E. Cluff, and K. Goshi. 1961. Studies on the pathogenesis of staphylococcal infection. I. The effect of repeated skin infections. J. Exp. Med. 113:235-248.

Johnson, K. 1986. Hemorrhagic fever-Hantaan virus. Pp. 193-207 in Viral and Mycoplasmal Infections of Laboratory Rodents: Effects on Biomedical Research. P. N. Bhatt, R. O. Jacoby, H. C. Morse III, and A. E. New, eds. Orlando, FL: Academic Press

Johnson, K. P. 1969. Mouse cytomegalovirus: Placental infection. J. Infect. Dis. 120:445-450.

Johnson, R. C., and S. Faine. 1984. Leptospiraceae. Pp. 62-70 in Bergey's Manual of Systematic Bacteriology, vol. I, N. R. Krieg and J. G. Holt, eds. Baltimore: Williams & Wilkins.

Jonas, A. M. 1965. Laboratory animal facilities. J. Am. Vet. Med. Assoc. 146:600-606.

Jonas, A. M. 1984. Notes on diagnostic problems. Pp. 3-4 in the Jackson Laboratory Animal Health and Genetic Quality Control Report, October 1983-March 1984. Bar Harbor, Maine: The Jackson Laboratory.

Jonas, A. M., J. Craft, C. L. Black, P. N. Bhatt, and D. Hilding. 1969. Sialodacryoadenitis in the rat, a light and electron microscopic study. Arch. Pathol. 88:613-622.

Jonas, A. M., D. Percy, and J. Craft. 1970. Tyzzer's disease in the rat. Arch. Pathol. 90:561-566.

Jones, R. L., C. M. Peterson, R. W. Grady, T. Kumbaraci, A. Cerami, and J. H. Graziano. 1977. Effects of iron chelators and iron overload on Salmonella infection. Nature 267:63-65.

Joo, I., E. S. Stanislavsky, M. I. Zhvanetskaya, G. M. Mashilova, and M. A. Gladus. 1982. Active and passive mouse-protecting capacity of *Pseudomonas aeruginosa* protein vaccines. Acta Microbiol. Hung. 29:267-275.

Jordan, J., and G. Mirick. 1965a. An infectious hepatitis of undetermined origin in mice. I. Description of the disease. J. Exp. Med. 102:601-616.

Jordan, J., and G. Mirick. 1965b. An infectious hepatitis of undetermined origin in mice. II. Characteristics of the infective agent. J. Exp. Med. 102:617-630.

Jordan, M. C. 1978. Interstitial pneumonia and subclinical infection after intranasal inoculation of murine cytomegalovirus. Infect. Immun. 21:275-280.

Jordan, M. C., J. L. Takagi, and J. G. Stevens. 1982. Activation of latent murine cytomegalovirus in vivo and in vitro. A pathogenetic role for acute infection. J. Infect. Dis. 145:699-705.

Jordan, S. W., and W. D. Doughty. 1969. Ultrastructural pathology of murine pneumonitis caused by K-papovavirus. Exp. Mol. Pathol. 11:1-7.

Juhr, N. C., and J. Horn. 1975. Modellinfektion mit *Corynebacterium kutscheri* bei der Maus. Z. Versuchstierkd. 17:129-141.

Juhr, von N. C., and S. Obi. 1970. Uterusinfektionen beimmeerschweinchen. Z. Versuchstierkd. 12:383-387.

Jungeblut, C. W., and H. Kodza. 1963. Interference between lymphocytic choriomeningitis virus and the leukemia-transmitting agent of L2C in guinea pigs. Arch. Ges. Virusforsch. 12:552-560.

Jure, M. N., S. S. Morse, and D. M. Stark. 1987. Serum albumin treatment to eliminate false-positive results with laboratory rodent specimens tested by rotazyme enzyme-linked immunosorbent assay. J. Clin. Microbiol. 25:2239-2240.

Kahan, B., R. Auerbach, B. J. Alter, and F. H. Bach. 1982. Histocompatibility and isozyme differences in commercially supplied "BALB/c" mice. Science 217:379-381.

Kajima, M., and M. Pollard. 1965. Detection of viruslike particles in germ-free mice. J. Bacteriol. 90:1448-1454.

Kaklamanis, E., and M. Pavlatos. 1972. The immunosuppressive effect of *Mycoplasma* infection. I. Effect on the humoral and cellular response. Immunology 22:695-702.

Kanazawa, K., and A. Imai. 1959. Pure culture of the pathogenic agent of Tyzzer's disease of mice. Nature 184:1810-1811.

Kaneko, J., H. Fujita, S. Matsuyama, H. Kojima, H. Saskura, Y. Nakamura, and T. Kodama. 1960. An outbreak of Tyzzer's disease in colonies of mice. Exp. Anim. 9:148-156.

Kaplan, H. S., and M. B. Brown. 1954. Development of lymphoid tumors in nonirradiated thymic grafts in thymectomized irradiated mice. Science 119:439-441.

Kappeler, V. R., S. Barandun, H. Luthi, and E. Weismann. 1961. Uber eine laboratoriunis Infektion mit *Leptospira ballum*, Orchitis als Komplikation. Schweiz. Med. Wochschr. 91:810-812.

Karr, H. V. 1943. Study of latent pneumotropic virus of mice. J. Infect. Dis. 72:108-116.

Katami, K., F. Taguchi, M. Nakayama, N. Goto, and K. Fujiwara. 1978. Vertical transmission of mouse hepatitis virus infection in mice. Jpn. J. Exp. Med. 48:481-490.

Kawamata, J., T. Yamanouchi, and H. W. Lee. 1980. Outbreaks of epidemic hemorrhagic fever in animal laboratories in Japan. Pp. 235-238 in Animal Quality and Models in Research, A. Spiegel, S. Erichsen, and H. A. Solleveld, eds. Stuttgart: Gustav Fischer Verlag.

Kawamata, J., T. Yamanouchi, K. Dohmae, H. Miyamoto, M. Takahaski, K. Yamaniski, T. Kurata, and H. W. Lee. 1987. Control of laboratory acquired hemorrhagic fever with renal syndrome (HFRS) in Japan. Lab. Anim. Sci. 37:431-436.

Kawamura, S., F. Taguchi, and K. Fujiwara. 1983. Plaque formation by Tyzzer's organism in primary monolayer culture of mouse hepatocytes. Microbiol. Immunol. 27:415-424.

Kay, M. M. B. 1978. Long term subclinical effects of parainfluenza (Sendai) infection on immune cells of aging mice. Proc. Soc. Exp. Biol. Med. 158:326-331.

Kay, M. M. B. 1979. Parainfluenza infection of aged mice results in autoimmune disease. Clin. Immunol. Immunopathol. 12:301-315.

Kay, M. M. B., J. Mendoza, S. Hausman, and B. Dorsey. 1979. Age related changes in the immune system of mice of eight medium and long lived strains and hybrids. II. Short- and long-term effects of natural infection with parainfluenza type 1 virus (Sendai). Mech. Aging Dev. 11:347-362.

Kaye, D., J. G. Merselis, Jr., and E. W. Hook. 1965. Influence of *Plasmodium berghei* infection on susceptibility to *Salmonella* infection. Proc. Soc. Exp. Biol. Med. 120:810-813.

Keast, D., and F. C. Chesterman. 1972. Changes in macrophage metabolism in mice heavily infected with *Hexamita muris*. Lab. Anim. 6:33-39.

Kellett, B. S., and J. E. C. Bywater. 1978. A modified India-ink immunoreaction for the detection of encephalitozoonosis. Lab. Anim. 12:59-60.

Kelsey, D. K., G. A. Olsen, J. C. Overall, Jr., and L. A. Glasgow. 1977. Alteration of host defense mechanisms by murine cytomegalovirus infection. Infect. Immun. 18:754-760.

Kenyon, A. J. 1983. Delayed wound healing in mice associated with viral alteration of macrophages. Am. J. Vet. Res. 44:652-656.

Kessler, W. R. 1943. Studies of experimental *Bartonella muris* anemia in the albino rat. J. Infect. Dis. 73:65-76.

Kessler, W. R., and R. L. Zwemer. 1944. Studies on experimental *Bartonella* anemia in the albino rat. J. Infect. Dis. 75:134-137.

Kijima, M., and M. Pollard. 1970. Ultrastructural pathology of glomerular lesions in gnotobiotic mice with congenital lymphocytic choriomeningitis (LCM) virus infection. Am. J. Pathol. 61:117-140.

Kilham, L. 1952. Isolation in suckling mice of a virus from C3H mice harboring Bittner milk agent. Science 116:391-392.

Kilham, L. 1961a. Mongolism associated with rat virus (RV) infection in hamsters. Virology 13:141-143.

Kilham, L. 1961b. Rat virus (RV) infections in hamsters. Proc. Soc. Exp. Biol. Med. 106:825-829.

Kilham, L. 1961c. Hemagglutination by K-virus. Virology 15:384-385.

Kilham, L. 1966. Viruses of laboratory and wild rats. Pp. 117-140 in Viruses of Laboratory Rodents, R. Holdenried, ed. National Cancer Institute Monograph 20. Washington, D.C.: U. S. Department of Health, Education, and Welfare.

Kilham, L., and V. H. Ferm. 1964. Rat virus (RV) infections of pregnant, fetal and newborn rats. Proc. Soc. Exp. Biol. Med. 117:874-879.

Kilham, L., and G. Margolis. 1966. Spontaneous hepatitis and cerebellar hypoplasia in suckling rats due to congenital infection with rat virus. Am. J. Pathol. 49:457-475.

Kilham, L., and G. Margolis. 1969. Transplacental infection of rats and hamsters induced by oral and parenteral inoculations of H-1 and rat viruses (RV). Teratology 2:111-123.

Kilham, L., and G. Margolis. 1970. Pathogenicity of minute virus of mice (MVM) for rats, mice, and hamsters. Proc. Soc. Exp. Biol. Med. 133:1447-1551.

Kilham, L., and G. Margolis. 1971. Fetal infections of hamsters, rats, and mice induced with the minute virus of mice (MVM). Teratology 4:43-62.

Kilham, L., and G. Margolis. 1974a. Transmission of rat virus in wild rats. J. Infect. Dis. 129:737-740.

Kilham, L., and G. Margolis. 1974b. Transmission of rat virus in milk of rats. J. Infect. Dis. 129:737-740.

Kilham, L., and G. Margolis. 1975. Problems of human concern arising from animal models of intrauterine and neonatal infections due to viruses: A review. I. Introduction and virologic studies. Prog. Med. Virol. 20:113-143.

Kilham, L., and J. B. Moloney. 1964. Association of rat virus and Moloney leukemia virus in tissues of inoculated rats. J. Natl. Cancer Inst. 32:523- 531.

Kilham, L., and H. W. Murphy. 1953. A pneumotropic virus isolated from C3H mice carrying the Bittner milk agent. Proc. Soc. Exp. Biol. Med. 82:133-137.

Kilham, L., and L. J. Olivier. 1959. A latent virus of rats isolated in tissue culture. Virology 7:428-437.

Kilham, L., C. E. Buckler, V. H. Ferm, and S. Baron. 1968. Production of interferon during rat virus infection. Proc. Soc. Exp. Biol. Med. 129:274-278.

Kilham, L., G. Margolis, and E. D. Colby. 1970. Enhanced proliferation of H-1 virus in livers of rats infected with *Cysticercus fasciolaris*. J. Infect. Dis. 121:648-652.

Kim, K. S., V. Sapienza, and R. I. Carp. 1975. Comparative characteristics of three cytomegaloviruses from rodents. Am. J. Vet. Res. 36:1495-1500.

Kimmig, W., and F. Lehmann-Grube. 1979. The immune response of the mouse to lymphocytic choriomeningitis virus. I. Circulating antibodies. J. Gen. Virol. 45:703-710.

Kimura, Y., H. Aoki, K. Shimokata, Y. Ito, M. Takana, N. Kirabayashi, and E. Norrby. 1979. Protection of mice against virulent virus infection by a temperature-sensitive mutant derived from an HVJ (Sendai virus) carrier culture. Arch. Virol. 61:297-304.

Kirchner, B. K., L. W. Dixon, R. H. Lentsch, and J. E. Wagner. 1982. Recovery and pathogenicity of several *Salmonella* species isolated from mice. Lab. Anim. Sci. 32:506-507.

Kitahara, Y., T. Ishibashi, Y. Harada, M. Takamoto, and K. Tanaka. 1981. Reduced resistance to *Pseudomonas* septicemia in diabetic mice. Clin. Exp. Immunol. 43:590-598.

Kitamura, T., C. Morita, T. Komatsu, K. Sugiyama, J. Arikawa, S. Shiga, H. Takeda, Y. Akao, K. Imaizumi, A. Oya, N. Hashimoto, and S. Urasawa. 1983. Isolation of a virus causing hemorrhagic fever with renal syndrome (HFRS) through a cell culture system. Jpn. J. Med. Sci. Biol. 36:17-25.

Kizaka, S., G. Goodman-Snitkoff, and J. J. McSharry. 1983. Sendai virus glycoproteins are T cell-dependent B cell mitogens. Infect. Immun. 40:592-600.

Klein, J. O., G. M. Green, J. G. Tilles, E. H. Kass, and M. Finland. 1969. Effect of intranasal reovirus infection on antibacterial activity of mouse lung. J. Infect. Dis. 119:43-50.

Klieneberger, E. 1935. The natural occurrence of pleuropneumonia-like organisms in apparent symbiosis with *Streptobacillus moniliformis* and other bacteria. J. Pathol. Bacteriol. 40:93-105.

Klieneberger, E. 1938. Pleuropneumonia-like organisms of diverse provenance. Some results of an inquiry into methods of differentiation. J. Hyg. 38:458-476.

Klieneberger, E. 1939. Studies on pleuropneumonia-like organisms: The L4 organism as the cause of Woglom's "pyogenic virus." J. Hyg. 39:260-265.

Klieneberger, E., and D. B. Steabben. 1937. On a pleuropneumonia-like organism in lung lesions of rats, with notes on the clinical and pathological features of the underlying condition. J. Hyg. 37:143-152.

Klieneberger, E., and D. B. Steabben. 1940. On the association of the pleuropneumonia-like organism L3 with bronchiectatic lesions in rats. J. Hyg. 40:223-227.

Klinge, O., and W. Siveke. 1971. Karyokinesis and karyogramm in the glandula orbitalis externa of rats. Virch. Arch. Zellpath. 9:235-259. (In German.)

Knobler, R. L., M. V. Haspel, and M.B.A. Oldstone. 1981. Mouse hepatitis virus type 4 (JHM strain)-induced fatal central nervous system disease. I. Genetic control and the murine neuron as the susceptible site of disease. J. Exp. Med. 153:832-843.

Kohn, D. F., and B. E. Kirk. 1969. Pathogencity of *Mycoplasma pulmonis* in laboratory rats. Lab. Anim. Care 19:321-330.

Kohn, D. F., and W. F. Mackenzie. 1980. Inner ear disease characterized by rolling in C3H mice. J. Am. Vet. Med. Assoc. 177:815-817.

Koi, M., M. Saito, T. Ebina, and N. Ishida. 1981. Lactate dehydrogenase- elevating agent is responsible for interferon induction and enhancement of natural killer cell activity by inoculation of Ehrlich ascites carcinoma cells into mice. Microbiol. Immunol. 25:565-574.

Kojima, A., F. Fujinami, A. Yasoshima, and A. Okaniwa. 1980. Isolation and properties of sialodacryoadenitis virus of rats. Exp. Anim. 29:409-418.

Kojima, A., H. Takada, H. Yamanaka, A. Okaniwa, K. Doi, and A. Yasoshima. 1983. Pathology of sialodacryoadenitis virus infection in newborn mice. Jpn. J. Vet. Sci. 45:297-304.

Koller, L. D. 1969. Spontaneous *Nosema cuniculi* infection in laboratory rabbits. J. Am. Vet. Med. Assoc. 155:1108-1114.

Kollmorgen, G. M., D. C. Cox, J. J. Killion, J. L. Cantrell, and W. A. Sansing. 1976. Immunotherapy of EL4 lymphoma with reovirus. Cancer Immunol. Immunother. 1:239-244.

Koopman, J. P., J. T. M. Van Der Logt, J. W. M. A. Mullink, F. W. A. Heessen, A. M. Stadhouders, H. M. Kennis, and W. J. I. Van Der Gulden. 1984. Tail lesions in C3H/He mice. Lab. Anim. 18:106-109.

Kournikakis, B., and L. A. Babiuk. 1987. Murine cytomegalovirus-*Pseudomonas* synergistic infections: comparison of virulent and attenuated virus. Can. J. Microbiol. 33:923-927.

Kovacs, J. A., J. C. Swan, J. Shelhamer, V. Gill, F. Ognibene, J. E. Parillo, and H. Masur. 1986. Prospective evaluation of a monoclonal antibody in diagnosis of *Pneumocystis carinii* pneumonia. Lancet 2:1-3.

Kowalchyk, K., and P.G.W. Plagemann. 1985. Cell surface receptors for lactate dehydrogenase-elevating virus subpopulation of macrophages. Virus Res. 2:211-229.

Kraft, L. M. 1957. Studies on the etiology and transmission of epidemic diarrhea of infant mice. J. Exp. Med. 106:743-755.

Kraft, L. M. 1958. Observations on the control and natural history of epidemic diarrhea in infant mice (EDIM). Yale J. Biol. Med. 31:121-137.

Kraft, L. M. 1961. Responses of the mouse to the virus of epidemic diarrhea of infant mice. Neutralizing antibodies and carrier state. Proc. Anim. Care Panel 11:125-136.

Kraft, L. M. 1962a. An apparently new lethal virus disease of infant mice. Science 137:282-283.

Kraft, L. M. 1962b. Two viruses causing diarrhea in infant mice. Pp. 115-130 in the Problems of Laboratory Animal Disease, R. J. C. Harris, ed. New York: Academic Press.

Kraft, L. M. 1966. Epizootic diarrhea of infant mice and lethal intestinal virus infection of infant mice. Pp. 55-63 in Viruses of Laboratory Rodents, R. Hold enried, ed. National Cancer Institute Monograph 20. Washington, D.C.: U.S. Department of Health, Education, and Welfare.

Kraft, L. M. 1982. Viral diseases of the digestive system. Pp. 159-191 in The Mouse in Biomedical Research. Vol. II: Diseases, H. L. Foster, J. D. Small, and J. G. Fox, eds. New York: Academic Press.

Kraft, V., and B. Meyer. 1986. Diagnosis of murine infections in relation to test method employed. Lab. Anim. Sci. 36:271-276.

Kraft, L. M., and A. E. Moore. 1961. A papular skin lesion of mice caused by a transmissible agent. Z. Versuchstierkd. 1:66-73.

Kraft, L. M., R. F. Pardy, D. A. Pardy, and H. Zwickel. 1964. Practical control of diarrheal disease in a commercial mouse colony. Lab. Anim. Care 14:16-20.

Kraft, L. M., E. D. D'Amelio, and F. E. D'Amelio. 1982. Morphological evidence for natural poxvirus infection in rats. Lab. Anim. Sci. 32:648-654.

Kraus, G. E., H. Soule, and J. Gruber. 1968. Uber Vorkommen, Diagnostik and Pathologie latenter Infektionen mit Killian-virus in laboratoriummausen. Arch. Exp. Veterinaermed. 22:1203-1210.

Kreier, J. P., and M. Ristic. 1968. Haemobartonellosis, eperythrozoonosis, grahamellosis and erhlichiosis. Pp. 387-472 in Infectious Blood Diseases of Man and Animals, D. Weinman and M. Ristic, eds. New York: Academic Press.

Krikun, V. A. 1977. Pox in rats: Isolation and identification of pox virus. Vopr. Virusol. 22:371-373.

Krzystyniak, K., and J. M. Dupuy. 1983. Immunodepression of lymphocyte response in mouse hepatitis virus 3 infection. Biomed. Pharmacother. 37:68-74.

Kunstyr, I. 1977. Infectious form of *Spironucleus* (*Hexamita*) *muris:* Banded cysts. Lab. Anim. 11:185-188.

Kunstyr, I. 1980. Laboratory animals as a possible source of dermatophytic infections in man. Zbl. Bakt. Med. Mycol. 8:361-367.

Kunstyr, I., and E. Ammerpohl. 1978. Resistance of faecal cysts of *Spironucleus muris* to some physical factors and chemical substances. Lab. Anim. 12:95-97.

Kunstyr, I., and K. T. Friedhoff. 1980. Parasitic and mycotic infections in laboratory animals. Pp. 181-192 in Animal Quality and Models in Research, A. Spiegel, S. Erichsen, and H. A. Solleveld, eds. Stuttgart: Gustav Fischer Verlag.

Kunstyr, I., and D. Hartman. 1983. *Pasteurella pneumotropica* and the prevalence of the AHP (*Actinobacillus*, *Haemophilus*, *Pasteurella*)-group in laboratory animals. Lab. Anim. 17:156-160.

Kunstyr, I., E. Ammerpohl, and B. Meyer. 1977a. Experimental spironucleosis (hexamitiasis) in the nude mouse as a model for immunologic and pharmacologic studies. Lab. Anim. Sci. 27:782-788.

Kunstyr, I., B. Meyer, and E. Ammerpohl. 1977b. Spironucleosis in nude mice: An animal model for immuno-parasitologic studies. Pp. 17-27 in Proceedings of the Second International Workshop on Nude Mice. Stuttgart: Gustav Fischer Verlag.

Kurata, T., T. F. Tsai, S. P. Bauer, and J. B. McCormick. 1983. Immunofluorescence studies of disseminated Hantaan Virus infection of suckling mice. Infect. Immun. 41:391-398.

Kutscher, D. 1894. Ein Beitrag zur Kentniss der bacillaren Pseudotuberculose der Nagethiere. Z. Hyg. Infekt. 18:327-342.

Kuttner, A. G., and S. H. Wang. 1934. The problem of the significance of the inclusion bodies found in the salivary glands of infants and the occurrence of inclusion bodies in the submaxillary glands of hamsters, white mice and wild rats (Peiping). J. Exp. Med. 60:773-789.

Kyriazis, A. P., L. DiPersio, J. G. Michaei, and A. J. Pesce. 1979. Influence of the mouse hepatitis virus (MHV) infection on the growth of human tumors in the athymic mouse. Int. J. Cancer 23:042-409.

Lackey, M. D., P. L. Eichman, and W. P. Havens. 1953. Hepatitis in laboratory mice. J. Infect. Dis. 93:14-20.

Lahdevirta, J. 1971. Nephropathia epidemica in Finland: a clinical, histological and epidemiological study. Ann. Clin. Res. 3 (Suppl. 8):12-17.

Lahdevirta, J., J. Saavola, M. Brummer-Korvenkontio, R. Berndt, R. Illikainen, and A. Vaheri. 1984. Clinical and serological diagnosis of nephropathia epidemica, the mild type of hemorrhagic fever with renal syndrome. J. Infect. 9:230-238.

Lahelle, O., and F. L. Horsfall, Jr. 1949. Hemagglutination with the GDVII strain of mouse encephalomyelitis virus. Proc. Soc. Exp. Biol. Med. 71:713-718.

Lai, W. C., S. P. Pakes, Y. S. Lu, and C. F. Brayton. 1987. *Mycoplasma pulmonis* infection augments natural killer cell activity in mice. Lab. Anim. Sci. 37:299-303.

Lai, Y. L., R. O. Jacoby, A. M. Jonas, and D. A. Papermaster. 1976. Keratoconjunctivitis associated with sialodacryoadenitis in rats. Invest. Ophthalmol. 15:538-541.

Lainson, R., P. C. C. Garnham, R. Killick-Kendrick, and R. G. Bird. 1964. Nosematosis, a microsporidial infection of rodents and other animals, including man. Br. Med. J. 2:470-472.

Lal, J. G., J. M. Lary, and D. L. Conover. 1980. Embryotoxicity of *Mycoplasma pulmonis* infection in rats (Abstract No. 84). Paper presented at the Annual Session of the Am. Assoc. Lab. Anim. Sci., Indianapolis, IN, October 5-10, 1980.

Laltoo, H., and L. S. Kind. 1979. Reduction in contact sensitivity reactions to oxazolone in mite-infested mice. Infect. Immun. 26:30-35.

Lancefield, R. C. 1972. Group A streptococcal infections in animals—natural and experimental. Pp. 313-326 in Streptococci and Streptococcal Diseases. Recognition, Understanding, and Management, L. W. Wannamaker and J. M. Matsen, eds. New York: Academic Press.

Lang, D. J., K. S. Cheung, J. N. Schwartz, C. A. Daniels, and S. E. Harwood. 1976. Cytomegalovirus replication and the host immune response. Yale J. Biol. Med. 49:45-58.

Lanken, P. N., M. Minda, G. G. Pietra, and A. P. Fishman. 1980. Alveolar response to experimental *Pneumocystis carinii* pneumonia in the rat. Am. J. Pathol. 99:561-578.

Lasfargues, E. Y., B. Kramarsky, J. C. Lasfargues, and D. H. Moore. 1974. Detection of mouse mammary tumor virus in cat kidney cells infected with purified B particles from RIII milk. J. Natl. Cancer Inst. 53:1831-1833.

Lattuada, C. P., R. M. Norberg, and H. P. Harlan. 1981. Large isolators for rearing rodents. Pp. 53-58 in Recent Advances in Germfree Research, S. Sasaki, A. Ozawa, and K. Hashimoto, eds. Tokyo: Tokai University Press.

Lavelle, G. C., and F. B. Bang. 1973. Differential growth of MHV (PRI) and MHV (C3H) in genetically resistant C3H mice rendered susceptible by eperythrozoan infection. Arch. Ges. Virusforsch. 41:175-184.

Lavelle, G. C., and T. J. Starr. 1969. Relationship of phagocytic activity to pathogenicity of mouse hepatitis virus as affected by triolein and cortisone. Br. J. Exp. Pathol. 50:475-480.

Law, L. W. 1965. Neoplasms in thymectomized mice following room infection with polyoma virus. Nature 205:672-673.

Lawrence, J. J. 1957. Infection of laboratory mice with *Corynebacterium murium*. Aust. J. Sci. 20:147.

Leader, R. W., I. Leader, and E. Witschi. 1970. Genital mycoplasmosis in rats treated with testosterone propionate to produce constant estrus. J. Am. Vet. Med. Assoc. 157:1923-1925.

LeDuc, J. W. 1987. Epidemiology of hantaan and related viruses. Lab. Anim. Sci. 37:413-418.

LeDuc, J. W., G. A. Smith, and K. M. Johnson. 1984. Hantaan-like viruses from domestic rats captured in the United States. Am. J. Trop. Med. 33:992-998.

LeDuc, J. W., G. A. Smith, F. P. Pinheiro, P. F. C. Vasconcelos, E.S.T. Rosa, and J. I. Maiztegui. 1985a. Isolation of a Hantaan-related virus from Brazilian rats and serologic evidence of its widespread distribution in South America. Am. J. Trop. Med. Hyg. 34:810-815.

LeDuc, J. W., G. A. Smith, M. Macy, and R. J. Hay. 1985b. Certified cell lines of rat origin appear free of infection with Hantavirus. J. Infect. Dis. 152:1082-1083.

Lee, C.-H., C. D. Bolinger, M. S. Bartlett, R. B. Kohler, C. E. Wilde III, and J. W. Smith. 1986. Production of monoclonal antibody against *Pneumocystis carinii* by using a hybrid of rat spleen and mouse myeloma cells. J. Clin. Microbiol. 23:505-508.

Lee, H. W. 1982. Korean hemorrhagic fever. Prog. Med. Virol. 28:96-113.

Lee, H. W., and K. M. Johnson. 1982. Laboratory-acquired infections with Hantaan virus , the etiologic agent of Korean hemorrhagic fever,. J. Infect. Dis. 146:645-651.

Lee, H. W., P. W. Lee, and K. M. Johnson. 1978. Isolation of the etiologic agent of Korean hemorrhagic fever. J. Infect. Dis. 137:298-308.

Lee, H. W., P. W. Lee, M. Tamura, T. Tamura, and Y. Okuno. 1979. Etiological relation between Korean hemorrhagic fever and epidemic hemorrhagic fever in Japan. Biken J. 22:41-45.

Lee, H. W., P. W. Lee, L. J. Baek, C. K. Song, and I. W. Seong. 1981. Intraspecific transmission of Hantaan virus, etiologic agent of Korean hemorrhagic fever, in the rodent *Apodemus agrarius*. Am. J. Trop. Med. Hyg. 30:1106-1112.

Lee, H. W., L. J. Baek, and K. M. Johnson. 1982. Isolation of Hantaan virus, the etiologic agent of Korean hemorrhagic fever, from wild urban rats. J. Infect. Dis. 146:638-644.

Lee, K. P., and H. J. Trochimowicz. 1982a. Pulmonary response to inhaled hexamethylphosphoramide in rats. Toxicol. Appl. Pharmacol. 62:90-103.

Lee, K. P., and H. J. Trochimowicz. 1982b. Induction of nasal tumors in rats exposed to hexamethylphosphoramide by inhalation. J. Natl. Cancer Inst. 68:157-171.

Lee, P. W., H. L. Amyx, C. J. Gibbs, Jr., D. C. Gajdusek, and H. W. Lee. 1981a. Propagation of Korean hemorrhagic fever virus in laboratory rats. Infect. Immun. 31:334-338.

Lee, P. W., C. J. Gibbs, Jr., D. C. Gajdusek, and A. Svedmyr. 1981b. Antibody to Korean hemorrhagic fever virus in man in parts of the world where hemorrhagic fever with renal syndrome is not known. Lancet ii:256 (letter).

Leftwich, W. B., and G. S. Mirick. 1949. The effect of diet on the susceptibility of the mouse to pneumonia virus of mice (PVM). I. Influence of pyridoxine in the period after inoculation of the virus. J. Exp. Med. 89:155-173.

Lehmann-Grube, F. 1982. Lymphocytic choriomeningitis virus. Pp. 231-266 in The Mouse in Biomedical Research. Vol. II: Diseases, H. L. Foster, J. D. Small, and J. G. Fox, eds. New York: Academic Press.

Lehmann-Grube, F., and J. Lohler. 1981. Immunopathologic alterations of lymphatic tissues of mice infected with lymphocytic choriomeningitis virus. II. Pathogenetic mechanisms. Lab. Invest. 44:205-213.

Lehmann-Grube, F., W. Slenczka, and R. Tees. 1969. A persistent inapparent infection of L cells with the virus of lymphocytic choriomeningitis. J. Gen. Virol. 5:63-82.

Lehmann-Grube, F., I. Niemeyer, and J. Lohler. 1972. Lymphocytic choriomeningitis of the mouse. IV. Depression of the allograft reaction. Med. Microbiol. Immunol. 158:16-25.

Lehmann-Grube, F., M. Kallay, B. Ibscher, and R. Schwartz. 1979. Serologic diagnosis of human infections with lymphocytic choriomeningitis virus: Comparative evaluation of seven methods. J. Med. Virol. 4:125-136.

Lehmann-Grube, F., L. M. Peralta, M. Bruns, and J. Lohler. 1983. Persistent infection of mice with the lymphocytic choriomeningitis virus. Pp. 43-103 in Virology, vol. 18, Virus-Host Interactions: Receptors, Persistence, and Neurological Disease, H. Fraenkel-Conrat and R. R. Wagner, eds. New York: Plenum Press.

LeMaistre, C., and R. Tompsett. 1952. The emergence of pseudotuberculosis in rats given cortisone. J. Exp. Med. 95:393-407.

LeMinor, L. 1984. Salmonella. Pp. 427-448 in Bergey's Manual of Systematic Bacteriology, vol. I, N. R. Krieg and J. G. Holt, eds. Baltimore: Williams & Wilkins.

Lentsch, R. H., and J. E. Wagner. 1980. Isolation of *Actinobacillus lignieresii* and *Actinobacillus equuli* from laboratory rodents. J. Clin. Microbiol. 12:351-354.

Lentsch, R. H., B. K. Kirchner, L. W. Dixon, and J. E. Wagner. 1983. A report of an outbreak of *Salmonella oranienburg* in a hybrid mouse colony. Vet. Microbiol. 8:105-109.

Lepine, P., and V. Sautter. 1936. Existence en France du virus murin de la choriomeningite lymphocytaire. C. R. Acad. Sci. 202:1624-1626.

Lerner, E. M., II, and E. Silverstein. 1957. Experimental infection of rats with *Streptobacillus moniliformis*. Science 126:208-209.

Lerner, E. M., II, and L. Sokoloff. 1959. The pathogenesis of bone and joint infections produced by *Streptobacillus moniliformis*. Arch. Pathol. 67:364-372.

Les, E. P. 1968. Effect of acidified-chlorinated water on reproduction in C3H/HeJ and C57BL/6J mice. Lab. Anim. Care 18:210-213.

Les, E. P. 1972. A disease related to cage population density: Tail lesions in C3H/HeJ mice. Lab. Anim. Sci. 22:56-60.

Leung, L. S. E., G. J. Szal, and R. H. Drachman. 1972. Increased susceptibility of splenectomized rats to infection with *Diplococcus pneumoniae*. J. Infect. Dis. 126:507-513.

Leung, W. C. T., and K. Hashimoto. 1986. Modification of susceptibility to *Klebsiella pneumonia* during murine cytomegalovirus infection. Microbial. Immunol. 30:761-776.

Levaditi, C., S. Nicolau, and R. Schoen. 1923a. L'etiologie de l'encephalite. C. R. Acad. Sci. 177:985-988.

Levaditi, C., S. Nicolau, and R. Schoen. 1923b. L'agent etiologique de l'encephalite epizootique du Lapin (*Encephalitozoon cuniculi*). C. R. Soc. Biol. 89:984-986.

Levaditi, C., S. Nicolau, and R. Schoen., 1924. L'etiologie de l'encephalite epizootique du lapin, dans ses rapports avec l'etude experimentale de l'encephalite lethargique *Encephalitozoon cuniculi* (nov. spec). Ann. Inst. Pasteur 38:651-712.

Levaditi, C., R. F. Selbie, and R. Schoen. 1932. La rhumatisme infectieux spontane de la souris provoque par le *Streptobacillus moniliformis*. Ann. Inst. Pasteur 48:308-343.

Levine, N. D. 1961. Protozoan Parasites of Domestic Animals and of Man. Minneapolis, Minn.: Burgess. 412 pp.

Levine, N. D. 1974. Diseases of laboratory animals—Parasitic. Pp. 209-327 in CRC Handbook of Laboratory Animal Science, vol. II, E. C. Melby and N. H. Altman, eds. Cleveland: CRC Press.

Levine, N. D., and V. Ivens. 1965. The Coccidian Parasites (Protozoa, Sporozoa) of Rodents. Urbana, Illinois: University of Illinois Press. 365 pp.

Levy, G. A., J. L. Leibowitz, and T. S. Edington. 1981. Induction of monocyte procoagulant activity by murine hepatitis virus type 3 parallels disease susceptibility in mice. J. Exp. Med. 154:1150-1163.

Levy-Leblond, E., and J. M. Dupuy. 1977. Neonatal susceptibility to MHV3 infection in mice. I. Transfer of resistance. J. Immunol. 118:1219-1222.

Lewis, A. M., Jr., W. P. Rowe, H. C. Turner, and R. J. Huebner. 1965. Lymphocytic choriomeningitis virus in hamster tumor: Spread to hamsters and humans. Science 150:363-364.

Liddle, C. G., J. P. Putnam, and O. H. Lewter. 1987. Effects of microwave exposure and temperature on survival of mice infected with *Streptococcus pneumoniae*. Bioelectromagnetics 8:295-302.

Lieber, M. M., and G. J. Todaro. 1975. Mammalian type C RNA viruses. Pp. 91-130 in Cancer: A Comprehensive Treatise, vol. II, F. F. Becker, ed. New York: Plenum Press.

Lieberman, M., and H. S. Kaplan. 1959. Leukemogenic activity of filtrates from radiation-induced lymphoid tumors of mice. Science 130:387-388.

Lieberman, M. M., H. L. Walker, E. Ayala, and I. Chapa. 1986. Active and passive immunization with *Pseudomonas aeruginosa* ribosomal vaccines and antisera in the burned rat model. J. Surg. Res. 40:138-144.

Lillie, R. D., and C. Armstrong. 1945. Pathology of lymphocytic choriomeningitis in mice. Arch. Pathol. 40:141-152.

Lilly, F., and A. Mayer. 1980. Genetic aspects of murine type-C viruses and their hosts in oncogenesis. Pp. 89-108 in Viral Oncology, G. Klein, ed. New York: Raven Press.

Lilly, F., and T. Pincus. 1973. Genetic control of murine viral leukemogenesis. Adv. Cancer Res. 17:231-277.

Lindsey, J. R. 1986. Prevalence of viral and mycoplasmal infections in laboratory rodents. Pp. 801-807 in Viral and Mycoplasma Infections of Laboratory Rodents: Effects on Biomedical Research, P. N. Bhatt, R. O. Jacoby, H. C. Morse III, and A. E. New, eds. New York: Academic Press.

Lindsey, J. R., and G. H. Cassell. 1973. Experimental *Mycoplasma pulmonis* infection in pathogen free mice. Models for studying mycoplasmosis of the respiratory tract. Am. J. Pathol. 72:63-90.

Lindsey, J. R., H. J. Baker, R. G. Overcash, G. H. Cassell, and C. E. Hunt. 1971. Murine chronic respiratory disease. Significance as a research complication and experimental production with *Mycoplasma pulmonis*. Am. J. Pathol. 64:675-716.

Lindsey, J. R., M. W. Conner, and H. J. Baker. 1978a. Physical, chemical and microbial factors affecting biologic response. Pp. 37-43 in Laboratory Animal Housing. Washington, D.C.: National Academy Press.

Lindsey, J. R., G. H. Cassell, and H. J. Baker. 1978b. Diseases due to mycoplasmas and rickettsias. Pp. 1481-1550 in Pathology of Laboratory Animals, vol. II, K. Benirschke, F. M. Garner, and T. C. Jones, eds. New York: Springer-Verlag.

Lindsey, J. R., G. H. Cassell, J. K. Davis, and M. K. Davidson. 1982. Mycoplasmal and other bacterial diseases of the respiratory system. Pp. 21-41 in The Mouse in Biomedical Research. Vol. II, H. L. Foster, J. D. Small, and J. G. Fox, eds. New York: Academic Press.

Lindsey, J. R., M. K. Davidson, T. R. Schoeb, and G. H. Cassell. 1985a. Murine mycoplasmal infections. Chapt. 5, pp. 91-121, in Complications of Viral and Mycoplasma Infections in Rodents to Toxicology Research and Testing. T. E. Hamm, Jr., ed. Washington, D.C.: Hemisphere Press.

Lindsey, J. R., M. K. Davidson, T. R. Schoeb, and G. H. Cassell. 1985b. *Mycoplasma pulmonis*-host relationships in a breeding colony of Sprague-Dawley rats with enzootic murine respiratory mycoplasmosis. Lab. Anim. Sci. 35:597-608.

Lindsey, J. R., D. B. Casebolt, and G. H. Cassell. 1986a. Animal health in toxicological research: An appraisal of past performance and future prospects. Pp. 155-171 in Managing Conduct and Data Quality of Toxicology Studies. Princeton, N.J.: Princeton Scientific.

Lindsey, J. R., M. K. Davidson, T. R. Schoeb, and G. H. Cassell. 1986b. Murine mycoplasmal infections. Pp. 91-121 in Complications of Viral and Mycoplasmal Infections in Rodents to Toxicology Research and Testing, T. E. Hamm, Jr., ed. Washington, D.C.: Hemisphere Press.

Lipman, N. S., C. E. Newcomer, and J. G. Fox. 1987. Rederivation of MHV and MEV antibody positive mice by cross-fostering and use of the microisolator caging system. Lab. Anim. Sci. 37:195-199.

Lipton, H. L. 1975. Theiler's virus infection in mice: An unusual biphasic disease process leading to demyelination. Infect. Immun. 11:1147-1155.

Lipton, H. L. 1978a. The relationship of Theiler's mouse encephalomyelitis virus plaque size with persistent infection. Pp. 679-689 in Persistent Viruses, J. G. Stevens, G. J. Todaro, and C. F. Fox, eds. New York: Academic Press.

Lipton, H. L. 1978b. Characterization of the TO strains of Theiler's mouse encephalomyelitis virus. Infect. Immun. 20:869-872.

Lipton, H. L. 1980. Persistent Theiler's murine encephalomyelitis virus infection in mice depends on plaque size. J. Gen. Virol. 46:169-177.

Lipton, H. L., and M. C. Dal Canto. 1976a. Theiler's virus-induced demyelination: Prevention by immunosuppression. Science 192:62-64.

Lipton, H. L., and M. C. Dal Canto. 1976b. Chronic neurologic disease in Theiler's virus infection of SJL/J mice. J. Neurol. Sci. 30:201-207.

Lipton, H. L., and M. C. Dal Canto. 1979a. The TO strains of Theiler's viruses cause "slow-virus-like" infections in mice. Ann. Neurol. 6:25-28.

Lipton, H. L., and M. C. Dal Canto. 1979b. Susceptibility of inbred mice to chronic central nervous system infection by Theiler's murine encephalomyelitis virus. Infect. Immun. 26:369-374.

Lipton, H. L., and R. T. Johnson. 1972. The pathogenesis of rat virus infection in the newborn hamster. Lab. Invest. 27:508-513.

Lipton, H. L., and E. J. Rozhon. 1986. The Theiler's murine encephalomyelitis viruses. Pp. 253-275 in Viral and Mycoplasmal Infections of Laboratory Rodents: Effects on Biomedical Research. P. N. Bhatt, R. O. Jacoby, H. C. Morse III, and A. E. New, eds. Orlando, FL: Academic Press.

Lipton, H., N. Nathanson, and J. Hodous. 1973. Enteric transmission of parvoviruses: Pathogenesis of rat virus infection in adult rats. Am. J. Epidemiol. 96:443-446.

Lipton, H. L., J. Kratochvil, P. Sethi, and M. C. Dal Canto. 1984. Theiler's virus antigen detected in mouse spinal cord 2 1/2 years after infection. Neurology 34:1117-1119.

Litterst, C. I. 1974. Mechanically self induced muzzle alopecia in mice. Lab. Anim. Sci. 24:806-809.

Little, L. M., and J. A. Shadduck. 1982. Pathogenesis of rotavirus infection in mice. Infect. Immun. 38:755-763.

Liu, J. J. and J. A. Shadduck. 1988. *Encephalitozoon cuniculi* infection in MRL/MPJ-LPR (lymphoproliferation) mice. Lab. Anim. Sci. 38:685-688.

Liu, J. J., E. H. Greeley, and J. A. Shadduck. 1988. Murine encephalitozoonois: The effect of age and mode of transmission on occurrence of infection. Lab. Anim. Sci. 38:675-679.

Ljungstrom, I., J. Holmgren, A.-M. Svennerholm, and A. Ferrante. 1985. Changes in intestinal fluid and muscosal immune responses to cholera toxin in *Giardia muris* infection and binding of cholera toxin to *Giardia muris* trophozoites. Infect. Immun. 50:243-249.

Lloyd, G., E. T. W. Bowen, N. Jones, and A. Pendry. 1984. HFRS outbreak associated with laboratory rats in UK. Lancet i:1175-1176.

Loew, F. M., and J. G. Fox. 1983. Animal health surveillance and health delivery systems. Pp. 69-82 in The Mouse in Biomedical Research. Vol. III: Normative Biology, Immunology, and Husbandry, H. L. Foster, J. D. Small, and J. G. Fox, eds. New York: Academic Press.

Loh, L., and J. B. Hudson. 1981. Murine cytomegalovirus infection in the spleen and its relationship to immunosuppression. Infect. Immun. 32:1067-1072.

Loh, L., and J. B. Hudson. 1982. Murine cytomegalovirus-induced immunosuppression. Infect. Immun. 36:89-95.

Lohler, J., and F. Lehmann-Grube. 1981. Immunopathologic alterations of lymphatic tissues of mice infected with lymphocytic choriomeningitis virus. I. Histopathologic findings. Lab. Invest. 44:193-204.

London, B. A., J. Kern, and W. D. Gehle. 1983. Detection of murine virus antibody by ELISA. Lab. Anim. 12:40-47.

Long, E. G., J. S. Smith, and J. L. Meier. 1986. Attachment of *Pneumocystis carinii* to rat pneumocytes. Lab. Invest. 54:609-615.

Long, S. Y. 1972. Hair-nibbling and whisker-trimming as indicators of social hierarchy in mice. Anim. Behav. 20:10-12.

Lucas, C., S. Frie, R. Peters, and J. Parker. 1987. A quantitative immunofluorescence test for detection of serum antibody to Sendai virus in mice. Lab. Anim. Sci. 37:51-54.

Luckey, T. D. 1963. Germfree Life and Gnotobiotics. New York: Academic Press. 512 pp.

Luethans, T. N., and J. E. Wagner. 1983. A naturally occurring intestinal mouse adenovirus infection associated with negative serologic findings. Lab. Anim. Sci. 33:270-272.

Lukas, V. S., W. W. Ruehl, and T. E. Hamm, Jr. 1987. An enzyme-linked immunosorbent assay to detect serum IgG in rabbits naturally exposed to cilia-associated respiratory bacillus. Lab. Anim. Sci. 37:533 (abstract).

Lukes, R. J. 1954. The pathology of thirty-nine fatal cases of epidemic hemorrhagic fever. Am. J. Med. 16:639-650.

Lum, G. S. 1970. In vitro studies of rat viruses. I. Effects of long-term culture. Oncology 24:401-415.

Lum, G. S., and A. W. Schreiner. 1963. Study of a virus isolated from a chloroleukemia Wistar rat. Cancer Res. 23:1742-1747.

Lusis, P. I., and M. A. Soltys. 1971. Immunization of mice and chinchillas against *Pseudomonas aeruginosa*. Can. J. Comp. Med. 35:60-66.

Lussenhop, N., B. Holmes, W. A. Cafruny, and P. G. W. Plagemann. 1982. Acute infection of mice with lactate dehydrogenase-elevating virus enhances Fc and complement receptor activity of peritoneal macrophages. J. Gen. Virol. 61:25-31.

Lussier, G. 1973. Encephalitis caused by murine cytomegalovirus in newborn and weanling mice. Vet. Pathol. 10:366-374.

Lussier, G. 1975. Effect of anti-thymocyte serum on murine cytomegalovirus encephalitis in weanling mice. Rev. Can. Biol. 34:1-10.

Lussier, G. 1976. Glomerulonephritis caused by murine cytomegalovirus. Vet. Pathol. 13:123-130.

Lussier, G., and J. P. Descoteaux. 1986. Prevalence of natural virus infections in laboratory mice and rats used in Canada. Lab. Anim. Sci. 36:145-148.

Lussier, G., and F. M. Loew. 1970. An outbreak of hexamitiasis in laboratory mice. Can. J. Comp. Med. 34:350-353.

Lussier, G., A. L. Smith, D. Guenette, and J. P. Descoteaux. 1987a. Serological relationship between mouse adenovirus strains FL and K87. Lab Anim. Sci. 37:55-57.

Lussier, G., D. Guenette, and J. P. Descoteaux. 1987b. Comparison of serological tests for the detection of antibody to natural and experimental murine cytomegalovirus. Can. J. Vet. Res. 51:249-252.

Lussier, G., D. Guenette, W. R. Shek, and J. P. Descoteaux. 1988a. Detection of antibodies to mouse thymic virus by enzyme-linked immunosorbent assay. Can. J. Vet. Res. 52:236-238.

Lussier, G., D. Guenette, W. R. Shek, and J. P. Descoteaux. 1988b. Evaluation of mouse thymic virus antibody detection techniques. Lab. Anim. Sci. 38:577-579.

Lutsky, I. I., and A. B. Organick. 1966. Pneumonia due to mycoplasma in gnotobiotic mice. I. Pathogenicity of *Mycoplasma pneumoniae*, *Mycoplasma salivarium* and *Mycoplasma pulmonis* for the lungs of conventional and gnotobiotic mice. J. Bacteriol. 92:1154-1163.

Lyngset, A. 1980. A survey of serum antibodies to *Encephalitozoon cuniculi* in breeding rabbits and their young. Lab. Anim. Sci. 30:558-561.

Lyon, H. W., J. J. Christian, and C. W. Miller. 1959. Cytomegalic inclusion disease of lacrimal glands in male laboratory rats. Proc. Soc. Exp. Biol. Med. 101:164-166.

Machii, K., H. Iwai, Y. Otsuka, K. Ueda, and N. Hirano. 1988. Reactivities of four murine coronavirus antigens with immunized or naturally infected rat sera by enzyme-linked immunosorbent assay. Exp. Anim. 37:251-255.

Mackenzie, D. W. R. 1961. *Trichophyton mentagrophytes* in mice; infections of humans and incidence amongst laboratory animals. Sabouraudia 1:178-182.

Mackenzie, W. F., L. S. Magill, and M. Hulse. 1981. A filamentous bacterium associated with respiratory disease in wild rats. Vet. Pathol. 18:836-839.

Mackie, T. J., C. E. Van Rooyen, and E. Gilroy. 1933. An epizootic disease occurring in breeding stock of mice: Bacteriological and experimental observations. Br. J. Exp. Pathol. 14:132-136.

Maddison, S. E., G. V. Hayes, S. B. Slemenda, L. G. Norman, and M. H. Ivey. 1982. Detection of specific antibody by enzyme linked immunosorbent assay and antigenemia by counterimmuno-electrophoresis in humans infected with *Pneumocystis carinii*. J. Clin. Microbiol. 15:1036-1043.

Madge, D. S. 1973. Small intestine carbohydrase activities in experimental *Salmonella enterocolitis* in mice. Life Sci. 12:535-542.

Maejima, K., K. Fujiwara, Y. Takagaki, M. Naiki, H. Kurashina, and Y. Tajima. 1965. Dietetic effects on experimental Tyzzer's disease of mice. Jpn. J. Exp. Med. 35:1-10.

Maenza, R. M., D. W. Powell, G. R. Plotkins, S. B. Formal, H. R. Jarvis, and H. Sprinz. 1970. Experimental diarrhea: *Salmonella enterocolitis* in the rat. J. Infect. Dis. 121:475-485.

Mahy, B. W. J., K. E. K. Rowson, C. W. Parr, and H. H. Salaman. 1965. Studies on the mechanisms of action of Riley virus. I. Action of substances affecting the reticuloendothelial system on plasma enzyme levels in mice. J. Exp. Med. 122:967-981.

Majborada, A. D., and Z. I. Lobanova. 1980. An asymptomatic form of rat pox in laboratory rats. Acta Mikrobiol. Epidemiol. Immunol. 2:106-109.

Majborada, A. D., Z. I. Lobanova, and V. A. Dushkin. 1980. Pathogenicity of rat pox virus for laboratory mice. Z. Versuchstierkd. 22:25-31.

Majeed, S. K., and A. J. Zubaidy. 1982. Histopathological lesions associated with *Encephalitozoon cuniculi* (nosematosis) infection in a colony of Wistar rats. Lab. Anim. 16:244-247.

Makino, S., S. Seko, H. Nakao, and K. Mikazuki. 1972. An epizootic of Sendai virus infection in a rat colony. Exp. Anim. 22:275-280.

Malherbe, H. H. 1978. Comments on the pathogenesis of rotaviral infections. J. Am. Vet. Med. Assoc. 173:546-547.

Mallucci, L. 1964. Mouse hepatitis virus and interferon production in normal and regenerating liver. Arch. Ges. Virusforsch. 15:91-97.

Manaker, R. A., C. W. Piczak, A. A. Miller, and M. F. Stanton. 1961. A hepatitis virus complicating studies with mouse leukemia. J. Natl. Cancer Inst. 27:29-45.

Manchee, R. J., and D. Taylor-Robinson. 1968. Haemadsorption and haemaggulination by mycoplasma. J. Gen. Microbiol. 50:465-478.

Mannini, A., and D. N. Medearis, Jr. 1961. Mouse salivary gland virus infections. Am. J. Hyg. 73:329-343.

Marchal, J. 1930. Infectious ectromelia. A hitherto undescribed virus disease of mice. J. Pathol. Bacteriol. 33:713-728.

Marennikova, S. S., and E. M. Shelukhina. 1976. White rats as a source of pox infection in carnivora of the family Felidae. Acta Virol. 20:422.

Marennikova. S. S., I. D. Ladnyj, Z. I. Ogorodnikova, E. M. Shelukhina, and N. N. Maltseva. 1978a. Identification and study of a poxvirus isolated from wild rodents in Turkmenia. Arch. Virol. 56:7-14.

Marennikova, S. S., E. M. Shelukhina, and V. A. Fimina. 1978b. Pox infection in white rats. Lab. Anim. 12:33-36.

Margard, W. L., and J. H. Litchfield. 1963. Occurrence of unusual Salmonella in laboratory mice. J. Bacteriol. 85:1451-1452.

Margard, W. L., and A. C. Peters. 1964. A study of gnotobiotic mice monocontaminated with *Salmonella typhimurium*. Lab. Anim. Care 14:200-206.

Margard, W. L., A. C. Peters, N. Dorko, J. H. Litchfield, and R. S. Davidson. 1963. Salmonellosis in mice-diagnostic procedures. Lab. Anim. Care 13:144-165.

Margileth, A. M., A. J. Strans, R. Chandra, R. Neafie, M. Blum, and R. M. McCully. 1973. Disseminated nosematosis in an immunologically compromised infant. Arch. Pathol. 95:145-150.

Margolis, G., and L. Kilham. 1968. In pursuit of an ataxic hamster, or virus-induced cerebellar hypoplasia. Pp. 157-183 in The Central Nervous System. International Academy of Pathology Monograph No. 9. Baltimore, Maryland: Williams & Wilkins.

Margolis, G., L. Kilham, and P. R. Ruffolo. 1968. Rat virus disease, an experimental model of neonatal hepatitis. Exp. Mol. Pathol. 8:1-20.

Margolis, G., and L. Kilham. 1970. Parvovirus infections, vascular endothelium and hemorrhagic encephalopathy. Lab. Invest. 22:478-488.

Margolis, G., L. Kilham, and R. H. Johnson. 1971. The parvoviruses and replicating cells: Insights into the pathogenesis of cerebellar hypoplasia. Pp. 168-201 in Progress in Neuropathology, vol. I., E. Zimmerman, ed. New York: Grune and Stratton.

Margolis, G., and L. Kilham. 1975. Problems of human concern arising from animal models of intrauterine and neonatal infections due to viruses: A review. II. Pathologic studies. Prog. Med. Virol. 20:144-179.

Margolis, G., L. R. Jacobs, and L. Kilham. 1976. Oxygen tension and the deletive tropism of K-virus for mouse pulmonary endothelium. Am. Rev. Respir. Dis. 114:45-51.

Marmorston-Gottesman, J., and D. Perla. 1930. Studies on *Bartonella muris* anemia of albino rats. I. *Trypanosoma lewisi* infection in normal albino rats associated with *Bartonella muris* anemia. II. Infection in adult normal rats. J. Exp. Med. 52:121-129.

Marmorston, J. 1935. Effect of splenectomy on a latent infection *Eperythrozoon coccoides* in white mice. J. Infect. Dis. 56:142-152.

Maronpot, R. R., and J.-M. Chavannes. 1977. Dacryoadenitis, conjunctivitis, and facial dermatitis of the mouse. Lab. Anim. Sci. 27:277-278.

Martin, M. L., H. Lindsey-Regnery, D. R. Sasso, J. B. McCormick, and E. Palmer. 1985. Distinction between Bunyaviridae genera by surface structure and comparison with Hantaan virus using negative stain electron microscopy. Arch. Virol. 86:17-28.

Martinez, D. 1979. Histocompatibility-linked genetic control of susceptibility to age-dependent polioencephalomyelitis in mice. Infect. Immun. 23:133-139.

Martinez, D., M. A. Brinton, T. G. Tachovsky, and A. H. Phelps. 1980. Identification of lactate dehydrogenase-elevating virus as the etiologic agent of genetically restricted age-dependent polioencephalomyelitis in mice. Infect. Immun. 27:979-987.

Martone, W. J., and C. M. Patton. 1981. Rat-bite fever. Pp. 581-586 in Diagnostic Procedures for Bacterial, Mycotic and Parasitic Infections, 6th ed., A. Balows and W. J. Hausler, Jr., eds. Washington, D.C.: American Public Health Association.

Maru, M., and K. Sato. 1982. Characterization of a coronavirus isolated from rats with sialoadenitis. Arch. Virol. 73:33-43.

Masur, H., and T. C. Jones. 1978. The interaction in vitro of *Pneumocystis carinii* with macrophages and L-cells. J. Exp. Med. 147:150-170.

Matsumoto, T. 1980. Early deaths after irradiation of mice contaminated by *Enterobacter cloacae*. Lab. Anim. 14:247-249.

Matsumoto, T. 1982. Influence of *Escherichia coli*, *Klebsiella pneumoniae* and *Proteus vulgaris* on the mortality pattern of mice after lethal irradiation with $\gamma$ rays. Lab. Anim. 16:36-39.

Matsushita, S. 1986. Spontaneous respiratory disease associated with cilia-associated respiratory (CAR) bacillus in a rat. Jpn. J. Vet. Sci. 48:437-440.

Matsushita, S., M. Kashima, and H. Joshima. 1987. Serodiagnosis of cilia-associated respiratory bacillus infection by the indirect immunofluorescence assay technique. Lab. Anim. 21:356-359.

Matsuya, Y., T. Kusano, S. Endo, N. Takahashi, and I. Yamane. 1978. Reduced tumorigenicity by addition in vitro of Sendai virus. Eur. J. Cancer 14:837-850.

Mattern, C. F. T., A. C. Allison, and W. P. Rowe. 1963. Structure and composition of K virus, and its relation to the "papovavirus" group. Virology 20:413-419.

Matthews, R. E. F. 1982. Classification and Nomenclature of Viruses. Fourth Report of the International Committee on Taxonomy of Viruses. Intervirology 17:1-199.

Mayer, M. 1921. Uber einige Bakterienahnliche Parasiten der Erythrozyten bei Menschen und Tieren. Arch. Schiffs Trop. Hyg. 25:150-151.

Mazanec, M. B., J. G. Nedrud, and M. E. Lamm. 1987. Immunoglobulin A monoclonal antibodies protect against Sendai virus. J. Virol. 61:2624-2626.

McCance, D. J. and C. A. Mims. 1977. Transplacental transmission of polyoma virus in mice. Infect. Immun. 18:196-202.

McCance, D. J., and C. A. Mims. 1979. Reactivation of polyoma virus in kidneys of persistently infected mice during pregnancy. Infect. Immun. 25:998-1002.

McCance, D. J., A. Sebesteny, B. E. Griffin, F. Balkwill, R. Tilly, and N. A. Gregson. 1983. A paralytic disease in nude mice associated with polyoma virus infection. J. Gen. Virol. 64:57-67.

McCluskie, J., and J. S. F. Niven. 1955. The blood changes in rats and mice after splenectomy. J. Pathol. Bacteriol. 9:185-196.

McConnell, S. J., D. L. Huxsoll, F. M. Garner, R. O. Spertzel, A. R. Warner, Jr., and R. H. Yager. 1964. Isolation and characterization of a neurotropic agent (MHG virus) from adult rats. Proc. Soc. Exp. Biol. Med. 115:362-367.

McCormick, J. B., D. R. Sasso, E. R. Palmer, and M. P. Kiley. 1982. Morphological identification of the agent of Korean hemorrhagic fever (Hantaan virus) as a member of the Bunyaviridae. Lancet i:765-768.

McCubrey, J., and R. Risser. 1982. Genetic interactions in the spontaneous production of endogenous murine leukemia virus in low leukemic mouse strains. J. Exp. Med. 156:337-349.

McDonald, T. L. 1983. Blocking of cell-mediated immunity to Moloney murine sarcoma virus-transformed cells by lactate dehydrogenase virus-antibody complex. J. Natl. Cancer Inst. 70:493-497.

McDougall, P. T., N. S. Wolf, W. A. Steinbach, and J. J. Trentin. 1967. Control of *Pseudomonas aeruginosa* in an experimental mouse colony. Lab. Anim. Care 17:204-215.

McGarrity, G. J., and L. L. Coriell. 1973. Mass air flow cabinet for control of airborne infection of laboratory rodents. Appl. Microbiol. 26:167-172.

McGarrity, G. J., and L. L. Coriell. 1976. Maintenance of axenic mice in open cages in mass air flow. Lab. Anim. Sci. 26:746-750.

McGarrity, G. J., and A. S. Dion. 1978. Detection of airborne polyoma virus. J. Hyg. 81:9-13.

McGarrity, G. J., L. L. Coriell, R. W. Schaedler, R. J. Mandle, and A. E. Greene. 1969. Medical applications of dust-free rooms. III. Use in an animal care laboratory. Appl. Microbiol. 18:142-146.

McGarrity, G. J., L. L. Coriell, and V. Ammen. 1976. Airborne transmission of polyomavirus. J. Natl. Cancer Inst. 56:159-162.

McGarrity, G. J., D. L. Rose, V. Kwiatkowski, A. S. Dion, D. M. Phillips, and J. G. Tully. 1983. *Mycoplasma muris*, a new species from laboratory mice. Int. J. Syst. Bacteriol. 33:350-355.

McKee, A. E. 1977. Personal communication to J. R. Lindsey.

McLaughlin, M. M., M. P. Dacquisto, D. P. Jacobus, and R. E. Horowitz. 1964. Effects of the germfree state on responses of mice to whole-body irradiation. Radiat. Res. 23:333-349.

McMaster, G. K., P. Beard, H. D. Engers, and B. Hirt. 1981. Characterization of an immunosuppressive parvovirus related to the minute virus of mice. J. Virol. 38:317-326.

McNeill, T. A., and M. Killen. 1971. Role of hemopoietic colony-forming cell responses in the pathogenesis of ectromelia. Infect. Immun. 4:331-336.

McPherson, C. W. 1963. Reduction of *Pseudomonas aeruginosa* and coliform bacteria in mouse drinking water following treatment with hydrochloric acid or chlorine. Lab. Anim. Care 13:737-744.

Medearis, D. N., Jr. 1964. Mouse cytomegalovirus infection. III. Attempts to produce intrauterine infections. Am. J. Hyg. 80:102-112.

Medina, D. 1982. Mammary tumors. Pp. 373-396 in The Mouse in Biomedical Research. Vol. IV: Experimental Biology and Oncology, H. L. Foster, J. D. Small, and J. G. Fox, eds. New York: Academic Press.

Meier, H. 1960. Spontaneous cytomegalic inclusion body disease involving lacrimal glands of caesarian-derived (so called) pathogen-free rats. Nature 188:506-507.

Meijer, H., P. H. J. Dormans, J. L. M. C. Geelen, and C. P. A. van Boven. 1984. Rat cytomegalovirus: Studies on the viral genome and the proteins of virions and nucleocapsids. J. Gen. Virol. 65:681-695.

Meiser, J., V. Kinzel, and O. Jirovec. 1971. Nosematosis as an accompanying infection to plasmacytoma ascites in Syrian golden hamsters. Pathol. Microbiol. 37:249-260.

Melnick, J. L., and J. T. Riordan. 1947. Latent mouse encephalomyelitis. J. Immunol. 57:331-342.

Mengeling, W. L., P. S. Paul, T. O. Bunn, and J. F. Ridpath. 1986. Antigenic relationships among autonomous parvoviruses. J. Gen. Virol. 67:2839-2844.

Mercer, J. A., C. A. Wiley and D. H. Spector. 1988. Pathogenesis of murine cytomegalovirus infection: Identification of infected cells in the spleen during acute and latent infections. J. Virol. 62:987-997.

Mergenhagen, S. E., A. L. Notkins, and S. F. Dougherty. 1967. Adjuvanticity of lactic dehydrogenase virus: Influence of virus infection on the establishment of immunologic tolerance to a protein antigen in adult mice. J. Immunol. 99:576-581.

Meruelo, D., and R. Bach. 1983. Genetics of resistance to virus-induced leukemias. Adv. Cancer Res. 40:107-188.

Meshorer, A. 1969. Hexmitiasis in laboratory mice. Lab. Anim. Care 19:33-37.

Meyers, D. D. 1973. Sensitivity to x-irradiation of mice infected with *Hexamita muris*. Abstr. 22. Presented at the 24th Annual Meeting of the American Association for Laboratory Animal Science held October 1-5, 1973, in Bal Harbour, Fla.

Michaelides, M. C., and S. Schlesinger. 1974. Effect of acute or chronic infection with lactic dehydrogenase virus (LDV) on the susceptibility of mice to plasmacytoma MOPC-315. J. Immunol. 112:1560-1564.

Michaelides, M. C., and E. S. Simms. 1980. Immune responses in mice infected with lactic dehydrogenase virus. Antibody response to a T-dependent and a T-independent antigen during acute and chronic LDV infection. Cell. Immunol. 50:253-260.

Michalides, R., A. Van Ooyen, and R. Nusse. 1983. Mammary tumor virus expression and mammary tumor development. Curr. Top. Microbiol. Immunol. 106:57-78.

Mielens, Z. E., and J. Rozitis, Jr. 1964. Acute periarticular inflammation induced in rats by oral 6-sulfanilamidoindazole. Proc. Soc. Exp. Biol. Med. 117:751-754.

Milder, J. E., P. D. Walzer, J. D. Coonrod, and M. E. Rutledge. 1980. Comparison of histological and immunological techniques for detection of *Pneumocystis carinii* in rat bronchial lavage fluid. J. Clin. Microbiol.11:409-417.

Miller, C. P., and M. Bohnhoff. 1962. A study of experimental *Salmonella* infection in the mouse. J. Infect. Dis. 111:107-116.

Millican, R. C. 1963. *Pseudomonas aeruginosa* infection and its effects in non-radiation stress. Lab. Anim. Sci. 13:11-19.

Mills, K. C., and A. R. Dochez. 1944. Specific agglutination of murine erythrocytes by a pneumonitis virus in mice. Proc. Soc. Exp. Biol. Med. 57:140-143.

Mills, K. C., and A. R. Dochez. 1945. Further observations on red cell agglutinating agent present in lungs of virus-infected mice. Proc. Soc. Exp. Biol. Med. 60:141-143.

Mims, C. A., and S. Wainwright. 1968. The immuno-depressive action of lymphocytic choriomeningitis virus in mice. J. Immunol. 101:717-724.

Mims, C. A., and F. A. Tosolini. 1969. Pathogenesis of lesions in lymphoid tissue of mice infected with lymphocytic choriomeningitis (LCM) virus. Br. J. Exp. Pathol. 50:584-592.

Mims, C. A., and J. Gould. 1979. Infection of salivary glands, kidneys, adrenals, ovaries, and epithelia by murine cytomegalovirus. J. Med. Microbiol. 12:113-122.

Minion, F. C., M. B. Brown, and G. H. Cassell. 1984. Identification of cross-reactive antigens between *Mycoplasma pulmonis* and *Mycoplasma arthritidis*. Infect. Immun. 43:115-121.

Mirick, G. S., and W. B. Leftwich. 1949. The effect of diet on the susceptibility of the mouse to pneumonia virus of mice (PVM). II. Influence of pyridoxine administered in the period before as well as after the inoculation of virus. J. Exp. Med. 89:175-184.

Mirick, G. S., C. P. Richter, I. G. Schaub, R. Franklin, R. MacCleary, G. Schipper, and J. Spitznagel. 1950. An epizootic due to *Pneumococcus* type II in laboratory rats. Am. J. Hyg. 52:48-53.

Mirick, G. S., J. M. Smith, C. I. Leftwich, Jr., and W. B. Leftwich. 1952. The enhancing effect of urethane on the severity of infection with pneumonia virus of mice (PVM). J. Exp. Med. 95:147-160.

Misra, V., M. T. Muller, J. K. Chantler, and J. B. Hudson. 1978. Regulation of murine cytomegalovirus gene expression. I. Transcription during productive infection. J. Virol. 17:263-268.

Mitruka, B. M. 1971. Biochemical aspects of *Diplococcus pneumoniae* infections in laboratory rats. Yale J. Biol. Med. 44:253-264.

Mokhtarian, F., and K. V. Shah. 1980. Role of antibody response in recovery from K-papovavirus infection in mice. Infect. Immun. 29:1169-1179.

Mokhtarian, F., and K. V. Shah. 1983. Pathogenesis of K-papovavirus infection in athymic nude mice. Infect. Immun. 41:434-436.

Molomut, N., and M. Padnos. 1965. Inhibition of transplantable and spontaneous tumors by the M-P virus. Nature 208:948-950.

Molomut, N., M. Padnos, and L. W. Smith. 1965. A lymphocytopenic filterable agent derived from tissue cell cultures of murine carcinoma. J. Natl. Cancer Inst. 34:403-413.

Moloney, J. B. 1960. Biological studies on a lymphoid leukemia virus extracted from sarcoma 137. I. Origin and introductory investigations. J. Natl. Cancer Inst. 24:933-951.

Montie, T. C., D. Doyle-Huntzinger, R. C. Craven, and I. A. Holder. 1982. Loss of virulence associated with absence of flagellum in an isogenic mutant of *Pseudomonas aeruginosa* in the burned-mouse model. Infect. Immun. 38:1296-1298.

Moon, H. W. 1972. Vacuolated villous epithelium of small intestine of young pigs. Vet. Pathol. 9:3-21.

Moon, H. W. 1978. Mechanisms in pathogenesis of diarrhea: A review. J. Am. Vet. Med. Assoc. 172:443-448.

Moore, G. J. 1979. Conjunctivitis in the nude rat (*rnu*/*rnu*). Lab. Anim. 13:35.

Moore, G. J., and P. Aldred. 1978. Treatment of *Pasteurella pneumotropica* abscesses in nude mice (*nu*/*nu*). Lab. Anim. 12:227-228.

Moore, D. H., R. H. Arison, H. Tanaka, W. T. Hall, and M. Chanowitz. 1965. Identity of the filterable hemolytic anemia agent of sacks with *Haemobartonella muris*. J. Bacteriol. 90:1669-1674.

Moore, R. N., B. A. Johnson, and L. J. Berry. 1977. Nutritional effects of salmonellosis in mice. Am. J. Clin. Nutr. 30:1289-1293.

Moore, T. D., A. M. Allen, and J. R. Ganaway. 1973. Latent *Pasteurella pneumotropica* infection of the intestine of gnotobiotic and barrier-held rats. Lab. Anim. Sci. 23:657-661.

Morello, J. A., T. A. DiGenio, and E. E. Baker. 1965. Significance of salmonellae isolated from apparently healthy mice. J. Bacteriol. 89:1460-1464.

Morita, C., Y. Matsuura, S. Morikawa, and T. Kitamura. 1985. Age-dependent transmission of hemorrhagic fever with renal syndrome (HFRS) virus in rats. Arch. Virol. 85:145-149.

Morrey, J. D., R. W. Sidwell, R. L. Noble, B. B. Barnett, and A. W. Mahoney. 1984. Effects of folic acid malnutrition on rotaviral infection in mice. Proc. Soc. Exp. Biol. Med. 176:77-83.

Morris, J. A., J. M. McCown, and R. E. Blount. 1956. Ascites and hepatosplenomegaly in mice associated with protozoan-like cytoplasmic structures. J. Infect. Dis. 98:306-311.

Morrow, D. T., L. R. Robinette, C. W. Saubert, and G. L. Van Hoosier, Jr. 1977. Poditis in the rat as a complication of experiments in exercise physiology. Lab. Anim. Sci. 27:579-681.

Morse, H. C., III, and J. W. Hartley. 1982. Expression of xenotropic murine leukemia virus. Curr. Top. Microbiol. Immunol. 98:17-26.

Morse, H. C., III, S. S. Cross, and P. J. Baker. 1976. Neonatal infection with mouse thymic virus: Effects on cells regulating the antibody response to type III pneumococcal polysaccharide. J. Immunol. 116:1613-1617.

Morse, S. S. 1987. Mouse thymic necrosis virus: A novel murine lymphotropic agent. Lab. Anim. Sci. 37:717-725.

Mosier, D. E., B. J. Mathieson, and P. S. Campbell. 1977. Ly phenotype and mechanism of action of neonatal suppressor T cells. J. Exp. Med. 146:59-73.

Moskophidis, D., and F. Lehmann-Grube. 1984. The immune response of the mouse to lymphocytic choriomeningitis virus. IV. Enumeration of antibody-producing cells in spleens during acute and persistent infection. J. Immunol. 133:3366-3370.

Moskophidis, D., S. P. Cobbold, H. Waldmann, and F. Lehmann-Grube. 1987. Mechanism of recovery from acute virus infection: Treatment of lymphocytic choriomeningitis virus-infected mice with monoclonal antibodies reveals that Lyt-$2^{+}$ T lymphocytes mediate clearance of virus and regulate the antiviral antibody response. J. Virol. 61:1867-1874.

Mosmann, T. R., and J. B. Hudson. 1973. Some properties of the genome of murine cytomegalovirus (MCMV). Virology 54:135-149.

Mosmann, T. R., and J. B. Hudson. 1974. Structural and functional heterogeneity of the murine cytomegalovirus genome. Virology 62:175-183.

Moudgil, G. C. 1973. Influence of halothane on mortality from murine hepatitis virus (MHV-3). Br. J. Anaesth. 45:1236.

Moulder, J. W. 1984. Order II. Chlamydiales. Pp. 729-739 in Bergey's Manual of Systematic Bacteriology, vol. I, N. R. Krieg and J. G. Holt, eds. Baltimore: Williams & Wilkins.

MRC-LAC (Medical Research Council Laboratory Animals Centre). 1974. The Accreditation and Recognition Schemes for Suppliers of Laboratory Animals, 2nd ed. Manual Series No. 1. Carshalton, England: Medical Research Council.

Much, D. H., and I. Zajac. 1978. Purification and characterization of epizootic diarrhea of infant mice virus. Infect. Immun. 6:1019-1024.

Mullink, J. W. M. A., E. J. Ruitenberg, and W. Kruzinga. 1980. Lack of effect of *Spironucleus* (*Hexamita*) *muris* on the immune response to tetanus toxoid in the rat. Lab. Anim. 14:127-128.

Mullink, M. W. M. A. 1968. Tyzzer's disease. Intestinal lesions in both S.P.F. and conventional mice. Z. Versuchstierkd. 10:271-284.

Murphy, F. A., and S. G. Whitfield. 1975. Morphology and morphogenesis of arenaviruses. Bull. W.H.O. 52:409-419.

Mutter, W., M. J. Redehase, F. W. Busch, H.-J. Buhring, and U. H. Koszinowski. 1988. Failure in generating hemopoietic stem cells is the primary cause of death from cytomegalovirus disease in the immunocompromised host. J. Exp. Med. 167:1645-1658.

Myers, D. D. 1980. Control of microbial and parasitic contamination in the production of laboratory rodents. Lab. Anim. Sci. 30:330-338.

Myhrman, G. 1951. Nephropathia epidemica: a new infectious disease in Northern Scandinavia. Acta Med. Scand. 140:52-56.

Nadel, E., and V. H. Haas. 1955. Inhibitory effect of virus of lymphocytic choriomeningitis on course of leukemia in guinea pigs. Fed. Proc. 14:414-415.

Naiki, M., Y. Takagaki, and K. Fujiwara. 1965. Note on the change of transaminases in the liver and the significance of the transaminase ratio in experimental Tyzzer's disease of mice. Jpn. J. Exp. Med. 35:305-309.

Nakagawa, M., M. Saito, E. Suzuki, K. Nakayama, J. Matsubara, and T. Muto. 1984. Ten years-long survey on pathogen status of mouse and rat breeding colonies. Exp. Anim. (Tokyo) 33:115-120.

Nakamura, T., R. Yangihara, C. J. Gibbs, Jr., and C. C. Gajdusek. 1985. Immune spleen cell-mediated protection against fatal Hantaan virus infection in infant mice. J. Infect. Dis. 151:681-697.

Namiki, M., H. Takayama, and K. Fujiwara. 1977. Viral growth in splenic megakaryocytes of mice experimentally infected with mouse hepatitis virus MHV-2. Jpn. J. Exp. Med. 47:41-48.

Naot, Y., J. G. Tully, and H. Ginsburg. 1977. Lymphocyte activation by various *Mycoplasma* strains and species. Infect. Immun. 18:310-317.

Naot, Y., S. Merchav, E. Ben-David, and H. Ginsburg. 1979a. Mitogenic activity of *Mycoplasma pulmonis*. I. Stimulation of rat B and T lymphocytes. Immunology 36:399-406.

Naot, Y., R. Simon-Tou, and H. Ginsburg. 1979b. Mitogenic activity of *Mycoplasma pulmonis*. II. Studies on the biochemical nature of the mitogenic factor. Eur. J. Immunol. 9:149-151.

Nathanson, N., G. A. Cole, R. A. Squire, and K. O. Smith. 1970. Viral hemorrhagic encephalopathy of rats. I. Isolation, identification, and properties of the HER strains of rat virus. Am. J. Epidemiol. 91:328-338.

Nawrocki, J. F., L. R. Pease, and W. H. Murphy. 1980. Etiologic role of lactic dehydrogenase virus infection in an age-dependent neuroparalytic disease in C58 mice. Virology 103:259-264.

Nedrud, J. G., X. Liang, N. Hague, and M. E. Lamm. 1987. Combined oral/nasal immunization protects mice from Sendai virus infection. J. Immunol. 139:3484-3492.

Needham, J. R., and J. E. Cooper. 1975. An eye infection in laboratory mice associated with *Pasteurella pneumotropica*. Lab. Anim. 9:197-200.

Needham, J. R., and J. E. Cooper. 1976. Bulbourethral gland infection in mice associated with *Staphylococcus aureus*. Lab. Anim. 10:311-315.

Nelson, J. B. 1937a. Infectious catarrh of mice. I. A natural outbreak of the disease. J. Exp. Med. 65:833-842.

Nelson, J. B. 1937b. Infectious catarrh of mice. II. The detection and isolation of coccobacilliform bodies. J. Exp. Med. 65:851-860..

Nelson, J. B. 1937c. Infectious catarrh of mice. III. The etiological significance of the coccobacilliform bodies. J. Exp. Med. 65:862-868.

Nelson, J. B. 1950a. Association of a special strain of pleuropneumonia-like organisms with conjunctivitis in a mouse colony. J. Exp. Med. 91:309-320.

Nelson, J. B. 1950b. The relation of pleuropneumonia-like organisms to the conjunctival changes occurring in mice of the Princeton strain. J. Exp. Med. 92:431-439.

Nelson, J. B. 1952a. Acute hepatitis associated with mouse leukemia. I. Pathological features and transmission of the disease. J. Exp. Med. 96:293-300.

Nelson, J. B. 1952b. Acute hepatitis associated with mouse leukemia. II. Etiology and host range of the causal agent in mice. J. Exp. Med. 96:301-305.

Nelson, J. B. 1953. Acute hepatitis associated with mouse leukemia. IV. The relationship of *Eperythrozoon coccoides* to the hepatitis virus of Princeton mice. J. Exp. Med. 98:441-450.

Nelson, J. B. 1954. Association of group A streptococci with an outbreak of cervical lymphadenitis in mice. Proc. Soc. Exp. Biol. Med. 86:542-545.

Nelson, J. B. 1957. The etiology and control of chronic respiratory disease in the rat. Proc. Anim. Care Panel 7:30-40.

Nelson, J. B. 1959. Emergence of hepatitis virus in mice injected with ascites tumor. Proc. Soc. Exp. Biol. Med. 102:357-360.

Nelson, J. B. 1960. The problems of disease and quality in laboratory animals. J. Med. Ed. 35:34-43.

Nelson, J. B. 1962. An intracellular parasite resembling a microsporidian associated with ascites in Swiss mice. Proc. Soc. Exp. Biol. Med. 109:714-717.

Nelson, J. B. 1964. Response of mice to reovirus type 3 in presence and absence of ascites tumour cells. Proc. Soc. Exp. Biol. Med. 116:1086-1089.

Nelson, J. B. 1967. Experimental transmission of a murine microsporidian in Swiss mice. J. Bacteriol. 94:1340-1345.

Nelson, J. B., and G. S. Tarnowski. 1960. An oncolytic virus recovered from Swiss mice during passage of an ascites tumour. Nature 188:866-867.

Nettesheim, P., D. C. Topping, and R. Jambasi. 1981. Host and environmental factors enhancing carcinogenesis in the respiratory tract. Ann. Rev. Pharmacol. Toxicol. 21:133-163.

Nettesheim, P., H. Schreiber, D. A. Cresia, and C. B. Richter. 1974. Respiratory infections in the pathogenesis of lung cancer. Recent Results Cancer Res. 44:138-157.

Nettleton, P. F., and M. M. Rweyemamu. 1980. The association of calf serum with the contamination of BHK 21 clone 13 suspension cells by a parvovirus serologically related to the minute virus of mice (MVM). Arch. Virol. 64:359-374.

Newberne, P. M., C. E. Hunt, and V. R. Young. 1968. The role of diet and the reticuloendothelial system in the response of rats to *Salmonella typhimurium*. Br. J. Exp. Pathol. 49:448-457.

Newman, L. E., and J. J. Kowalski. 1973. Fresh sawdust bedding a possible source of *Klebsiella* organisms. Am. J. Vet. Res. 34:979-980.

Newsome, P. M., and K. A. Coney. 1985. Synergistic rotavirus and *Escherichia coli* diarrheal infection of mice. Infect. Immun. 47:573-574.

Newton, W. L. 1965. Methods in germfree animal research. Pp. 215-273 in Methods of Experimentation, vol. I, W. I. Gay, ed. New York: Academic Press.

Nicklas, W., M. Giese, R. Zawatzky, H. Kirchner, and P. Eaton. 1988. Contamination of a monoclonal antibody with LDH-virus causes interferon induction. Lab. Anim. Sci. 38:152-154.

Niederkorn, J. Y., J. A. Shadduck, and E. C. Schmidt. 1981. Susceptibility of selected inbred strains of mice to *Encephalitozoon cuniculi*. J. Infect. Dis. 144:249-253.

Niederkorn, J. Y. 1985. Enhanced pulmonary natural killer cell activity during murine encephalitozoonosis. J. Parasitol. 71:70-74.

Niederkorn, J. Y., J. A. Brieland, and E. Mayhew. 1983. Enhanced natural killer cell activity in experimental murine encephalitozoonosis. Infect. Immun. 41:302-307.

Nigg, C. 1942. Unidentified virus which produces pneumonia and systemic infection in mice. Science 95:49-50.

Nigg, C., and M. D. Eaton. 1944. Isolation from normal mice of a pneumotropic virus which forms elementary bodies. J. Exp. Med. 79:497-510.

Niven, J. S. F., A. W. Gledhill, G. W. A. Dick, and C. H. Andrewes. 1952. Further light on mouse hepatitis. Lancet ii:1061.

Njaa, L. R., F. Utne, and O. R. Brackkan. 1957. Effect of relative humidity on rat breeding and ringtail. Nature 180:585-587.

Noble, R. L., R. W. Sidwell, A. W. Mahoney, B. B. Barnett, and R. S. Splendlove. 1983. Influence of malnutrition and alterations in dietary protein on murine rotaviral disease. Proc. Soc. Exp. Biol. Med. 173:417-426.

Notkins, A. L. 1965. Lactic dehydrogenase virus. Bacteriol. Rev. 29:143-160.

Notkins, A. L., and C. Scheele. 1963. Studies on the transmission and the excretion of the lactic dehydrogenase agent. J. Exp. Med. 118:7-12.

Notkins, A. L., and C. Scheele. 1964. Impaired clearance of plasma enzyme in normal and lactate dehydrogenase agent infected mice. Proc. Soc. Exp. Biol. Med. 117:350-353.

Notkins, A. L., S. E. Mergenhagen, A. A. Rizzo, C. Scheele, and T. A. Waldman. 1966. Elevated *r*-globulin and increased antibody production in mice infected with lactic dehydrogenase virus. J. Exp. Med. 123:347-364.

Notkins, A. L., M. Mage, W. K. Ashe, and S. Mahar. 1968. Neutralization of sensitized lactic dehydrogenase virus by anti-*r*-globulin. J. Immunol. 100:314-320.

Novotny, J. F., and F. M. Hetrick. 1970. Pathogenesis and transmission of Kilham rat virus infecion in rats. Infect. Immun. 2:298-303.

NRC (National Research Council). 1985. Models for Biomedical Research: A New Perspective. A report of the Board on Basic Biology Committee on Models for Biomedical Research. Washington, D.C.: National Academy Press. 180 pp.

Nunoya, T., M. Itabashi, S. Kudow, M. Hayashi, and M. Tajima. 1977. An epizootic outbreak of sialodacryoadenitis in rats. Jpn. J. Vet. Sci. 39:445-450.

O'Brien, A. D., D. L. Rosenstreich, E. S. Metcalf, and I. Scher. 1980. Differential sensitivity of inbred mice to *Salmonella typhimurium*: A model for genetic regulation of innate resistance to bacterial infection. Pp. 101-114 in Genetic Control of Natural Resistance to Infection and Malignancy, E. Skamene, ed. New York: Academic Press.

O'Neill, H. C., and M. Brenan. 1987. A role for early cytotoxic T cells in resistance to ectromelia virus infection in mice. J. Gen. Virol. 68:269-273.

O'Neill, S., E. Lesperance, and D. J. Klass. 1984. Rat lung lavage surfactant enhances bacterial phagocytosis and intracellular killing by alveolar macrophages. Am. Rev. Resp. Dis. 130:225-230.

Oeding, P. 1983. Taxonomy and identification. Pp. 1-31 in Staphylococci and Staphylococcal Infections, vol. 1, C. S. F. Easmon and C. Adlam, eds. New York: Academic Press.

Offor, E., M. Riepenhoff-Talty, and P. L. Ogra. 1985. Effect of malnutrition on rotavirus infection in suckling mice: Kinetics of early infection. Proc. Soc. Exp. Biol. Med. 178:85-90.

Ogino, K. 1978. *Pneumocystis carinii:* Experimental pulmonary infection in rats. Jpn. J. Parasit. 27:77-89.

Old, L. J., and E. Stockert. 1977. Immunogenetics of cell surface antigens of mouse leukemia. Annu. Rev. Genet. 17:127-160.

Oldham, J. N. 1967. Helminths, ectoparasites and protozoa in rats and mice. Pp. 641-678 in Pathology of Laboratory Rats and Mice, E. Cotchin and F. J. C. Roe, eds. Oxford: Blackwell Scientific.

Oldstone, M. B. A., and F. J. Dixon. 1967. Lymphocytic choriomeningitis: Production of antibody by "tolerant" infected mice. Science 158:1193-1195.

Oldstone, M. B. A., and F. J. Dixon. 1969. Pathogenesis of chronic disease associated with persistent lymphocytic choriomeningitis viral infection. I. Relationship of antibody production to disease in neonatally infected mice. J. Exp. Med. 129:483-505.

Oldstone, M. B. A., and F. J. Dixon. 1970. Pathogenesis of chronic disease associated with persistent lymphocytic choriomeningitis viral infection. II. Relationship of the antilymphocytic choriomeningitis immune response to tissue injury in chronic lymphocytic choriomeningitis disease. J. Exp. Med. 131:1-19.

Oldstone, M. B. A., and F. J. Dixon. 1972. Inhibition of antibodies to nuclear antigen and to DNA in New Zealand mice infected with lactate dehydrogenase virus. Science 175:784-786.

Oldstone, M. B. A., M. J. Buchmeier, M. V. Doyle, and A. Tishon. 1980. Virus-induced immune complex disease: Specific anti-viral antibody and C1q binding material in the circulation during persistent lymphocytic choriomeningitis virus infection. J. Immunol. 124:831-838.

Oldstone, M. B. A., A. Tishon, and M. J. Buchmeier. 1983. Virus-induced immune complex disease: Genetic control of C1q binding complexes in the circulation of mice persistently infected with lymphocytic choriomeningitis virus. J. Immunol. 130:912-918.

Olitsky, P. K. 1940. A transmissible agent (Theiler's virus) in the intestines of normal mice. J. Exp. Med. 72:113-127.

Olson, L. D., and R. D. Ediger. 1972. Histopathologic study of the heads of circling mice infected with *Pseudomonas aeruginosa*. Lab. Anim. Sci. 22:522-527.

Ondera, T., A. B. Jenson, J.-W. Yoon, and A. L. Notkins. 1978. Virus-induced diabetes mellitus: Reovirus infection of pancreatic b cells in mice. Science 201:529-531.

Orskov, I. 1957. Biochemical types in the *Klebsiella* group. Acta Pathol. Microbiol. Scand. 40:155-162.

Orskov, I. 1984. Genus V. *Klebsiella*. Pp. 461-465 in Bergey's Manual of Systematic Bacteriology, vol. I, N. R. Kreig and J. G. Holt, eds. Baltimore: Williams & Wilkins.

Orvell, C., and M. Grandien. 1982. The effects of monoclonal antibodies on biologic activities of structural proteins of Sendai virus. J. Immunol. 129:2779-2787.

Osborn, J. E. 1982. Cytomegalovirus and other herpesviruses. Pp. 267-292 in The Mouse in Biomedical Research. Vol. II: Diseases, H. L. Foster, J. D. Small, and J. G. Fox, eds. New York: Academic Press.

Osborn, J. E., and D. N. Medearis, Jr. 1967. Suppression of interferon and antibody and multiplication of Newcastle disease virus in cytomegalovirus infected mice. Proc. Soc. Exp. Biol. Med. 124:347-353.

Osborn, J. E., and N. T. Shahidi. 1973. Thrombocytopenia in murine cytomegalovirus infection. J. Lab. Clin. Med. 81:53-56.

Osborn, J. E., A. A. Blazkovec, and D. L. Walker. 1968. Immunosuppression during acute murine cytomegalovirus infection. J. Immunol. 100:835-844.

Osborne, M. P., S. J. Haddon, A. J. Spencer, W. G. Starkey, T. S. Wallis, G. J. Clarke, K. J. Worton, D. C. A. Candy, and J. Stephen. 1988. J. Pediat. Gastroenterol. and Nutr. 7:236-248.

Osterhaus, A. D. M. E., J. S. Teppema, R. M. S. Wirahadiredja, and G. van Steenis. 1981. Mousepox in the Netherlands. Lab. Anim. Sci. 31:704-706.

Ostrom, C. A. 1958. Studies of the oral flora in experimental airborne infection: *Klebsiella pneumoniae* as an indicator organism. J. Infect. Dis. 103:12-18.

Ott, K. J., and L. A. Stauber. 1967. *Eperythrozoon coccoides:* Influence on course of infection of *Plasmodium chabaudi* in the mouse. Science 155:1546-1548.

Otten, J. A., and R. W. Tennant. 1982. Mouse adenovirus. Pp. 335-340 in The Mouse in Biomedical Research. Vol. II: Diseases, H. L. Foster, J. D. Small, and J. G. Fox, eds. New York: Academic Press.

Overcash, R. G., J. R. Lindsey, G. H. Cassell, and H. J. Baker. 1976. Enhancement of natural and experimental respiratory mycoplasmosis in rats by hexamethylphosphoramide. Am. J. Pathol. 82:171-189.

Owen, D. 1972. Common Parasites of Laboratory Rodents and Lagomorphs. MRC Laboratory Animals Centre Handbook No. 1. London: Medical Research Council. 140 pp.

Owen, D. G. 1982. *Haemobartonella muris:* Case report and investigation of transplacental transmission. Lab. Anim. 16:17-19.

Owen, R. L., P. C. Nemanic, and D. P. Stevens. 1979. Ultrastructural observations on giardiosis in a murine model. I. Intestinal distribution and relationship to the immune system of *Giardia muris*. Gastroenterology 76:751-769.

Padnos, M., and N. Molomut. 1973. Inhibition of mouse tumors and viruses by the M-P strain of LCM virus. Pp. 151-163 in Lymphocytic Choriomeningitis Virus and Other Arenaviruses, F. Lehmann-Grube, ed. New York: Springer-Verlag.

Page, D. L., and G. G. Glenner. 1972. Social interaction and wounding in the genesis of "spontaneous" murine amyloidosis. Am. J. Pathol. 67:555-570.

Pakes, S. P., J. A. Shadduck, and R. G. Olsen. 1972. A diagnostic skin test for encephalitozoonosis (nosematosis) in rabbits. Lab. Anim. Sci. 22:870-877.

Pakes, S. P., Y. S. Lu, and P. C. Meunier. 1984a. Factors that complicate animal research. Pp. 649-665 in Laboratory Animal Medicine, J. G. Fox, B. J. Cohen, and F. M. Loew, eds. New York: Academic Press.

Pakes, S. P., J. A. Shadduck, D. B. Feldman, and J. A. Moore. 1984b. Comparison of tests for the diagnosis of spontaneous encephalitozoonosis in rabbits. Lab. Anim. Sci. 34:356-359.

Palleroni, N. J. 1984. Pseudomonadaceae. Pp. 141-219 in Bergey's Manual of Systematic Bacteriology, vol. I, N. R. Krieg and J. G. Holt, eds. Baltimore: Williams & Wilkins.

Papadimitriou, J. M. 1966. Ultrastructural features of chronic murine hepatitis after reovirus type 3 infection. Br. J. Exp. Pathol. 47:624-631.

Papadimitriou, J. M. 1968. The biliary tract in acute murine reovirus 3 infection. Am. J. Pathol. 52:595-611.

Papadimitriou, J. M., and T. A. Robertson. 1976. Acute murine adrenalitis induced by reovirus 3. Am. J. Pathol. 85:595-608.

Papadimitriou, J. M., and M. N. I. Walters. 1967. Studies on the exocrine pancreas. II. Ultrastructural investigation of reovirus pancreatitis. Am. J. Pathol. 51:387-403.

Papadimitriou, J. M., G. R. Shellam, and J. E. Allan. 1982. The effect of the beige mutation on infection with murine cytomegalovirus. Histopathologic studies. Am. J. Pathol. 108:299-309.

Papenheimer, A. M., and F. S. Cheever. 1948. Epidemic diarrheal disease of suckling mice. IV. Cytoplasmic inclusion bodies in intestinal epithelium in relation to the disease. J. Exp. Med. 88:317-324.

Papenheimer, A. M., and J. F. Enders. 1947. An epidemic diarrheal disease of suckling mice. II. Inclusions in the intestinal epithelial cells. J. Exp. Med. 85:417-423.

Paradisi, F., L. Graziano, and G. Maio. 1972. Histochemistry of glutamicoxalo-acetic transaminase in mouse liver during MHV3 infection. Experimentia 28:551-552.

Parke, L. M., C. A. Long, and W. P. Weidanz. 1986. A method for freeing murine plasmodia of contaminating lactate dehydrogenase elevating virus. J. Parasitol. 72:956-958.

Parker, J. C. 1980. The possibilities and limitations of virus control in laboratory animals. Pp. 161-172 in Animal Quality and Models in Research. A. Spiegel, S. Erichsen, and H. A. Solleveld, eds. New York: Gustave Fischer Verlag.

Parker, J. C. 1983. ELISA: An Introduction. Lab. Anim. 12:15-17.

Parker, J. C., and R. K. Reynolds. 1968. Natural history of Sendai virus infection in mice. Am. J. Epidemiol. 88:112-125.

Parker, J. C., and C. B. Richter. 1982. Viral diseases of the respiratory system. Pp. 109-158 in The Mouse in Biomedical Research. Vol. II, H. L. Foster, J. D. Small, and J. G. Fox, eds. New York: Academic Press.

Parker, J. C., R. W. Tennant, and T. G. Ward. 1966. Prevalence of viruses in mouse colonies. Pp. 25-36 in Viruses of Laboratory Rodents, R. Holdenried, ed. National Cancer Institute Monograph 20. Washington, D.C.: U.S. Department of Health, Education, and Welfare.

Parker, J. C., S. S. Cross, M. J. Collins, Jr., and W. P. Rowe. 1970a. Minute virus of mice. I. Procedures for quantitation and detection. J. Natl. Cancer Inst. 45:297-303.

Parker, J. C., M. J. Collins, Jr., S. S. Cross, and W. P. Rowe. 1970b. Minute virus of mice. II. Prevalence, epidemiology, and occurrence as a contaminant of transplanted tumors. J. Natl. Cancer Inst. 45:305-310.

Parker, J. C., S. S. Cross, and W. P. Rowe. 1970c. Rat coronavirus (RCV): A prevalent, naturally occurring pneumotropic virus of rats. Arch. Gesamte Virusforsch. 31:239-302.

Parker, J. C., M. L. Vernon, and S. S. Cross. 1973. Classification of mouse thymic virus as a herpesvirus. Infect. Immun. 7:305-308.

Parker, J. C., H. J. Igel, R. K. Reynolds, A. M. Lewis, Jr., and W. P. Rowe. 1976. Lymphocytic choriomeningitis virus infection in fetal, newborn, and young adult Syrian hamsters (*Mesocricetus auratus*). Infect. Immun. 13:967-981.

Parker, J. C., M. D. Whiteman, and C. B. Richter. 1978. Susceptibility of inbred and outbred mouse strains to Sendai virus and prevalence of infection in laboratory rats. Infect. Immun. 19:123-130.

Parker, J. C., A. J. O'Beirne, and M. J. Collins, Jr. 1979. Sensitivity of the enzyme-linked immunosorbent assay, complement fixation, and hemagglutination-inhibition serologic tests for detection of Sendai virus antibody in laboratory mice. J. Clin. Microbiol. 9:444-447.

Parsons, D. F. 1963. Morphology of K virus and its relation to the papova group of viruses. Virology 20:385-387.

Paturzo, F. X., R. O. Jacoby, P. N. Bhatt, A. L. Smith, D. J. Gaertner, and R. B. Ardito. 1987. Persistence of rat virus in seropositive rats as detected by explant culture. Arch. Virol. 95:137-142.

Paulini, K., and W. Mohr. 1975. Hormone-dependent polyploidy in the glandula orbitalis externa and infraorbitalis of animals of different age. Beitr. Pathol. 156:65-74.

Paulini, K., G. Beneke, and R. Kulka. 1972a. Age- and sex-dependent changes in glandular cells. I. Histological and chemical investigations on the glandula lacrimalis, glandula orbitalis externa, and glandula infraorbitalis of the rat. Gerontologia 18:131-146. (In German)

Paulini, K., W. Mohr, G. Beneke, and R. Kulka. 1972b. Age- and sex-dependent changes in glandular cells. II. Cytophotometric and autoradiographic investigations on the glandula lacrimalis, glandula infraorbitalis, and glandula orbitalis externa of the rat. Gerontologia 18:147-156. (In German)

Pavlovskis, O. R., D. C. Edman, S. H. Leppla, B. Wretlind, L. R. Lewis, and K. E. Martin. 1981. Protection against experimental *Pseudomonas aeruginosa* infection in mice by active immunization with exotoxin A toxiods. Infect. Immun. 32:681-689.

Pawanda, M. C., R. W. Wannemacher, Jr., and G. L. Cockerell. 1972. Nitrogen metabolism and protein synthesis during pneumococcal sepsis in rats. Infect. Immun. 6:266-271.

Payment, P., and J.-P. Descoteaux. 1978. Enzyme-linked immunosorbent assay for the detection of antibodies to pneumonia virus of mice in rat sera. Lab. Anim. Sci. 28:676-679.

Pearson, C. M. 1959. Development of arthritis in the rat following injection with adjuvant. Pp. 647-671 in Mechanisms of Hypersensitivity, J. H. Shafer, G. A. LoGrippo, and M. W. Chase, eds. Boston: Little, Brown.

Pearson, D. J., and G. Taylor. 1975. The influence of the nematode *Syphacia obvelata* on adjuvant arthritis in rats. Immunology 29:391-396.

Peck, R. M., G. J. Eaton, E. B. Peck, and S. Litwin. 1983. Influence of Sendai virus on carcinogenesis in strain A mice. Lab. Anim. Sci. 33:154-156.

Penney, J. G., Jr., and J. S. Wolinsky. 1979. Neuronal and oligodendroglial infection by the WW strain of Theiler's virus. Lab. Invest. 40:324-330.

Pennington, J. E., and R. M. Williams. 1979. Influence of genetic factors on natural resistance of mice to *Pseudomonas aeruginosa*. J. Infect. Dis. 139:396-400.

Percy, D. H., P. E. Hanna, F. Paturzo, and P. N. Bhatt. 1984. Comparison of strain susceptibility to experimental sialodacryoadenitis in rats. Lab. Anim. Sci. 34:255-260.

Percy, D. H., J. A. Lynch, and J. P. Descoteaux. 1986. Central nervous system lesions in suckling mice and rats inoculated intranasally with sialodacryoadenitis virus. Vet. Pathol. 23:42-49.

Percy, D. H., S. J. Bond, J. I. MacInnes, and J. P. Descoteaux. 1988a. Experimental sialodacryoadenitis virus infection in athymic CD-1 mice. Can. J. Vet. Res. 52:370-374.

Percy, D. H., M. A. Hayes, T. E. Kocal, and Z. W. Wojcinski. 1988b. Depletion of salivary gland epidermal growth factor by sialodacryoadenitis virus infection in the Wistar rat. Vet. Pathol. 25:183-192.

Pereira, C. A., G. Mercier, D. Oth, and J. M. Dupuy. 1984. Induction of natural killer cells and interferon during mouse hepatitis virus infection of resistant and susceptible inbred mouse strains. Immunobiology 166:35-44.

Perlman, S., R. Schelper, and D. Ries. 1987. Maternal antibody-modulated MHV-JHM infection in C57BL/6 and BALB/c mice. Adv. Exp. Med. Biol. 218:297-305.

Perlman, S., G. Jacobsen, and S. Moore. 1988. Regional localization of virus in the central nervous system of mice persistently infected with murine coronavirus JHM. Virology 166:328-338.

Perrin, T. L. 1943a. Spontaneous and experimental encephalitozoon infection of laboratory animals. Arch. Pathol. 36:559-567.

Perrin, T. L. 1943b. Toxoplasma and encephalitozoon in spontaneous and in experimental infections in animals—A comparative study. Arch. Pathol. 36:568-578.

Pesanti, E. 1982. Effects of bacterial pneumonitis on development of pneumocystosis in rats. Am. Rev. Resp. Dis. 125:723-728.

Peters, R. L., and M. J. Collins. 1981. Use of mouse hepatitis virus antigen in an enzyme-linked immunosorbent assay for rat coronaviruses. Lab. Anim. Sci. 31:472-475.

Peters, R. L., and M. J. Collins, Jr. 1983. The enzyme-linked immunosorbent assay for mouse hepatitis and rat coronaviruses. Lab. Anim. 12:18-25.

Peters, R. L., M. J. Collins, A. J. O'Bierne, P. A. Howton, S. L. Hourihan, and S. F. Thomas. 1979. Enzyme-linked immunosorbent assay for detection of antibodies to murine hepatitis virus. J. Clin. Microbiol. 10:595-597.

Peters, W. 1965. Competitive relationship between *Eperythrozoon coccoides* and *Plasmodium berghei* in the mouse. Exp. Parasitol. 16:158-166.

Petri, M. 1965. A cytolytic parasite in the cells of transplantable, malignant tumors. Nature 105:302-303.

Petri, M. 1966. The occurrence of *Nosema cuniculi* (*Encephalitozoon cuniculi*) in the cells of transplantable, malignant ascites tumors and its effect upon tumor and host. Acta Pathol. Microbiol. Scand. 66:13-30.

Petri, M. 1967. Persistence and possibility of late recurrence of tumour tissue in rats with Nosema-infected Yoshida sarcoma. Acta Pathol. Microbiol. Scand. 187(Suppl.):86 (abstr.).

Petri, M. 1968. High incidence of intraperitoneal rhabdomyosarcomas in rats after growth and regression of *Nosema cuniculi*-infected Yoshida ascites sarcoma. Acta Pathol. Microbiol. Scand. 73:1-12.

Petri, M. 1969. Studies on *Nosema cuniculi* found in transplantable ascites tumors with a survey of microsporidiosis in mammals. Acta Pathol. Microbiol. Scand. 204(Suppl.):1-91.

Petri, M., and T. Schiodt. 1966. On the ultrastructure of *Nosema cuniculi* in the cells of Yoshida rat ascites sarcoma. Acta Pathol. Microbiol. Scand. 66:437-446.

Pfau, C. J., J. K. Valenti, S. Jacobson, and D. C. Pevear. 1982. Cytotoxic T-cells are induced in mice infected with lymphocytic choriomeningitis virus strains of markedly different properties. Infect. Immun. 36:598-602.

Phillips, B. P. 1960. Parasitological survey of Lobund germfree animals. Lobund Reports 3:172-175.

Piazza, M., F. Piccianino, and F. Matano. 1965. Haematological changes in viral (MHV-3) murine hepatitis. Nature 205:1034-1035.

Piccinino, F., B. Galanti, and G. Giusti. 1966. Lack of transplacental transmissibility of MHV-3 virus. Arch. Gesamte Virusforsch. 18:327-332.

Pierce-Chase, C. H., M. Fauve, and R. Dubos. 1964. Corynebacterial pseudotuberculosis in mice. I. Comparative susceptibility of mouse strains to experimental infection with *Corynebacterium kutscheri*. J. Exp. Med. 120:267-281.

Pierson, C. L., A. G. Johnson, and I. Feller. 1976. Effect of cyclophosphamide on the immune response to *Pseudomonas aeruginosa* in mice. Infect. Immun. 14:168-177.

Pifer, L. L. 1983. *Pneumocystis carinii*: a diagnostic dilemma. Pediat. Infect. Dis. 2:177-183.

Pifer, L. L. 1984. *Pneumocystis carinii* in germ-free rats. J. Infect. Dis. 150:619.

Pifer, L. L., W. T. Hughes, and M. J. Murphy, Jr. 1977. Propagation of *Pneumocystis carinii* in vitro. Pediat. Res. 11:305-316.

Pifer, L. L., C. P. Lattuada, C. C. Edwards, D. R. Woods, and D. R. Owens. 1984. *Pneumocystis carinii* infection in germ-free rats: implications for human patients. Diag. Microbiol. Infect. Dis. 2:23-36.

Pike, R. M. 1979. Laboratory-associated infections: Incidence, fatalities, causes, and prevention. Annu. Rev. Microbiol. 33:41-66.

Plagemann, P. G. W., and H. E. Swim. 1963. Studies of the plasma lactic dehydrogenase-elevating virus (PLDEV) of mice. Proc. Am. Assoc. Cancer Res. 4:53. (abstr.)

Plagemann, P. G. W., and H. E. Swim. 1966. Relationship between the lactic dehydrogenase-elevating virus and transplantable murine tumors. Proc. Soc. Exp. Biol. Med. 121:1142-1146.

Plagemann, P. G. W., K. F. Gregory, H. E. Swim, and K. K. W. Chan. 1963. Plasma lactic dehydrogenase elevating agent of mice: Distribution in tissues and effect on lactic dehydrogenase isozyme patterns. Can. J. Microbiol. 9:75-86.

Poiesz, B. J., F. W. Ruscetti, M. S. Reitz, V. S. Kalyanaraman, and R. C. Gallo. 1981. Isolation of a new type C retrovirus (HTLV) in primary uncultured cells of a patient with Sezary T-cell leukemia. Nature 294:268-271.

Poiley, S. M. 1967. The development of an effective method for control of epizootic diarrhea in infant mice. Lab. Anim. Care 17:501-511.

Pollard, M., and N. Sharon. 1969. Immunoproliferative effects of lymphocytic choriomeningitis virus in germfree mice. Proc. Soc. Exp. Biol. Med. 132:242-246.

Pollard, M., and N. Sharon. 1973. Congenital LCM virus infection in "germ-free" Haas strain mice. Pp. 121-127 in Lymphocytic Choriomeningitis Virus and Other Arenaviruses, F. Lehmann-Grube, ed. New York: Springer-Verlag.

Pomerat, C. M., E. H. Frienden, and E. Yeager. 1947. Reticuloendothelial immune serum (REIS). V. An experimental anemia in *Bartonella* infected rats produced by anti-blood immune serum. J. Infect. Dis. 80:154-163.

Pope, J. H. 1961. Studies of a virus isolated from a wild house mouse, *Mus musculus,* and producing splenomegaly and lymph node enlargement in mice. Aust. J. Exp. Biol. Med. Sci. 39:521-536.

Pope, J. H., and W. P. Rowe. 1964. Identification of WMI as LDH virus and its recovery from wild mice in Maryland. Proc. Soc. Exp. Biol. Med. 116:1015-1019.

Porter, D. D., and H. G. Porter. 1971. Deposition of immune complexes in the kidneys of mice infected with lactic dehydrogenase virus. J. Immunol. 106:1264-1266.

Povar, M. L. 1965. Ringworm (*Trichophyton mentagrophytes*) infection in a colony of albino Norway rats. Lab. Anim. Care 15:264-265.

Pratt, H. D., and K. S. Littig. 1961. Lice of Public Health Importance and Their Control. Insect Control Series: Part VIII. PHS Publ. No. 772. Washington, D.C.: U.S. Department of Health, Education, and Welfare. 16 pp.

Pratt, H. D., and J. S. Wiseman. 1962. Fleas of Public Health Importance and Their Control. Insect Control Series: Part VIII. PHS Publ. No. 772. Washington, D.C.: U.S. Department of Health, Education, and Welfare.

Preston, W. S. 1942. Arthritis in rats caused by pleuropneumonia-like microorganisms and the relationship of similar organisms to human rheumatism. J. Infect. Dis. 70:180-184.

Price, P., J. G. Winter, S. Nikoletti, J. B. Hudson, and G. R. Shellam. 1987. Functional changes in murine macrophages infected with cytomegalovirus related to H-2- determined sensitivity to infection. J. Virol. 61:3602-3606.

Priscott, P. K., and D. A. J. Tyrrell. 1982. The isolation and partial characterization of a cytomegalovirus from the brown rat, *Rattus norvegicus.* Arch. Virol. 73:145-160.

Profitt, M. R., and C. C. Congdon. 1970. The effect of a large dose of LDH virus on mouse lymphatic tissue. Fed. Proc. 29:559. (abstr.)

Profitt, M. R., C. C. Congdon, and R. L. Tyndall. 1972. The combined action of Rauscher leukemia virus and lactic dehydrogenase virus on mouse lymphatic tissue. Int. J. Cancer 9:193-211.

Proust, J. J., M. A. Buchholz, and A. A. Nordin. 1985. A "lymphokine-like" soluble product that induces proliferation and maturation of B cells appears in the serum-free supernatant of a T cell hybridoma as a consequence of mycoplasmal contamination. J. Immunol. 134:390-396.

Pye, D., and J. C. Cox. 1977. Isolation of *Encephalitozoon cuniculi* from urine samples. Lab. Anim. 11:233-234.

Quie, P. G., G. S. Giebink, and J. A. Winkelstein, eds. 1981. The pneumococcus. Rev. Infect. Dis. 3:183-395.

Quie, P. G., E. L. Mills, K. L. Cates, J. S. Abramson, W. E. Regelmann, and P. K. Peterson. 1983. Functional defects of granulocytes and susceptibility to staphylococcal disease. Pp. 243-273 in Staphylococci and Staphylococcal Infections, vol. 1, C. S. F. Easmon and C. Adlam, eds. New York: Academic Press.

Quinnan, G. V., and J. E. Manischewitz. 1979. The role of natural killer cells and antibody-dependent cell-mediated cytotoxicity during murine cytomegalovirus infection. J. Exp. Med. 150:1549-1554.

Quinnan, G. V., and J. E. Manischewitz. 1987. Genetically determined resistance to lethal murine cytomegalovirus infection is mediated by interferon-dependent and -independent restriction of virus replication. J. Virol. 61:1875-1881.

Quinnan, G. V., J. E. Manischewitz, and F. A. Ennis. 1978. Cytotoxic T-lymphocyte response to murine cytomegalovirus infection. Nature 273:541-543.

Quinnan, G. V., J. E. Manischewitz, and F. A. Ennis. 1980. Role of cytotoxic T lymphocytes in murine cytomegalovirus infection. J. Gen. Virol. 47:503-508.

Quinnan, G. V., and J. E. Manischewitz, and N. Kirmani. 1982. Involvement of natural killer cells in the pathogenesis of murine cytomegalovirus interstitial pneumonitis and the immune response to infection. J. Gen. Virol. 58:173-180.

Rabson, A. S., J. H. Edgcomb, F. Y. Legallais, and S. A. Tyrrell. 1969. Isolation and growth of rat cytomegalovirus in vitro. Proc. Soc. Exp. Biol. Med. 131:923-927.

Rabstein, M. M. 1958. The practical establishment and maintenance of Salmonella free mouse colonies. Proc. Anim. Care Panel 8:67-74.

Ramig, R. F., and B. N. Fields. 1977. Reoviruses. Pp. 383-431 in The Molecular Biology of Animal Viruses, vol. I, D. P. Nayak, ed. New York: Marcel Dekker.

Ramquist, T., D. O. Pallas, J. DeAnda, L. Ahrlund-Richter, G. Reinholdsson, T. M. Roberts, B. S. Schaffhausen, and T. Dalianis. 1988. Immunization against the polyoma tumor-specific transplantation antigen (TSTA) with polyoma T antigens. Int. J. Cancer. 42:123-128.

Ratcliffe, H. L. 1949. Spontaneous diseases of laboratory rats. Pp. 515-530 in The Rat in Laboratory Investigation, 2nd ed., E. J. Farris and J. Q. Griffith, eds. Philadelphia: Lippincott.

Rauscher, F. J. 1962. A virus-induced disease of mice characterized by erythropoiesis and lymphoid leukemia. J. Natl. Cancer Inst. 29:515-543.

Rawls, W. E., and M. Buchmeier. 1975. Arenaviruses: Purification and physicochemical nature. Bull. W.H.O. 52:393-399.

Rawls, W. E., and W.C. Leung. 1979. Arenaviruses. Pp. 157-192 in Comprehensive Virology, vol. 14, H. Fraenkel-Conrat and R. R. Wagner, eds. New York: Plenum Press.

Razin, S., and E. A. Freundt. 1984. The mycoplasmas. Pp. 740-793 in Bergey's Manual of Systematic Bacteriology. Vol. I, N. R. Krieg and J. G. Holt, eds. Baltimore: Williams & Wilkins.

Reddehase, M. J., W. Mutter, K. Munch, H.J. Buhring, and U. H. Koszinowski. 1987. CD8-positive lymphocytes specific for murine cytomegalovirus immediate-early antigens mediate protective immunity. J. Virol. 61:3102-3108.

Reddehase, M.J., S. Jonjic, F. Weiland, W. Mutter, and U. H. Koszinowski. 1988. Adoptive immunotherapy of murine cytomegalovirus adrenalitis in the immunocompromised host: CD4-helper-independent antiviral function of CD8-positive memory T lymphocytes derived from latently infected donors. J. Virol. 62:1061-1065.

Refai, M., and A. H. Ali. 1970. Laboratory acquired infection with *Keratinomyces ajelloi*. Mykosen 13:317-318.

Reith, von H. 1968. Spontane and experimentelle Pilzerkrankungen bei Mausen. Z. Versuchstierkd. 10:75-81.

Rekers, P. E. 1951. The effect of x-irradiation on rats with and without *Bartonella muris*. J. Infect. Dis. 88:224-229.

Reyniers, J. A. 1957a. The control of contamination in colonies of laboratory animals by use of germfree techniques. Proc. Anim. Care Panel 7:9-29.

Reyniers, J. A. 1957b. The production and use of germfree animals in experimental biology and medicine. Am. J. Vet. Res. 68:678-687.

Richter, C. B. 1970. Application of infectious agents to the study of lung cancer: Studies on the etiology and morphogenesis of metaplastic lung lesions in mice. P. Nettesheim, M. V. Hanna, Jr., and J. W. Deatherage, Jr., eds. U. S. Atomic Energy Commission Symposium Series 21:365-382.

Richter, C. B. 1973. Experimental pathology of Sendai virus infection in mice. J. Am. Vet. Med. Assoc. 163:1204.

Richter, C. B., J. E. Thigpen, C. S. Richter, and J. M. Mackenzie, Jr. 1988. Fatal pneumonia with terminal emaciation in nude mice caused by pneumonia virus of mice. Lab. Anim. Sci. 38:255-261.

Riepenhoff-Talty, M., P. C. Lee, P. J. Carmody, H. J. Barrett, and P. L. Ogra. 1982. Age dependent rotavirus-enterocyte interactions. Proc. Soc. Exp. Biol. Med. 170:146-154.

Riepenhoff-Talty, M., T. Dharakul, E. Kowalski, S. Michalak, and P. L. Ogra. 1987a. Persistent rotavirus infection in mice with severe combined immunodeficiency. J. Virol. 61:3345-3348.

Riepenhoff-Talty, M., T. Dharakul, E. Kowalski, D. Sterman, and P. L. Ogra. 1987b. Rotavirus infection in mice: Pathogenesis and immunity. Adv. Exp. Med. Biol. 216B: 1015-1023.

Riet, F., S. V. D. De, and L. B. Kahn. 1973. Isolation of a murine hepatitis virus from Swiss mice treated with antilymphocyte serum. Arch. Gesamte Virusforsch. 42:1-8.

Rights, F. L., E. B. Jackson, and F. E. Smadel. 1947. Observations on Tyzzer's disease in mice. Am. J. Pathol. 23:627-635.

Riley, V. 1964. Synergism between a lactate dehydrogenase elevating virus and *Eperythrozoon coccoides*. Science 146:921-922.

Riley, V. 1966. Spontaneous mammary tumors: Decrease of incidence in mice infected with an enzyme-elevating virus. Science 153:1657-1658.

Riley, V. 1968. Lactate dehydrogenase in the normal and malignant state in mice and the influence of a benign enzyme-elevating virus. Methods Cancer Res. 4:493-618.

Riley, V. 1974. Persistence and other characteristics of the lactate dehydrogenase-elevating virus (LDH-virus). Prog. Med. Virol. 18:198-213.

Riley, V., and F. Wroblewski. 1960. Serial lactic dehydrogenase activity in plasma of mice with growing or regressing tumors. Science 132:151-152.

Riley, V., F. Lilly, E. Huerto, and D. Bardell. 1960. Transmissible agent associated with 26 types of experimental mouse neoplasms. Science 132:545-547.

Riley, V., J. D. Loveless, and M. A. Fitzmaurice. 1964. Comparison of a lactate dehydrogenase elevating virus-like agent and *Eperythrozoon coccoides*. Proc. Soc. Exp. Biol. Med. 116:486-490.

Riley, V., H. A. Campbell, and C. C. Stock. 1970. Asparaginase clearance: Influence of the LDH-elevating virus. Proc. Soc. Exp. Biol. Med. 133:38-42.

Riley, V., W. Braun, M. Ishizuka, and D. Spackman. 1975. Antibody-producing cells: Virus-induced alteration of response to antigen. Proc. Natl. Acad. Sci. USA 73:1707-1711.

Rinaldo, C. R., Jr., B. C. Cole, J. C. Overall, Jr., and L. A. Glasgow. 1974. Induction of interferon in mice by mycoplasmas. Infect. Immun. 10:1296-1301.

Ringold, G. M. 1983. Regulation of mouse mammary tumor virus gene expression by glucocorticoid hormones. Curr. Top. Microbiol. Immunol. 106:79-103.

Risser, R., J. M. Horowitz, and J. McCubrey. 1983. Endogenous mouse leukemia viruses. Annu. Rev. Genet. 17:85-121.

Ristic, M., and J. P. Kreier. 1984. Family III. Anaplasmataceae. Pp. 719-739 in Bergey's Manual of Systematic Bacteriology, vol. I, N. R. Krieg and J. G. Holt, eds. Baltimore: Williams & Wilkins.

Riviere, Y., I. Gresser, J. C. Guillon, M. T. Bandu, P. Ronco, L. Morel-Maroger, and P. Verroust. 1980. Severity of lymphocytic choriomeningitis virus disease in different strains of suckling mice correlates with increasing amounts of endogenous interferon. J. Exp. Med. 152:633-640.

Robb, J. A., and C. W. Bond. 1979. Coronaviridae. Pp. 193-247 in Comprehensive Virology, vol. 14, H. Fraenkel-Conrat and R. R. Wagner, eds. New York: Plenum Press.

Roberts, J. A. 1962a. Histopathogenesis of mousepox. I. Respiratory infection. Br. J. Exp. Pathol. 43:451-461.

Roberts, J. A. 1962b. Histopathogenesis of mousepox. II. Cutaneous infection. Br. J. Exp. Pathol. 43:462-468.

Roberts, J. A. 1963. Histopathogenesis of mousepox. III. Ectromelia virulence. Br. J. Exp. Pathol. 44:465-472.

Roberts, N. J. 1982. Different effects of influenza virus, respiratory syncytial virus, and Sendai virus on human lymphocytes and macrophages. Infect. Immun. 35:1142-1146.

Roberts, S. A., and B. J. Gregory. 1980. Facultative *Pasteurella ophthalmitis* in hooded Lister rats. Lab. Anim. (London) 14:323-324.

Roberts-Thomson, I. C., and G. F. Mitchell. 1978. Giardiasis in mice. I. Prolonged infections in certain mouse strains and hypothymic (nude) mice. Gastroenterology 75:42-46.

Roberts-Thomson, I. C., and G. F. Mitchell. 1979. Protection of mice against *Giardia muris* infection. Infect. Immun. 24:971-973.

Roberts-Thomson, I. C., D. E. Grove, D. P. Stevens, and K. S. Warren. 1976a. Suppression of giardiasis during the intestinal phase of trichinosis in the mouse. Gut 17:953-958.

Roberts-Thomson, I. C., D. P. Stevens, A. A. F. Mahmoud, and K. S. Warren. 1976b. Giardiosis in the mouse: An animal model. Gastroenterology 71:57-61.

Roberts-Thomson, I. C., G. F. Mitchell, R. F. Anders, B. D. Tait, P. Kerlin, A. Kerr-Grant, and P. Cavanach. 1980. Genetic studies in human and murine giardiasis. Gut 21:397-401.

Robey, R. E., D. R. Woodman, and F. M. Hetrick. 1968. Studies on the natural infection of rats with Kilham rat virus. Am. J. Epidemiol. 88:139-142.

Robinson, G. W., N. Nathanson, and J. Hodous. 1974. Seroepidemiological study of rat virus infection in a closed laboratory colony. Am. J. Epidemiol. 94:91-100.

Robinson, T. W. E., R. J. R. Cureton, and R. B. Heath. 1968. The pathogenesis of Sendai virus infection in the mouse lung. J. Med. Microbiol. 1:89-95.

Robinson, T. W. E., R. J. R. Cureton, and R. B. Heath. 1969. The effect of cyclophosphamide on Sendai virus infection of mice. J. Med. Microbiol. 2:137-145.

Rodriguez, M., M. J. Buchmeier, M. B. A. Oldstone, and P. W. Lampert. 1983. Ultrastructural localization of viral antigens in the CNS of mice persistently infected with lymphocytic choriomeningitis virus (LCMV). Am. J. Pathol. 110:95-100.

Rodriquez, M., J. L. Leibowitz, and P. W. Lampert. 1983. Persistent infection of oligodendrocytes in Theiler's virus-induced encephalomyelitis. Ann. Neurol. 13:426-433.

Ronco, P., D. Woodrow, Y. Riviere, J. Moss, P. Verroust, J. C. Guillon, I. Gresser, J. C. Sloper, and L. Morel-Maroger. 1980. Further studies on the inhibition of lymphocytic choriomeningitis-induced glomerulonephritis by antiinterferon globulin. Circulating immune complexes and ultrastructural studies. Lab. Invest. 43:37-46.

Ronco, P., Y. Riviere, Y. Thouas, M. T. Bandu, J. C. Guillon, P. Verroust, and L. Morel-Maroger. 1981. Lymphocytic choriomeningitis virus infection in the nude mouse. An immunopathological study. Immunology 43:763-770.

Rose, R. M., C. Crumpacker, J. L. Waner, and J. D. Brain. 1982. Murine cytomegalovirus pneumonia. Description of a model and investigation of pathogenesis. Am. Rev. Respir. Dis. 125:568-573.

Rosen, L. 1960. Serologic grouping of reoviruses by hemagglutination-inhibition. Am. J. Hyg. 71:242-249.

Rosen, D. D., and R. S. Berk. 1977. *Pseudomonas* eye infections in cyclophosphamide treated mice. Invest. Ophthalmol. Vis. Sci. 16:649-652.

Ross, C. R., J. E. Wagner, S. R. Wightman, and S. E. Dill. 1980. Experimental transmission of *Syphacia muris* among rats, mice, hamsters, and gerbils. Lab. Anim. Sci. 30:35-37.

Roughgarden, J. W. 1965. Antimicrobial therapy of rat-bite fever. Arch. Intern. Med. 116:39-54.

Rowe, W. P. 1961. The epidemiology of mouse polyoma infection. Bacteriol. Rev. 25:18-31.

Rowe, W. P., and W. I. Capps. 1961. A new mouse virus causing necrosis of the thymus in newborn mice. J. Exp. Med. 113:831-844.

Rowe, W. P., J. W. Hartley, I. Brodsky, R. J. Huebner, and L. W. Law. 1958. Observations on the spread of mouse polyomavirus infection. Nature 182:1617.

Rowe, W. P., J. W. Hartley, J. D. Estes, and R. J. Huebner. 1959a. Studies of mouse polyoma virus infection. I. Procedures for quanitation and detection of virus. J. Exp. Med. 109:379-391.

Rowe, W. P., J. W. Hartley, L. W. Law, and R. J. Huebner. 1959b. Studies of mouse polyomavirus infection. III. Distribution of antibody in laboratory mouse colonies. J. Exp. Med. 109:449-462.

Rowe, W. P., J. W. Hartley, J. D. Estes, and R. J. Huebner. 1960. Growth curves of polyoma in mice and hamsters. J. Natl. Cancer Inst. Monogr. No. 4:189-206.

Rowe, W. P., J. W. Hartley, and R. J. Huebner. 1961. Polyoma and other indigenous mouse viruses. Pp. 131-142 in The Problems of Laboratory Animal Disease. New York: Academic Press.

Rowe, W. P., J. W. Hartley, and W. I. Capps. 1963. Mouse hepatitis virus infection as a highly contagious prevalent, enteric infection of mice. Proc. Soc. Exp. Biol. Med. 112:161-165.

Rowe, W. P., J. W. Hartley, and R. J. Huebner. 1963. Polyoma and other mouse viruses. Lab. Anim. Care 13:166-175.

Rowson, K. E. K. 1963. Riley virus in wild mice, effect of drugs on replication of Riley viruses. Br. Emp. Cancer Campaign Annu. Rep. 41:222-223.

Rowson, K. E. K., and B. W. J. Mahy. 1975. Lactic dehydrogenase virus. Virol. Monogr. 13:1-121.

Rowson, K. E. K., and B. W. J. Mahy. 1985. Lactate dehydrogenase-elevating virus. J. Gen. Virol 66:2297-2312.

Rubino, M. J., and D. Walker. 1988. Immunosuppression and murine polyomavirus infection. Virus Res. 9:1-10.

Rudnick, P., and J. W. Hollingsworth. 1959. Life span of rat erythrocyte parasitized by *Bartonella*. J. Infect. Dis. 104:24-27.

Ruebner, B. H., and T. Hirano. 1965. Viral hepatitis in mice. Changes in oxidative enzymes and phosphatases after murine hepatitis virus (MHV-3) infection. Lab. Invest. 14:157-168.

Ruffolo, P. R., G. Margolis, and L. Kilham. 1966. The induction of hepatitis by prior partial hepatectomy in resistant adult rats infected with H-1 virus. Am. J. Pathol. 49:795-824.

Ruitenberg, E. J., and B. C. Kruyt. 1975. Effect of intestinal flagellates on immune response in mice. Parasitology 71:30 (abstr).

Ruitenberg, E. J., P. A. M. Guinee, B. C. Kruyt, and J. M. Berkvens. 1971. Salmonella pathogenesis in germ-free mice. A bacteriological and histological study. Br. J. Exp. Pathol. 52:192-197.

Runner, M. N., and J. Palm. 1953. Factors associated with the incidence of infantile diarrhea in mice. Proc. Soc. Exp. Biol. Med. 82:147-150.

Sabesin, S. M. 1972. Isolation of a latent murine hepatitis virus from cultured mouse liver cells. Am. J. Gastroenterol. 58:259-274.

Sabin, A. B. 1938a. Isolation of a filterable, transmissible agent with "neurolytic" properties from toxoplasma infected tissues. Science 88:189-191.

Sabin, A. B. 1938b. Identification of the filterable, transmissible neurolytic agent isolated from toxoplasma infected tissues as a new pleuropneumonia-like microbe. Science 88:575-576.

Sabin, A. B. 1939. Mice as carriers of pathogenic pleuropneumonia-like microorganisms. Science 90:18-19.

Sabin, A. B., and B. Johnson. 1940. Pathogenic pleuropneumonia-like microorganisms in tissues of normal mice and isolation of new immunological types. Proc. Soc. Exp. Biol. Med. 44:569-571.

Sacks, H. J., and R. H. Egdahl. 1960. Protective effects of immunity and immune serum on the development of hemolytic anemia and cancer in rats. Surg. Forum 10:22-25.

Sacks, J. H., R. F. Clark, and R. H. Egdahl. 1960. Induction of tumor immunity with a new filterable agent. Surgery 48:244-260.

Sacquet, E. 1965. Pathogen-free animals. Food Cosmet. Toxicol. 3:47-55.

Sahli, R., G. K. McMaster, and B. Hirt. 1985. DNA sequence comparison between two tissue-specific variants of the autonomous parvovirus, minute virus of mice. Nucleic Acids Res. 13:3617-3633.

Saito, S., and M. Tsukamura. 1976. Mycobacterium intracellulare from public bath water. Jpn. J. Microbiol. 20:561-563.

Saito, M., M. Nakagawa, K. Kinoshita, and K. Imaizumi. 1978. Etiological studies on natural outbreaks of pneumonia in mice. Jpn. J. Vet. Sci. 40:283-290.

Saito, M., M. Nakagawa, E. Suzuki, K. Kinoshita, and K. Imaizumi. 1981. Synergistic effect of Sendai virus on *Mycoplasma pulmonis* infection in mice. Jpn. J. Vet. Sci. 43:43-50.

Saito, M., K. Nakayama, T. Muto, and M. Nakagawa. 1982. Effects of gaseous ammonia on *Mycoplasma pulmonis* infection in mice and rats. Exp. Anim. 31:203-206.

Sakazaki, R. 1984. Genus *Citrobacter*. Pp. 458-461 in Bergey's Manual of Systematic Bacteriology, vol. 1, N. R. Krieg and J. G. Holt, eds. Baltimore: Williams & Wilkins.

Saltzgaber-Muller, J., and B. A. Stone. 1986. Detection of *Corynebacterium kutscheri* in animal tissues by DNA-DNA hybridization. J. Clin. Microbiol. 24:759-763.

Sansing, W. A., J. J. Killion, and G. M. Kollmorgen. 1977. Evaluation of time and dose in treating mammary adenocarcinoma with immunostimulants. Cancer Immunol. Immunother. 2:63-68.

Santisteban, G. A., V. Riley, and M. A. Fitzmaurice. 1972. Thymolytic and adrenal cortical responses to the LDH-elevating virus. Proc. Soc. Exp. Biol. Med. 139:202-206.

Saron, M.F., Y. Riviere, A. G. Hovanessian, and J. C. Guillon. 1982. Chronic production of interferon in carrier mice congenitally infected with lymphocytic choriomeningitis virus. Virology 117:253-256.

Sass, B., and T. B. Dunn. 1979. Classification of mouse mammary tumors in Dunn's miscellaneous group including recently reported types. J. Natl. Cancer Inst. 62:1287-1293.

Sato, H., and H. Miyata. 1986. Detection of lymphocytic choriomeningitis virus antibodies in colonies of laboratory animals in Japan. Exp. Anim. 35:189-192.

Savage, D. C. 1971. Defining the gastrointestinal microflora of laboratory mice. Pp. 60-73 in Defining the Laboratory Animal. A symposium organized by the International Committee on Laboratory Animals and the Institute of Laboratory Animal Resources. Washington, D.C.: National Academy of Sciences.

Savage, N. 1984. Genus *Streptobacillus*. Pp. 598-600 in Bergey's Manual of Systematic Bacteriology, vol. I, N. R. Krieg and J. G. Holt, eds. Baltimore: Williams & Wilkins.

Savage, N. L. 1972. Host-parasite relationships in experimental *Streptobacillus moniliformis* arthritis in mice. Infect. Immun. 5:183-190.

Savage, N. L., G. N. Joiner, and D. W. Florey. 1981. Clincial, microbiological, and histological manifestations of *Streptobacillus moniliformis* induced arthritis in mice. Infect. Immun. 34:605-609.

Sawicki, L. 1961. Influence of age of mice on the recovery from experimental Sendai virus infection. Nature 192:1258-1259.

Sawicki, L. 1962. Studies on experimental Sendai virus infection in laboratory mice. Acta Virol. 6:347-351.

Sawicki, L., H. M. Bruce, and C. H. Andrewes. 1962. *Streptobacillus moniliformis* as a probable cause of arrested pregnancy and abortion in laboratory mice. Br. J. Exp. Pathol. 43:194-197.

Scheff, G. J., I. M. Scheff, and G. Eiseman. 1956. Concerning the mechanism of *Bartonella* anemia in the splenectomized rat. J. Infect. Dis. 98:113-120.

Scheid, M. P., G. Goldstein, and E. A. Boyse. 1975. Differentiation of T-cells in nude mice. Science 10:1211-1213.

Schell, K. 1960a. Studies on the innate resistance of mice to infection with mousepox. I. Resistance and antibody production. Aust. J. Exp. Biol. Med. Sci. 38:271-288.

Schell, K. 1960b. Studies on the innate resistance of mice to infection with mousepox. II. Route of inoculation and resistance; and some observations on the inheritance of resistance. Aust. J. Exp. Biol. Med. Sci. 38:289-299.

Schiffman, G., R. M. Douglas, M. J. Bonner, M. Roberts, and R. Austrian. 1980. A radioimmunoassay for immunologic phenomena in pneumococcal disease and for the antibody response to pneumococcal vaccines. I. Method for the radioimmunoassay of anticapsular antibodies and comparison with other techniques. J. Immunol. Meth. 33:133-144.

Schilt, U. 1987. Murine cytomegalovirus. Immunobiology 174:10-19.

Schindler, L., G. Streissle, and H. Kirchner. 1981. Protection of mice against mouse hepatitis virus by *Corynebacterium parvum*. Infect. Immun. 32:1128-1131.

Schindler, L., H. Engles, and H. Kirchner. 1982. Activation of natural killer cells and induction of interferon after injection of mouse hepatitis virus type 3 in mice. Infect. Immun. 35:869-873.

Schindler, L., J. Brucher, and H. Kirchner. 1984. Protection of mice against infection with mouse hepatitis virus type 3 by injection of silica. Immunobiology 166:62-71.

Schlom, J. 1980. Type B and type D retroviruses. Pp. 447-484 in Molecular Biology of RNA Tumor Viruses, J. R. Stephenson, ed. New York: Academic Press.

Schmaljohn, C. S., and J. M. Dalrymple. 1983. Analysis of Hantaan virus RNA: Evidence for a new genus of Bunyaviridae. Virology 131:482-491.

Schmaljohn, C. S., S. E. Hasty, S. A. Harrison, and J. M. Dalrymple. 1983. Characterization of Hantaan virions, prototype virus of hemorrhagic fever with renal syndrome. J. Infect. Dis. 148:1005-1012.

Schmaljohn, C. S., S. E. Hasty, J. M. Dalrymple, J. W. LeDuc, H. W. Lee, C.H. von Bonsdorff, M. Brummer-Korvenkontio, A. Vaheri, T. F. Tsai, H. L. Regnery, D. Goldgaber, and P.W. Lee. 1985. Antigenic and genetic properties of viruses linked to hemorrhagic fever with renal syndrome. Science 227:1041-1044.

Schmidt, E. C., and J. A. Shadduck. 1983. Murine encephalitozoonosis model for studying the host-parasite relationship of a chronic infection. Infect. Immun. 40:936-942.

Schneemilch, H. D. 1976. A naturally acquired infection of laboratory mice with *Klebsiella* capsule type 6. Lab. Anim. 10:305-310.

Schneider, H. A., and G. R. Collins. 1966. Successful prevention of infantile diarrhea of mice during an epizootic by means of a new filter cage unopened from birth to weaning. Lab. Anim. Care 16:60-71.

Schoeb, T. R., and J. R. Lindsey. 1987. Exacerbation of murine respiratory mycoplasmosis by sialodacryoadenitis virus infection in gnotobiotic F344 rats. Vet. Pathol. 24:392-399.

Schoeb, T. R., M. K. Davidson, and J. R. Lindsey. 1982. Intracage ammonia promotes growth of *Mycoplasma pulmonis* in the respiratory tract of rats. Infect. Immun. 38:212-217.

Schoeb, T. R., K. C. Kervin, and J. R. Lindsey. 1985. Exacerbation of murine respiratory mycoplasmosis in gnotobiotic F344/N rats by Sendai virus infection. Vet. Pathol. 22:272-282.

Schook, L. B., L. Carrick, Jr., and R. S. Berk. 1977. Experimental pulmonary infection in mice by tracheal intubation of *Pseudomonas aeruginosa:* The use of antineoplastic agents to overcome natural resistance. Can. J. Microbiol. 23:823-826.

Schoolman, H. M., W. Spurrier, S. O. Schwartz, and P. B. Szants. 1957. Studies in leukemia. VII. The induction of leukemia in Swiss mice by means of cell-free filtrates of leukemic mouse brain. Blood 12:694-700.

Schrieber, H., P. Nettesheim, W. Lijinsky, C. B. Richter, and H. E. Walburg, Jr. 1972. Induction of lung cancer in germ free, specific pathogen free and infected rats by N-nitroso-heptamethyleneimine: Enhancement of respiratory infection. J. Natl. Cancer Inst. 4:1107-1114.

Schwimmbeck, P. L., T. Dyrberg, and M. B. A. Oldstone. 1988. Abrogation of diabetes in BB rats by acute virus infection. Association of viral-lymphocyte interactions. J. Immunol. 140:3394-3400.

Scott, J. P., and E. Fredericson. 1951. The causes of fighting in mice and rats. Physiol. Zool. 24:273-309.

Scott, J. K., and J. N. Stannard. 1954. Relationship between *Bartonella muris* infection and acute radiation effects in the rat. J. Infect. Dis. 95:302-308.

Seamer, J., A. W. Gledhill, J. L. Barlow, and J. Hotchin. 1961. Effect of *Eperythrozoon coccoides* upon lymphocytic choriomeningitis in mice. J. Immunol. 86:512-515.

Sebesteny, A. 1969. Pathogenicity of intestinal flagellates in mice. Lab. Anim. 3:71-77.

Sebesteny, A. 1973. Abscesses of the bulbourethral glands of mice due to *Pasteurella pneumotropica*. Lab. Anim. 7:315-317.

Sebesteny, A., and A. C. Hill. 1974. Hepatitis and brain lesions due to mouse hepatitis virus accompanied by wasting in nude mice. Lab. Anim. 8:317-326.

Sebesteny, A., R. Tilly, F. Balkwill, and D. Trevan. 1980. Demyelination and wasting associated with polyomavirus infection in nude (*nu*/*nu*) mice. Lab. Anim. 14:337-345.

Sedlacek, R. S., and K. A. Mason. 1977. A simple and inexpensive method for maintaining a defined flora mouse colony. Lab. Anim. Sci. 27:667-670.

Sedlacek, R. S., R. P. Orcutt, H. D. Suit, and E. F. Rose. 1981. A flexible barrier at cage level for existing colonies: Production and maintenance of a limited stable anaerobic flora in a closed inbred mouse colony. Pp. 65-69 in Recent Advances in Germfree Research, S. Sasaki, A. Ozawa, and K. Hashimoto, eds. Tokyo: Tokai University Press.

Selgrade, M. K., A. Ahmed, K. W. Sell, M. E. Gershwin, and A. D. Steinberg. 1976. Effect of murine cytomegalovirus on the in vitro responses of T and B cells to mitogens. J. Immunol. 116:1459-1465.

Seronde, J. 1954. Resistance of rats to inoculation with *Corynebacterium* pathogenic in pantothenate deficiency. Proc. Soc. Exp. Biol. Med. 85:521-524.

Seronde, J., L. M. Zucker, and T. F. Zucker. 1955. The influence of duration of pantothenate deprivation upon natural resistance of rats to a *Corynebacterium*. J. Infect. Dis. 97:35-38.

Seronde, J., T. F. Zucker, and L. M. Zucker. 1956. Thiamine, pyridoxine and pantothenic acid in the natural resistance of the rat to a *Corynebacterium* infection. J. Nutr. 59:287-298.

Serrano, L. J. 1971. Defined mice in a radiobiological experiment. Pp. 13-43 in Defining the Laboratory Animal. A symposium organized by the International Committee on Laboratory Animals and the Institute of Laboratory Animal Resources. Washington, D.C.: National Academy of Sciences.

Shackelford, P. G., and R. D. Feigin. 1973. Periodicity of susceptibility to pneumococcal infection. Influence of light and adrenocortical secretions. Science 182:285-287.

Shadduck, J. A. 1969. *Nosema cuniculi:* In vitro isolation. Science 24:516-517.

Shadduck, J. A., and M. J. Geroulo. 1979. A simple method for the detection of antibodies to *Encephalitozoon cuniculi* in rabbits. Lab. Anim. Sci. 29:330-334.

Shadduck, J. A., and S. P. Pakes. 1971. Encephalitozoonosis (nosematosis) and toxoplasmosis. Am. J. Pathol. 64:657-674.

Shadduck, J. A., R. Bender, and G. T. Robinson. 1978. Isolation of the causative organism of canine encephalitozoonosis. Vet. Pathol. 15:459-460.

Shadduck, J. A., W. T. Watson, S. P. Pakes, and A. Cali. 1979. Animal infectivity of *Encephalitozoon cuniculi*. J. Parasitol. 65:123-129.

Shah, K. V., and C. Christian. 1986. Mouse polyoma and other papovaviruses. Pp. 505-527. in Viral and Mycoplasmal Infections of Laboratory Rodents: Effects on Biomedical Research. P. N. Bhatt, R. O. Jacoby, H. C. Morse III, and A. E. New, eds. Orlando, FL: Academic Press.

Shambaugh, G. E., III, and W. R. Beisel. 1966. Alterations in thyroid physiology during pneumococcal septicemia in the rat. Endocrinology 79:511-523.

Shanley, J. D., and E. L. Pesanti. 1980. Replication of murine cytomegalovirus in lung macrophages: Effect on phagocytosis of bacteria. Infect. Immun. 29:1152-1159.

Shanley, J. D., M. C. Jordan, M. L. Cook, and T. G. Steven. 1979. Pathogenesis of reactivated latent murine cytomegalovirus infection. Am. J. Pathol. 95:67-78.

Shanley, J. D., E. L. Pesanti, and K. M. Nugent. 1982. The pathogenesis of penumonitis due to murine cytomegalovirus. J. Infect. Dis. 146:388-396.

Sharpe, A. H., and B. N. Fields. 1984. Reovirus cytopathology: Effects on cellular macromolecular synthesis and cytoskeleton. Pp. 431-464 in Comprehensive Virology, vol. 19, H. Fraenkel-Conrat and R. R. Wagner, eds. New York: Plenum Press.

Sharpe, A. H., and B. N. Fields. 1985. Pathogenesis of viral infections. Basic concepts derived from the reovirus model. N. Engl. J. Med. 312:486-497.

Shechmeister, J. L., and F. L. Adler. 1953. Activation of pseudotuberculosis in mice exposed to sublethal total body radiation. J. Infect. Dis. 92:228-239.

Sheedy, J. A., H. F. Froeb, H. A. Batson, C. C. Conley, J. P. Murphy, R. B. Hunter, D. W. Cugell, R. B. Giles, S. C. Bershady, J. W. Vester, and R. H. Yoe. 1954. The clinical course of epidemic hemorrhagic fever. Am. J. Med. 16:628-629.

Sheena, S., and C. J. Meade. 1978. Mice bearing the ob/ob mutation have impaired immunity. Int. Arch. Allergy Appl. Immunol. 57:263-268.

Sheets, P., K. V. Shah, and F. B. Bang. 1978. Mouse hepatitis virus (MHV) infection in thymectomized C3H mice. Proc. Soc. Exp. Biol. Med. 159:34-38.

Shellam, G. R., J. E. Allan, J. M. Papadimitriou, and G. J. Bancroft. 1981. Increased susceptibility to cytomegalovirus infection in beige mutant mice. Proc. Natl. Acad. Sci. USA 78:5104-5108.

Sheridan, J. F., and S. Vonderfecht. 1986. Mouse rotavirus. Pp. 217-243 in Viral and Mycoplasmal Infections of Laboratory Rodents: Effects on Biomedical Research. P. N. Bhatt, R. O. Jacoby, H. C. Morse III, and A. E. New, eds. Orlando, FL: Academic Press.

Sheridan, J. F., R. S. Eydelloth, S. L. Vonderfacht, and L. Aurelian. 1983. Virus-specific immunity in neonatal and adult mouse rotavirus infection. Infect. Immun. 39:917-927.

Sheridan, J. F., C. C. Smith, M. M. Manak, and L. Aurelian. 1984. Prevention of rotavirus-induced diarrhea in neonatal mice born to dams immunized with empty capsids of simian rotavirus SA-11. J. Infect. Dis. 149:434-438.

Shif, I., and F. B. Bang. 1970. In vitro interaction of mouse hepatitis virus and macrophages from genetically resistant mice. I. Adsorption of virus and growth curves. J. Exp. Med. 131:343-350.

Shiota, T. 1986. Simultaneous demonstration of cyst walls and intracystic bodies of *Pneumocystis carinii* in paraffin embedded lung sections using Gomori's methenamine silver nitrate and Giemsa stain. J. Clin. Pathol. 39:1269-1274.

Shope, R. E. 1954. Report of the Committee on Infectious Ectromelia of Mice. J. Natl. Cancer Inst. 15:405-408.

Shu-heh, W. C., K. J. Welch, E. S. Murray, and D. M. Hegsted. 1976. Effect of iron deficiency on susceptibility to *Streptococcus pneumoniae* in the rat. Nutr. Rep. Int. 14:605-609.

Shultz, F. S., P. C. Estes, J. A. Franklin, and C. B. Richter. 1973. Staphylococcal botryomycosis in a specific-pathogen-free mouse colony. Lab. Anim. Sci. 23:36-42.

Siegl, G., R. C. Bates, I. Berns, B. J. Carter, D. C. Kelly, E. Kurstak, and P. Tattersall. 1985. Characteristics and taxonomy of Parvoviridae. Intervirology 23:61-73.

Silverman, J., F. Paturzo, and A. L. Smith. 1982. Effects of experimental infection of the deer mouse (*Peromyscus maniculatus*) with mouse hepatitis virus. Lab. Anim. Sci. 32:273-274.

Simmons, D. J., and W. Simpson. 1977. Staphylococcal kidney abscesses in rats treated with corticosteroids. Lab. Anim. 11:259-260.

Simmons, D. J. C., and W. Simpson. 1980. *Salmonella montevideo* salmonellosis in laboratory mice: Successful treatment of the disease by oral oxytetracycline. Lab. Anim. (London) 14:217-219.

Simmons, M. L., C. B. Richter, R. W. Tennant, and J. Franklin. 1967. Production of specific-pathogen-free rats in plastic germfree isolator rooms. Pp. 38-47 in Advances in Germfree Research and Gnotobiology, M. Miyakawa and T. D. Luckey, eds. Cleveland, Ohio: CRC Press.

Simon, P. C. 1977. Isolation of *Bacillus piliformis* from rabbits. Can. Vet. J. 18:46-48.

Simpson, W., and D. J. C. Simmons. 1980. Two *Actinobacillus* species isolated from laboratory rodents. Lab. Anim. 14:15-16.

Simpson, W., and D. J. C. Simmons. 1981. *Salmonella livingstone* salmonellosis in laboratory mice: Successful containment and treatment of the disease. Lab. Anim. 15:261-262.

Singer, S. H., M. Ford, and R. L. Kirschstein. 1972. Respiratory diseases in cyclophosphamide treated mice. Increased virulence of *Mycoplasma pulmonis*. Infect. Immun. 5:953-956.

Singh, S. B., and C. M. Lang. 1984. Enzyme-linked immunosorbent assay in the diagnosis of Kilham rat virus infection in rats. Lab. Anim. 18:364-370.

Skinner, H. H., and E. H. Knight. 1969. Studies on murine lymphocytic choriomeningitis within a partially infected colony. Lab. Anim. 3:175-184.

Skinner, H. H., and E. H. Knight. 1971. Monitoring mouse stocks for lymphocytic choriomeningitis virus—a human pathogen. Lab. Anim. 5:73-87.

Skinner, H. H., E. H. Knight, and R. Grove. 1977. Murine lymphocytic choriomeningitis: The history of a natural cross-infection from wild to laboratory mice. Lab. Anim. 11:219-222.

Sklar, J. 1985. DNA hybridization in diagnostic pathology. Hum. Pathol. 16:654-658.

Smadel, J. E. 1953. Epidemic hemorrhagic fever. Am. J. Public Health. 43:1327-1330.

Small, J. D. 1984. Rodent and lagomorph health surveillance-quality assurance. Pp. 709-723 in Laboratory Animal Medicine, J. G. Fox, B. J. Cohen, and F. M. Loew, eds. New York: Academic Press.

Small, J. D., and A. E. New. 1981. Prevention and control of mousepox. Lab. Anim. Sci. 31:616-632.

Smith, A. L. 1983a. Response of weanling random-bred mice to inoculation with minute virus of mice. Lab. Anim. Sci. 33:37-39.

Smith, A. L. 1983b. An immunofluorescence test for detection of serum antibody to rodent coronaviruses. Lab. Anim. Sci. 33:157-160.

Smith, A. L. 1986a. Detection methods for rodent viruses. Pp. 123-142 in Complications of Viral and Mycoplasmal Infections in Rodents to Toxicology Research and Testing. T. E. Hamm, Jr., ed. Washington, D.C.: Hemisphere Press.

Smith, A. L. 1986b. Serologic tests for detection of antibody to rodent viruses. Pp. 731-751 in Viral and Mycoplosmal Infections of Laboratory Rodents: Effects on Biomedical Research. P. N. Bhatt, R. O. Jacoby, H. C. Morse III, and A. E. New, eds. Orlando, FL: Academic Press.

Smith, A. L. 1986c. Methods for potential application to rodent virus isolation and identification. Pp. 753-776 in Viral and Mycoplasmal Infections of Laboratory Rodents: Effects on Biomedical Research. P. N. Bhatt, R. O. Jacoby, H. C. Morse III, and A. E. New, eds. Orlando, FL: Academic Press.

Smith, A. L., and S. W. Barthold. 1987. Factors influencing susceptibility of laboratory rodents to infection with mouse adenovirus strains K 87 and FL. Arch. Virol. 95:143-148.

Smith, A. L., D. L. Knudson, J. F. Sheridan, and F. X. Paturzo. 1983. Detection of antibody to epizootic diarrhea of infant mice (EDIM) virus. Lab. Anim. Sci. 33:442-445.

Smith, A. L., V. A. Carrano, and D. G. Brownstein. 1984a. Response of weanling random-bred mice to infection with pneumonia virus of mice (PVM). Lab. Anim. Sci. 34:35-37.

Smith, A. L., F. X. Paturzo, E. P. Gardner, S. Morgenstern, G. Cameron, and H. Wadley. 1984b. Two epizootics of lymphocytic choriomeningitis virus occurring in laboratory mice despite intensive monitoring programs. Can. J. Comp. Med. 48:335-337.

Smith, A. L., D. F. Winograd, and T. G. Burrage. 1986. Comparative biological characterization of mouse adenovirus strains FL and K87 and seroprevalence in laboratory rodents. Arch. Virol. 91:233-246.

Smith, C. B., M. M. Griffiths, and L. S. Wei. 1986. Rat cytomegalovirus infection enhances type II collagen arthritis in rats. Arth. Rheum. 29:1263-1268.

Smith, M. S., R. E. Click, and P. G. W. Plagemann. 1984. Control of MHV replication in macrophages by a recessive gene on chromosome 7. J. Immunol. 133:428-432.

Smorodintsev, A.A., V.G. Chudakov, and A.V. Churilov. 1959. Hemorrhagic Nephrosonephritis. 120 pp. Translated from Russian by Catherine Mathews. New York: Pergamon.

Solleveld, H. A. 1978. Types and quality of animals in cancer research. Acta Zool. Pathol. Antverpiensia 72:5-18.

Sommers, H. M., and R. C. Good. 1985. *Mycobacterium*. Pp. 216-248 in Manual of Clinical Microbiology, 4th ed. E. H. Lennette, A. Balows, W. J. Hausler, Jr., and H. J. Shadomy, eds. Washington, D.C.: American Society for Microbiology.

Song, G., C.-S. Hang, X.-Z. Qui, D.-S. Ni, H.-X. Liao, G.-Z. Gao, Y.-L. Du, J.-K. Xu, Y.S. Wu, J.-N. Zhao, B.-X. Kong, Z.-S. Wang, Z.-Q. Zhang, H.-K. Shen, and N. Zhou. 1983. Etiologic studies of epidemic hemorrhagic fever (hemorrhagic fever with renal syndrome). J. Infect. Dis. 147:654-659.

Spalholz, B. A., and P. Tattersall. 1983. Interaction of minute virus of mice with differentiated cells: Strain-dependent target cell specificity is mediated by intracellular factors. J. Virol. 46:937-943.

Sparrow, S. 1976. The microbiological and parasitological status of laboratory animals from accredited breeders in the United Kingdom. Lab. Anim. 10:365-373.

Speckman, D., and V. Riley. 1975. Stress effects of the LDH-virus in altering the Gardner tumor in mice. Proc. Am. Assoc. Cancer Res., abstract no. 678.

Specter, S. C., M. Bendinelli, W. S. Ceglowski, and H. Friedman. 1978. Macrophage-induced reversal of immunosuppression by leukemia viruses. Fed. Proc. 37:97-101.

Squire, R. A., D. G. Goodman, M. G. Valerio, T. Frederickson, J. D. Strandberg, M. H. Levitt, C. H. Lingeman, J. C. Harshbarger, and C. J. Dawe. 1978. Pp. 1051-1283 in Pathology of Laboratory Animals, vol. II, K. Benirschke, F. M. Garner, and T. C. Jones, eds. New York: Springer-Verlag.

St-Pierre, Y., E. F. Potworowski, and G. Lussier. 1987. Transmission of mouse thymic virus. J. Gen. Virol. 68:1173-1176.

Stachan, R., and I. Kunstyr. 1983. Minimal infectious doses and prepatent periods in *Giardia muris, Spironucleus muris* and *Tritrichomonas muris*. Z. Bakt. Hyg. A256:249-256.

Stanley, N. F. 1961. Relationship of hepato-encephalomyelitis virus and reoviruses. Nature 189:687.

Stanley, N. F. 1974. The reovirus murine models. Prog. Med. Virol. 18:257-272.

Stanley, N. F., and R. A. Joske. 1975a. Animal model of human disease. Active chronic hepatitis; animal model; chronic murine hepatitis induced by reovirus type 3. Am. J. Pathol. 80:181-184.

Stanley, N. F., and R. A. Joske. 1975b. Animal model of human disease. Chronic biliary obstruction caused by reovirus type 3. Am. J. Pathol. 80:185-187.

Stanley, N. F., D. C. Dorman, and J. Ponsford. 1953. Studies on the pathogenesis of a hitherto undescribed virus (hepato-encephalomyelitis) producing unusual symptoms in suckling mice. Aust. J. Exp. Biol. Med. Sci. 31:147-180.

Stanley, N. F., D. C. Dorman, and J. Ponsford. 1954. Studies on the hepato-encephalomyelitis virus (HEV). Aust. J. Exp. Biol. Med. Sci. 32:543-562.

Stanley, N. F., P. J. Leak, M. N. Walter, and R. A. Joske. 1964. Murine infection with reovirus. II. The chronic disease following reovirus type 3 infection. Br. J. Exp. Med. 45:142-149.

Stansly, P. G., and C. F. Neilson. 1965. Relationship between spleen weight increase factor (SWIF) of mice and *Eperythrozoon coccoides*. Proc. Soc. Exp. Biol. Med. 119:1059-1063.

Stansly, P. G., and C. F. Neilson. 1966. Sedimentation of *Eperythrozoon coccoides*. Proc. Soc. Exp. Biol. Med. 121:363-365.

Stansly, P. G., D. S. Ramsey, and C. F. Neilson. 1962. A transmissible spleen weight increase factor (SWIF) of mice. Proc. Soc. Exp. Biol. Med. 109:265-267.

Starkey, W. G., J. Collins, T. S. Wallis, G. J. Clarke, A. J. Spencer, S. J. Haddon, M. P. Osborne, D.C.A. Candy, and J. Stephen. 1986. Kinetics, tissue specificity and pathological changes in murine rotavirus infection of mice. J. Gen. Virol. 67:2625-2634.

Starr, S. E., and A. C. Allison. 1977. Role of T lymphocytes in recovery from murine cytomegalovirus infection. Infect. Immun. 17:458-462.

Starr, T. J., and M. Pollard. 1958. Susceptibility of cortisone treated mice to infection with mouse hepatitis virus. Proc. Soc. Exp. Biol. Med. 99:108-110.

Stedham, M. A., and T. J. Bucci. 1970. Spontaneous Tyzzer's disease in a rat. Lab. Anim. Care 20:743-746.

Steeves, R. 1974. Murine oncornaviruses. Pp. 4-11 in Handbook of Laboratory Animal Science, vol. II, E. C. Melby, Jr., and N. H. Altman, eds. Cleveland: CRC Press.

Steeves, R., and F. Lilly. 1977. Interactions between host and viral genomes in mouse leukemia. Annu. Rev. Genet. 11:277-296.

Steffen, E. K., and J. E. Wagner. 1983. *Salmonella enteritidis* serotype amsterdam in a commercial rat colony. Lab. Anim. Sci. 33:454-456.

Steuckemann, J. A., D. M. Ritzi, M. Holth, M. S. Smith, W. J. Swart, W. A. Cafruny, and P. G. W. Plagemann. 1982a. Replication of lactate dehydrogenase-elevating virus in macrophages. I. Evidence for cytocidal replication. J. Gen. Virol. 59:245-262.

Steuckemann, J. A., M. Holth, W. J. Swart, K. Kowalchyk, M. S. Smith, A. J. Wolstenholme, W. A. Cafruny, and P. G. W. Plagemann. 1982b. Replication of lactate dehydrogenase-elevating virus in macrophages. 2. Mechanisms of persistent infection in mice and cell culture. J. Gen. Virol. 59:263-272.

Stevens, D. P. 1982. Giardiasis: Immunity, immunopathology and immunodiagnosis. Pp. 192-203 in Immunology of Parasitic Infections, 2nd ed., S. Cohen and K. S. Warren, eds. Oxford: Blackwell Scientific.

Stevens, D. P., and D. M. Frank. 1978. Local immunity giardiasis: Is milk protective at the expense of maternal gut? Trans. Assoc. Am. Phys. 91:268-272.

Stevens, D. P., and I. C. Roberts-Thomson. 1978. Animal model of human disease: Giardiasis. Am. J. Pathol. 90:529-532.

Stevens, D. P., D. M. Frank, and A. A. F. Mahmoud. 1978. Thymus dependency of host resistance to *Giardia muris* infection: Studies in nude mice. J. Immunol. 120:680-682.

Stewart, D. D., and G. E. Buck. 1975. The occurrence of *Mycoplasma arthritidis* in the throat and middle ear of rats with chronic respiratory disease. Lab. Anim. Sci. 25:769-775.

Stewart, D. D., G. E. Buck, E. D. McConnell, and R. L. Amster. 1975. An epizootic of necrotic dermatitis in laboratory mice caused by Lancefield group G streptococci. Lab. Anim. Sci. 25:296-302.

Stewart, S. E., and V. H. Haas. 1956. Lymphocytic choriomeningitis virus in mouse neoplasms. J. Natl. Cancer Inst. 17:233-245.

Stewart, S. W. 1953. Leukemia in mice produced by filterable agent present in AKR leukemic tissue with notes on a sarcoma produced by the same agent. Anat. Rec. 117:532. (abstr.)

Stewart, S. W., B. E. Eddy, A. M. Gochenour, N. G. Borgese, and G. G. Grubbs. 1957. The induction of neoplasms with a substance released from mouse tumors by tissue culture. Virology 3:380-400.

Stieritz, D. D., and I. A. Holder. 1975. Experimental studies of the pathogenesis of infections due to *Pseudomonas aeruginosa:* description of a burned mouse model. J. Infect. Dis. 131:688-691.

Stoenner, H. G., E. F. Grimes, F. B. Thrailkill, and E. Davis. 1959. Elimination of *Leptospira ballum* from a colony of Swiss albino mice by use of chlortetracycline hydrochloride. Am. J. Trop. Med. Hyg. 7:423-426.

Stoenner, H. G., and D. Maclean. 1958. Leptospirosis (ballum) contracted from Swiss albino mice. Arch. Intern. Med. 101: 606-610.

Stohlman, S. A., and L. P. Weiner. 1978. Stability of neurotropic mouse hepatitis virus (JHM strain) during chronic infection of neuroblastoma cells. Arch. Virol. 57:53-61.

Stott, J. A., J. E. Hodgson, and J. C. Chaney. 1975. Incidence of salmonellae in animal feed and the effect of pelleting on content of enterobacteriaceae. J. Appl. Bacteriol. 39:41-46.

Strangeways, W. I. 1933. Rats as carriers of *Streptobacillus moniliformis*. J. Pathol. Bacteriol. 37:45-51.

Streilein, J. W., J. A. Shadduck, and S. P. Pakes. 1981. Effects of splenectomy and Sendai virus infection on rejection of male skin isografts by pathogen free C57BL/6 female mice. Transplantation 32:34-37.

Stroop, W. G., and J. R. Baringer. 1981. Biochemistry of Theiler's murine encephalomyelitis virus isolated from acutely infected mouse brain: Identification of a previously unreported polypeptide. Infect. Immun. 32:769-777.

Stroop, W. G., and M. A. Brinton. 1983. Mouse strain-specific central nervous system lesions associated with lactate dehydrogenase-elevating virus infection. Lab. Invest. 49:334-345.

Stroop, W. G., J. R. Baringer, and M. Brahic. 1981. Detection of Theiler's virus RNA in mouse central nervous system by in situ hybridization. Lab. Invest. 45:504-509.

Stuart, A. E. 1960. Chemical splenectomy. Lancet 2:896-897.

Stuhlman, R. A., and J. E. Wagner. 1971. Ringtail in *Mystromys albicaudatus:* A case report. Lab. Anim. Sci. 21:585-587.

Sturman, L. S., and K. V. Holmes. 1983. The molecular biology of coronaviruses. Adv. Virus Res. 28:35-112.

Sturman, L. S., and I. Tamm. 1966. Host dependence of GDVII virus: Complete or abortive multiplication in various cell lines. J. Immunol. 97:885-896.

Sugiyama, K., and Y. Amano. 1981. Morphological and biological properties of a new coronavirus associated with diarrhea in infant mice. Arch. Virol. 67:241-251.

Sugiyama, T., K. Hashimoto, and S. Sasaki. 1967. An adenovirus isolated from the feces of mice. II. Experimental infection. Jpn. J. Microbiol. 11:3342.

Sulzer, C. R., and W. L. Jones. Undated. Leptospirosis: Methods in Laboratory Diagnosis, revised ed. U.S. Department of Health, Education, and Welfare Publ. No. (CDC) 78-8275. Atlanta, Ga.: Centers for Disease Control. 40 pp.

Suzuki, E., J. Matsubara, M. Saito, T. Muto, M. Nakagawa, and K. Imaizumi. 1982. Serological survey of laboratory rodents for infection with Sendai virus, mouse hepatitis virus, reovirus type 3, and mouse adenovirus. Jpn. J. Med. Sci. Biol. 35:249-254.

Suzuki, E., K. Mochida, and M. Nakagawa. 1988. Naturally occurring subclinical *Corynebacterium kutscheri* infection in laboratory rats: strain and age related antibody response. Lab. Anim. Sci. 38:42-45.

Syverton, J. T., and C. L. Larson. 1947. Intranuclear inclusion bodies in the kidneys of wild rats. Arch. Pathol. 43:541-552.

Taffs, L. F. 1974. Some diseases in normal and immunosuppressed experimental animals. Lab. Anim. 8:149-154.

Taguchi, F., M. Aiuchi, and K. Fujiwara. 1977. Age-dependent response of mice to a mouse hepatitis virus, MHV-S. Jpn. J. Exp. Med. 47:109-115.

Taguchi, F., Y. Goto, M. Aiuchi, T. Hayashi, and K. Fujiwara. 1979a. Pathogenesis of mouse hepatitis virus infection. The role of nasal epithelial cells as a primary target of low virulence virus, MHV-S. Microbiol. Immunol. 23:249-262.

Taguchi, F., A. Yamada, and K. Fujiwara. 1979b. Asymptomatic infection of mouse hepatitis virus in the rat. Arch. Virol. 59:275-279.

Taguchi, F., A. Yamada, and K. Fujiwara. 1979c. Factors involved in the age-dependent resistance of mice infected with low virulence mouse hepatitis virus. Arch. Virol. 62:333-340.

Taguchi, F., S. Kawamura, and K. Fujiwara. 1983. Replication of mouse hepatitis virus with high and low virulence in cultured hepatocytes. Infect. Immun. 39:955-959.

Tajima, T., E. Suzuki, H. Ushijima, K. Araki, B. Kim, T. Shinozaki, and R. Fujii. 1984. Isolation of murine rotavirus in cell cultures. Arch. Virol. 82:119-123.

Takagaki, Y., and K. Fujiwara. 1968. Bacteremia in experimental Tyzzer's disease in mice. Jpn. J. Microbiol. 12:129-143.

Takagaki, Y., M. Ito, M. Naiki, K. Fujiwara, M. Okugi, K. Maejima, and Y. Tajima. 1966. Experimental Tyzzer's disease in different species of laboratory animals. Jpn. J. Exp. Med. 36:519-534.

Takagaki, Y., M. Naiki, M. Ito, G. Noguchi, and K. Fujiwara. 1967. Checking of corynebacteriosis and Tyzzer's disease in mice by cortisone treatment. Exp. Anim. 16:12-19.

Takemoto, K. F., and P. Fabisch. 1970. Transformation of mouse cells by K-papovavirus. Virology 40:135-143.

Takenaka, S., and K. Fujiwara. 1975. Effect of carbon tetrachloride on experimental Tyzzer's disease of mice. Jpn. J. Exp. Med. 45:393-402.

Takeuchi, A., and K. Hashimoto. 1976. Electron microscopy study of experimental enteric adenovirus infection in mice. Infect. Immun. 13:569-580.

Takeyama, H., K. Kawashima, K. Yamada, and Y. Ito. 1979. Induction of tumor resistance in mice by L1210 leukemia cells persistently infected with HVJ (Sendai virus). Gann 70:493-501.

Tamura, H., C. Ishihara, A. Sasama, M. Tajima, I. Kuwamizu, and K. Maejima. 1981. Efficacy of hemadsorption for rapid identification of *Mycoplasma pulmonis*. Lab. Anim. Sci. 31:713-714.

Tamura, M. 1964. Occurrence of epidemic hemorrhagic fever in Osaka City: first cases found in Japan with characteristic feature of marked proteinuria. Biken J. 7:79-94.

Tamura, T., and K. Fujiwara. 1979. IgM and IgG response to sheep red blood cells in mouse hepatitis virus infected nude mice. Microbiol. Immunol. 23:177-183.

Tamura, T., F. Taguchi, F. Ueda, and K. Fujiwara. 1977. Persistent infection with mouse hepatitis virus of low virulence in nude mice. Microbiol. Immunol. 21:683-691.

Tamura, T., K. Ueda, T. Furuta, Y. Goto, and K. Fujiwara. 1978a. Electron microscopy of spontaneous pneumocystosis in a nude mouse. Jpn. J. Exp. Med. 48:363-368.

Tamura, T., K. Machii, K. Ueda, and K. Fujiwara. 1978b. Modification of immune response in nude mice infected with mouse hepatitis virus. Microbiol. Immunol. 22:557-564.

Tamura, T., C. Kai, C., Sakaguchi, T. Ishida, and K. Fujiwara. 1979. The role of macrophages in the early resistance to mouse hepatitis virus infection in nude mice. Microbiol. Immunol. 23:965-974.

Tamura, T., A. Sakaguchi, C. Kai, and K. Fujiwara. 1980. Enhanced phagocytic activity of macrophages in mouse hepatitis virus infected nude mice. Microbiol. Immunol. 24:243-247.

Tanaka, H., W. T. Hall, J. B. Sheffield, and D. H. Moore. 1965. Fine structure of *Haemobartonella muris* as compared with *Eperythrozoon coccoides* and *Mycoplasma pulmonis*. J. Bacteriol. 90:1735-1749.

Tannock, G. W., and J. M. B. Smith. 1971. A *Salmonella* carrier state involving the upper respiratory tract of mice. J. Infect. Dis. 123:502-506.

Tannock, G. W., and J. M. B. Smith. 1972. The effect of food and water deprivation (stress) on salmonella-carrier mice. J. Med. Microbiol. 5:283-289.

Tardieu, M., C. Hery, and J. M. Dupuy. 1980. Neonatal susceptibility to MHV-3 infection in mice. II. Role of natural effector marrow cells in transfer to resistance. J. Immunol. 124:418-423.

Tashiro, M., and M. Homma. 1983. Evidence of proteolytic activation of Sendai virus in mouse lungs. Arch. Virol. 77:127-137.

Tashiro, M., and M. Homma. 1985. Protection of mice from wild-type Sendai virus infection by a trypsin-resistant mutant, TR-2. J. Virol. 53:228-234.

Tashiro, M., Y. Fujii, K. Nakamura, and M. Homma. 1988. Cell-mediated immunity induced in mice after vaccination with a protease activation mutant, TR-2, of Sendai virus. J. Virol. 62:2490-2497.

Tattersall, P., and J. Bratton. 1983. Reciprocal productive and restrictive virus-cell interactions of immunosuppressive and prototype strains of minute virus of mice. J. Virol. 46:944-955.

Tattersall, P., and S. F. Cotmore. 1986. The rodent parvoviruses. Pp. 305-348 in Viral and Mycoplasmal Infections of Laboratory Rodents: Effects on Biomedical Research. P. N. Bhatt, R. O. Jacoby, H. C. Morse III, and A. E. New, eds. Orlando, Fla: Academic Press.

Taubler, J. H. 1968. Staphylococcal delayed hypersensitivity in mice. I. Induction and in vivo demonstration of delayed hypersensitivity. J. Immunol. 101:546-549.

Taubler, J. H., and S. Mudd. 1968. Staphylococcal delayed hypersensitivity in mice. II. In vitro demonstration of specificity of delayed hypersensitivity. J. Immunol. 101:550-555.

Taurog, J. D., S. L. Leary, M. A. Cremer, M. L. Mahowald, G. P. Sandberg, and P. J. Manning. 1984. Infection with *Mycoplasma pulmonis* modulates adjuvant- and collagen-induced arthritis in Lewis rats. Arth. Rheum. 27:943-946.

Taylor, C. E., W. Y. Weisser, and F. B. Bang. 1981. In vitro macrophage manifestation of cortisone-induced decrease in resistance to mouse hepatitis virus. J. Exp. Med. 153:732-737.

Taylor, D. M., and D. L. Neal. 1980. An infected eczematous condition in mice: Methods of treatment. Lab. Anim. 14:325-328.

Tennant, J. R. 1962. Derivation of a murine lymphoid leukemia virus. J. Natl. Cancer Inst. 28:1291-1301.

Tennant, R. W., J. C. Parker, and T. G. Ward. 1965. Virus studies with germfree mice. II. Comparative responses of germfree mice to virus infection. J. Natl. Cancer Inst. 34:381-387.

Tennant, R. W., J. C. Parker, and T. C. Ward. 1966. Respiratory virus infections of mice. Pp. 93-104 in Viruses of Laboratory Rodents, R. Holdenried, ed. National Cancer Institute Monograph 20. Washington, D.C.: U.S. Department of Health, Education, and Welfare.

Teramoto, Y. A., P. H. Hand, R. Callahan, and J. Schlom. 1980. Detection of novel murine mammary tumor viruses by interspecies immunoassays. J. Natl. Cancer Inst. 64:967-975.

Theiler, M. 1934. Spontaneous encephalomyelitis of mice—a new virus disease. Science 80:122.

Theiler, M. 1937. Spontaneous encephalomyelitis of mice. A new virus disease. J. Exp. Med. 65:705-719.

Theiler, M. 1941. Studies on poliomyelitis. Medicine 20:443-460.

Theiler, M., and S. Gard. 1940a. Encephalomyelitis of mice. I. Characteristics and pathogenesis of the virus. J. Exp. Med. 72:49-67.

Theiler, M., and S. Gard. 1940b. Encephalomyelitis of mice. III. Epidemiology. J. Exp. Med. 72:79-90.

Theiss, J. C., G. D. Stoner, and A. K. Kniazeff. 1978. Effect of reovirus infection on pulmonary tumor response to urethan in strain A mice. J. Natl. Cancer Inst. 61:131-134.

Theiss, J. C., M. B. Shimkin, G. D. Stoner, A. J. Kniazeff, and R. D. Hoppenstand. 1980. Effect of lactate dehydrogenase virus on chemically induced mouse lung tumorigenesis. Cancer Res. 40:64-66.

Thigpen, J. E., and P. W. Ross. 1983. Viral cross contamination of rats maintained in a fabric-walled mass air flow system. Lab. Anim. Sci. 33:446-450.

Thigpen, J. E., and J. A. Tortorich. 1980. Recommended goals for microbiological quality control for laboratory animals used in the National Toxicology Program (NTP). Pp. 229-233 in Animal Quality and Models in Biomedical Research, A. Spiegel, S. Erichsen, and H. A. Solleveld, eds. Stuttgart: Gustav Fischer Verlag.

Thirkill, C. E., and D. S. Gregerson. 1982. *Mycoplasma arthritidis*-induced ocular inflammatory disease. Infect. Immun. 36:775-781.

Thomas, L. 1967. The neurotoxins of *M. neurolyticum* and *M. gallisepticum*. Ann. N.Y. Acad. Sci. 143:218-224.

Thomas, L., and M. W. Bitensky. 1966. Studies of PPLO infection. IV. The neurotoxicity of intact mycoplasmas and their production of toxin in vivo and in vitro. J. Exp. Med. 124:1089-1098.

Thomas, L., F. Aleu, M. W. Bitensky, M. Davidson, and B. Gesner. 1966. Studies of PPLO infection. II. The neurotoxin of *Mycoplasma neurolyticum*. J. Exp. Med. 124:1067-1082.

Thomas, T. B., C. M. Pomerat, and E. H. Frieden. 1949. Cellular reactions in *Haemobartonella* infected rats with anemia produced by anti-blood immune serum. J. Infect. Dis. 84:169-186.

Thompson, M. J. 1932. Intranuclear inclusions in the submaxillary gland of the rat. J. Infect. Dis. 50:162-170.

Thompson, R., V. M. Harrison, and F. P. Myers. 1951. A spontaneous epizootic of mouse encephalomyelitis. Proc. Soc. Exp. Biol. Med. 77:262-266.

Thompson, R. B., Jr., and T. F. Smith. 1982. Acridine orange staining of *Pneumocystis carinii*. J. Clin. Microbiol. 16:191-192.

Thompson, W. L., and R. W. Wannemacher, Jr. 1980. Effects of infection and endotoxin on rat hepatic RNA production and distribution. Am. J. Physiol. 238:6303 6311.

Thomsen, A. C., and S. Rosendal. 1974. Mycoplasmosis: Experimental pyelonephritis in rats. Acta Pathol. Microbiol. Scand. 82:94-98.

Thomsen, A. R., K. Bro-Jorgensen, and B. L. Jensen. 1982. Lymphocytic choriomeningitis virus-induced immunosuppression: Evidence for viral interference with T-cell maturation. Infect. Immun. 37:981-986.

Thornburg, L. P., H. D. Stowe, and J. F. Pick. 1973. The pathogenesis of alopecia due to hair chewing in mice. Lab. Anim. Sci. 23:843-850.

Thunert, A. 1984. Is it possible to cultivate the agent of Tyzzer's disease (*Bacillus piliformis*) in cellfree media? Z. Versuchstierkd. 26:145-150.

Thunert, A., L. C. Jonas, S. Rehm, and E. Sickel. 1985. Transmission and course of Tyzzer's disease in euthymic and thymus aplastic nude Han: RNU rats. Z. Versuchtierk. 27:241-248.

Thurston, J. P. 1955. Observations on the course of *Eperythrozoon coccoides* infection in mice, and the sensitivity of the parasite to external agents. Parasitology 45:141-151.

Tiensiwakul, P., and S. S. Husain. 1979. Effect of mouse hepatitis virus infection on iron retention in the mouse liver. Br. J. Exp. Pathol. 60:161-166.

Tinghitella, T. J., and J. Booss. 1979. Enhanced immune response late in primary cytomegalovirus infection in mice. J. Immunol. 122:2442-2446.

Tisdale, W. A. 1963. Potentiating effect of K-virus on mouse hepatitis virus (MHV-S) in weanling mice. Proc. Soc. Exp. Biol. Med. 114:774-777.

Tishon, A., P. J. Southern, and M. B. A. Oldstone. 1988. Virus-lymphocyte interactions. II. Expression of viral sequences during the course of persistent lymphocytic choriomeningitis virus infection and their localization to the L3T4 lymphocyte subset. J. Immunol. 140:1280-1284.

Toolan, H. W. 1960. Experimental production of mongoloid hamsters. Science 131:1446-1448.

Toolan, H. W. 1961. A virus associated with transplantable human tumors. Bull. N. Y. Acad. Med. 37:305-310.

Toolan, H. W. 1968. The Picodna Viruses: H, RV, and AAV. Int. Rev. Exp. Pathol. 6:135-180.

Toolan, H. W., and N. Ledinko. 1968. Inhibition by H-1 virus of the incidence of tumors produced by adenovirus 12 in hamsters. Virology 35:475-478.

Toolan, H. W., G. Dalldorf, M. Barclay, S. Chandra, and A. E. Moore. 1960. An unidentified filterable agent isolated from transplanted human tumors. Proc. Natl. Acad. Sci. USA 46:1256-1259.

Toolan, H. W., S. L. Rhode III, and J. F. Gierthy. 1982. Inhibition of 7, 12-dimethylbenz(a)anthracene tumors in Syrian hamsters by prior infection with H-1 parvoviruses. Cancer Res. 42:2552-2555.

Topley, W. W. C., and G. S. Wilson. 1920. The spread of bacterial infection. The problem of herd immunity. J. Hyg. 21:243-249.

Topp, W. C., D. Lane, and R. Pollack. 1980. Transformation by SV40 and polyoma virus. Pp. 205-296 in Molecular Biology of Tumor Viruses, 2nd ed. Part 2:DNA Tumor Viruses, J. Tooze, ed. New York: Cold Spring Harbor Laboratory.

Toriumi, W., S. Kawamura, and K. Fujiwara. 1986. Application of enzyme-linked immunosorbent assay (ELISA) to detection of antibodies against Tyzzer's organism *Bacillus piliformis* in mice. Jpn. J. Vet. Sci. 48:1241-1244.

Totton, M. 1958. Ringtail in newborn Norway rats—A study of the effect of environmental temperature and humidity on incidence. J. Hyg. 56:190-196.

Traina-Dorge, V., and J. C. Cohen. 1983. Molecular genetics of mouse mammary tumor virus. Curr. Top. Microbiol. Immunol. 106:55-56.

Tram, C., J. C. Guillon, and I. Chouroulinkov. 1970. Isolement de mycoplasmes de foetus de rats obtenus par cesarienne aseptique. C. R. Soc. Biol. 164:2470-2471.

Traub, E. 1935. A filterable virus recovered from white mice. Science 81:298-299.

Traub, E. 1939. Epidemiology of lymphocytic choriomeningitis in a mouse stock observed for four years. J. Exp. Med. 69:801-817.

Traub, E. 1973. LCM virus research, retrospect and prospects. Pp. 3-10 in Lymphocytic Choriomeningitis Virus and Other Arenaviruses, F. Lehmann-Grube, ed. New York: Springer-Verlag.

Trentin, J. J., and B. A. Briody. 1953. An outbreak of mousepox (infectious ectromelia) in the U.S. II. Definitive diagnosis. Science 117:227-228.

Trentin, J. J., and M. A. Ferrigno. 1959. Control of mousepox by immunization with vaccinia virus. J. Natl. Cancer Inst. 18:757-767.

Trentin, J. J., G. L. Van Hoosier, Jr., J. Shields, K. Stepens, and W. A. Stenback. 1966. Establishment of a caesarean-derived gnotobiotic foster nursed inbred mouse colony with observations on the control of *Pseudomonas*. Lab. Anim. Care 12:109-118.

Trexler, P. C. 1963. An isolator system for the control of contamination. Lab. Anim. Care 13:572-581.

Trexler, P. C. 1983. Gnotobiotics. Pp. 1-16 in The Mouse in Biomedical Research. Vol. III: Normative Biology, Immunology, and Husbandry, H. L. Foster, J. D. Small, and J. G. Fox, eds. New York: Academic Press.

Trexler, P. C., and E. D. Barry. 1958. Development of inexpensive germ-free animal rearing equipment. Proc. Anim. Care Panel 8:75-77.

Trexler, P. C., and L. I. Reynolds. 1957. Flexible film apparatus for the bearing and use of germ-free animals. Appl. Microbiol. 5:406-412.

Tsai, T. F. 1985. Serological and virological evidence of a Hantaan virus-related enzootic in the United States. J. Infect. Dis. 152:126-136.

Tsai, T. F. 1987a. Hemorrhagic fever with renal syndrome: Mode of transmission to humans. Lab. Anim. Sci. 37:428-430.

Tsai, T. F. 1987b. Hemorrhagic fever with renal syndrome: Clinical aspects. Lab. Anim. Sci. 37:419-427.

Tsuchitani, M., T. Umemura, and I. Narama. 1983. Naturally occurring Tyzzer's disease in a clean mouse colony: High mortality with coincidental cardiac lesions. J. Comp. Pathol. 93:499-507.

Tsukui, M., H. Ito, M. Tada, M. Nakata, H. Miyajima, and K. Fujiwara. 1982. Protective effect of inactivated virus vaccine on Sendai virus infection in rats. Lab. Anim. Sci. 32:143-146.

Tuazon, C. U., T. Nash, A. Cheever, F. Neva, and L. Lininger. 1986. Influence of *Salmonella* and other gram-negative bacteria on the survival of mice infected with *Schistosoma japonicum*. J. Infect. Dis. 154:179-182.

Tucek, P. C. 1971. Case Report. Diplococcal pneumonia in the laboratory rat. Lab. Anim. Dig. 7:32-36.

Tuchi, K. T. Matthiesen, and F. Helm. 1977. Sialadenitis in spontaneously hypertensive rats. Z. Versuchstierkd. 19:40-46.

Tuffery, A. A. 1956. Laboratory mouse in Great Britain. IV. Intercurrent infection (Tyzzer's disease). Vet. Rec. 68:511-515.

Tuffery, A. A. 1958. Vaccination in the control of ectromelia in mouse colonies. Lab. Pract. 7:412-415.

Tully, J. G. 1964. Production and biological characteristics of an extracellular neurotoxin from *Mycoplasma neurolyticum*. J. Bacteriol. 88:381-388.

Tully, J. G., and R. Rask-Nielsen. 1967. *Mycoplasma* in leukemic and nonleukemic mice. Ann. N.Y. Acad. Sci. 143:345-352.

Tully, J. G., and I. Ruchman. 1964. Recovery, identification, and neurotoxicity of Sabin's type A and C mouse mycoplasma (PPLO) from lyophilized cultures. Proc. Soc. Exp. Biol. Med. 115:554-558.

Turk, M. A. M., A. M. Gallina, and L. E. Perryman. 1981. *Bacillus piliformis* infection (Tyzzer's disease) in foals in northwestern United States: A retrospetive study of 21 cases. J. Am. Vet. Med. Assoc. 178:279-281.

Turner, L. H. 1967. Leptospirosis I. Trans. R. Soc. Trop. Med. Hyg. 61:842-855.

Turner, L. H. 1968. Leptospirosis II. Trans. R. Soc. Trop. Med. Hyg. 62:880-899.

Turner, L. H. 1970. Leptospirosis III. Trans. R. Soc. Trop. Med. Hyg. 64:623-646.

Turner, W., P. S. Ebert, R. Bassin, G. Spahn, and M. A. Chirigos. 1971. Potentiation of murine sarcoma virus (Harvey) (Maloney) oncogenicity in lactic dehydrogenase-elevating virus-infected mice. Proc. Soc. Exp. Biol. Med. 136:1314-1318.

Tvedten, H. W., C. K. Whitehair, and R. F. Langham. 1973. Influence of vitamins A and E on gnotobiotic and conventionally maintained rats exposed to *Mycoplasma pulmonis*. J. Am. Vet. Med. Assoc. 163:605-612.

Tyzzer, E. E. 1917. A fatal disease of the Japanese waltzing mouse caused by spore-bearing bacillus (*Bacillus piliformis* N. sp.). J. Med. Res. 37:307-338.

Ueda, K., S. Yamazaki, and S. Someya. 1976. Experimental mycobacterial infection in congenitally athymic "nude" mice. J. Reticuloendothel. Soc. 19:77-90.

Ueda, K., U. Goto, S. Yamazaki, and K. Fujiwara. 1977a. Chronic fatal pneumocytosis in nude mice. Jpn. J. Exp. Med. 47:475-482.

Ueda, K., T. Tamura, K. Machii, and K. Fujiwara. 1977b. An outbreak of Sendai virus infection in a nude mouse colony. Proc. Internat. Workshop Nude Mice 2:61-69

Umehara, K., M. Hirakawa, and K. Hashimoto. 1984. Fluctuation of antiviral resistance in the intestinal tracts of nude mice infected with a mouse adenovirus. Microbiol. Immunol. 28:679-690.

Umenai, T., P. W. Lee, T. Toyoda, K. Yoshinaga, T. Horiuchi, H. W. Lee, T. Saito, M. Hongo, T. Nobunaga, and N. Ishida. 1979. Korean hemorrhagic fever in staff in an animal laboratory. Lancet i:1314-1316.

Urano, T., and K. Maejima. 1978. Provocation of pseudomoniasis with cyclophosphamide in mice. Lab. Anim. 12:159-161.

Utsumi, K. T. Maeda, H. Tatsumi, and K. Fijiwara. 1978. Some clinical and epizootological observations of infectious sialoadenitis in rats. Exp. Anim. 27:283-287.

Utsumi, K., T. Ishikawa, T. Maeda, S. Shimizu, H. Tatsumi, and K. Fujiwara. 1980. Infectious sialodacryoadenitis and rat breeding. Lab. Anim. 14:303-307.

Van Der Logt, J. T. M. 1986. Serological study on the prevalence of murine viruses in laboratory animal colonies, in France and in the Netherlands (1981-1984). Sci. Tech. Anim. Lab: 11:197-203.

Van der Shaaf, A., J. W. M. A. Mullink, R. J. Nikkels, and J. Goudswaard. 1970. *Pasteurella pneumotropica* as a causal microorganism of multiple subcutaneous abscesses in a colony of Wistar rats. Z. Versuchstierkd. 12:356-362.

Van der Veen, J., and A. Mes. 1973. Experimental infection with mouse adenovirus in adult mice. Arch. Gesamte Virusforsch. 42:235-241.

Van der Veen, J., and A. Mes. 1974. Serological classification of two mouse adenoviruses. Arch. Gesamte Virusforsch. 45:386-387.

van der Veen, J., Y. Poort, and D. J. Birchfield. 1970. Experimental transmission of Sendai virus infection in mice. Arch. Gesamte Virusforsch. 31:237-246.

van der Veen, J., Y. Poort, and D. J. Birchfield. 1972. Effect of relative humidity on experimental transmission of Sendai virus in mice. Proc. Soc. Exp. Biol. Med. 140:1437-1440.

van der Waaij, D., and A. H. Andreas. 1971. Prevention of airborne contamination and cross-contamination in germ-free mice by laminar flow. J. Hyg. 69:83-89.

van der Zeijst, B. A. M., B. E. Noyes, M.-E. Mirault, B. Parker, A. D. M. E. Osterhaus, E. A. Swyryd, N. Bleumink, M. C. Horzinek, and G. R. Stark. 1983. Persistent infection of some standard cell lines by lymphocytic choriomeningitis virus: Transmission of infection by an intracellular agent. J. Virol. 48:249-261.

Van Hoosier, G. L., Jr., J. J. Trentin, J. Shields, K. Stephens, W. A. Stenback, and J. C. Parker. 1966. Effect of cesarean derivation gnotobiote foster nursing and barrier maintenance of an inbred mouse colony on enzootic virus status. Lab. Anim. Sci. 16:119-128.

Van Kruiningen, H. J., D. R. Knibbs, and C. N. Burke. 1978. Hexamitiasis in laboratory mice. J. Am. Vet. Med. Assoc. 173:1202-1204.

van Nie, R. 1967. Behavior and morphology of pregnancy responsive mammary tumors in mice. Pathol. Eur. 2:357-373.

van Nie, R., and J. Hilgers. 1976. Genetic analysis of mammary tumor induction and expression of mammary tumor virus antigen in hormone-treated ovariectomized GR mice. J. Natl. Cancer Inst. 56:27-32.

Van Rooyen, C. R. 1936. The biology, pathogenesis and classification of *Streptobacillus moniliformis*. J. Pathol. Bacteriol. 43:455-472.

van Ypersele de Strihou, C. 1979. Acute oliguric interstitial nephritis. Kidney Int. 16:751-765.

van Zwieten, M. J., H. A. Solleveld, J. R. Lindsey, F. G. deGroot, C. Zurcher, and C. F. Hollander. 1980a. Respiratory disease in rats associated with a filamentous bacterium. Lab. Anim. Sci. 30:215-221.

van Zwieten, M. J., H. A. Solleveld, J. R. Lindsey, F. G. deGroot, C. Zurcher, and C. F. Hollander. 1980b. Respiratory disease in rats associated with a long rod-shaped bacterium; preliminary results of a morphologic study. Pp. 243-247 in Animal Quality and Models in Research. A. Spiegel, S. Erichsen, and H. A. Solleveld, eds. New York: Gustave Fischer Verlag.

Vella, P. P., and T. J. Starr. 1965. Effect of x-irradiation and cortisone on mouse hepatitis virus infection in mice. J. Infect. Dis. 115:271-277.

Verhoef, J., and H. A. Verbrugh. 1981. Host determinants in staphylococcal disease. Annu. Rev. Med. 32:107-122.

Vincent, J. G., R. C. Veomett, and R. F. Riley. 1955. Relation of the indigenous flora of the small intestine of the rat to post-irradiation bacteremia. J. Bacteriol. 69:38-44.

Virelizier, J. L., A. M. Virelizier, and A. C. Allison. 1976. The role of circulating interferon in the modifications of immune responsiveness by mouse hepatitis virus (MHV3). J. Immunol. 117:748-753.

Visscher, M. B., R. G. Green, and J. J. Bittner. 1942. Characterization of milk influence in spontaneous mammary carcinoma. Proc. Soc. Exp. Biol. Med. 49:94-96.

Vogelzang, A. A. 1975. The survival of *Mycoplasma pulmonis* in drinking water and in other materials. Z. Versuchstierkd. 17:S240-246.

von Magnus, H., and P. von Magnus. 1948. Breeding of a colony of white mice free of encephalomyelitis virus. Acta Pathol. Microbiol. Scand. 26:175-177.

von Matthiesen, T., I. Kunstyr, and K. Tuch. 1976. *Hexamita muris*-Infektionbei Mausen und Feldhamstern in einem Versuchstierbestand. Z. Versuchstierkd. 18:S113-S120.

Vonderfecht, S. L., A. C. Huber, J. J. Eiden, L. C. Mader, and R. H. Yolken. 1984. Infectious diarrhea of infant rats produced by a rotavirus-like agent. J. Virol. 52:94-98.

Vonderfecht, S. L., R. L. Miskuff, J. J. Eiden, and R. H. Yoklen. 1985. Enzyme immunoassay inhibition assay for the detection of rat rotavirus-like agent in intestinal and fecal specimens obtained from diarrheic rats and humans. J. Clin. Microbiol. 22:726-730.

Vonderfecht, S. L., J. J. Eiden, R. L. Miskuff, and R. H. Yolken. 1988. Kinetics of intestinal replication of group B rotavirus and relevance to diagnostic methods. J. Clin. Microbiol. 26:216-221.

Voravuthikunchai, S. P., and A. Lee. 1987. Cecectomy causes long-term reduction of colonization resistance in the mouse gastrointestional tract. Infect. Immun. 55:995-999.

Vossen, M. E. M. H., P. J. A. Beckers, T. H. E. T. Meuwissen, and A. M. Stadhouders. 1978. Developmental biology of *Pneumocystis carinii*, an alternate view on the life cycle of the parasite. Z. Parasitenkd. 55:101-118.

W.H.O. (World Health Organization). 1983. Hemorrhagic fever with renal syndrome: Memorandum from a WHO meeting. Bull. W.H.O. 61:269-275.

Waggie, K. S., C. T. Hansen, J. R. Ganaway, and T. S. Spencer. 1981. A study of mouse strain susceptibility to *Bacillus piliformis* (Tyzzer's disease): The association of B-cell function and resistance. Lab. Anim. Sci. 31:139-142.

Waggie, K. S., J. E. Wagner, and R. H. Lentsch. 1983a. A naturally occurring outbreak of *Mycobacterium avium-intracellulare* infections in C57BL/6N mice. Lab. Anim. Sci. 33:249-253.

Waggie, K. S., J. E. Wagner, and R. H. Lentsch. 1983b. Experimental murine infections with a *Mycobacterium avium-intracellulare* complex organism isolated from mice. Lab. Anim. Sci. 33:254-257.

Waggie, K. S., J. R. Ganaway, J. E. Wagner, and T. H. Spencer. 1984. Experimentally induced Tyzzer's disease in Mongolian gerbils (*Meriones unquiculatus*). Lab. Anim. Sci. 34:53-57.

Waggie, K. S., T. H. Spencer, and A. M. Allen. 1987. Cilia associated respiratory (CAR) bacillus infection in New Zealand White rabbits. Lab. Anim. Sci. 37:533 (abstract).

Wagner, J. E. 1969. Control of mouse ectoparasites with resin vaporizer strips containing vapona. Lab. Anim. Care 19:804-807.

Wagner, J. E. 1970. Control of mouse pinworms, *Syphacia obvelata*, utilizing dichlorovos. Lab. Anim. Care 20:39-44.

Wagner, J. E., R. G. Garrison, D. R. Johnson, and T. J. McGuire. 1969. Spontaneous conjunctivitis and dacryoadenitis of mice. J. Am. Vet. Med. Assoc. 155:1211-1217.

Wagner, J. E., R. E. Doyle, N. C. Ronald, R. G. Garrison, and J. A. Schmitz. 1974. Hexamitiasis in laboratory mice, hamsters, and rats. Lab. Anim. Sci. 24:349-354.

Wagner, J. E., D. R. Owens, M. C. LaRegina, and G. A. Volger. 1977. Self-trauma and *Staphylococcus aureus* in ulcerative dermatitis in rats. J. Am. Vet. Med. Assoc. 171:839-841.

Wagner, M. 1985. Absence of *Pneumocystis carinii* in Lobund germfree and conventional rat colonies. Pp. 51-54 in Germfree Research: Microflora Control and Its Application to the Biomedical Sciences. B. S. Wostmann, ed. New York: Alan R. Liss.

Wainberg, M. A., and E. Israel. 1980. Viral inhibition of lymphocyte mitogenesis. I. Evidence for the nonspecificity of the effect. J. Immunol. 124:64-70.

Waksman, B. H. and R. D. Adams. 1956. A comparative study of experimental allergic neuritis in the rabbit, guinea pig, and mouse. J. Neuropathol. Exp. Neurol. 15:293-334.

Walker, R. 1958. Age changes in the rat's exorbital lacrimal gland. Anat. Rec. 132:49-69.

Wallace, G. D., and R. M. L. Buller. 1985. Kinetics of ectromelia virus (mousepox) transmission and clinical response in C57BL/6J, BALB/cByJ and AKR/J inbred mice. Lab. Anim. Sci. 35:41-46.

Wallace, G. D., and R. M. L. Buller. 1986. Ectromelia virus (mousepox): biology, epizooitology, prevention and control. Chapt. 23, pp. 539-556 in Viral and Mycoplasmal Infections of Laboratory Rodents: Effects on Biomedical Research. P. N. Bhatt, R. O. Jacoby, H. C. Morse III, and A. E. New, eds. Orlando, Fla. Academic Press.

Wallace, G. D., R. M. Werner, P. L. Galway, D. M. Hernandez, D. W. Alling, and D. A. George. 1981. Epizootiology of an outbreak of mousepox at the National Institutes of Health. Lab. Anim. Sci. 31:609-615.

Wallace, G. D., R. M. L. Buller, and H. C. Morse III. 1985. Genetic determinants of resistance to ectromelia (mousepox) virus-induced mortality. J. Virol. 55:890-891.

Waller, T. 1975. Growth of *Nosema cuniculi* in established cell lines. Lab. Anim. 9:61-68.

Waller, T. 1977. The India-ink immunoreaction: A method for the rapid diagnosis of encephalitozoonosis. Lab. Anim. 11:93-97.

Waller, T., B. Morein, and E. Tabiansson. 1978. Humoral immune response to infection with *Encephalitozoon cuniculi* in rabbits. Lab. Anim. 12:145-148.

Walters, M. N.-I., R. A. Joske, P. J. Leak, and N. F. Stanley. 1963. Murine infection with reovirus. I. Pathology of the acute phase. Br. J. Exp. Pathol. 44:427-436.

Walters, M. L., N. F. Stanley, R. L. Dawkins, and M. P. Alpers. 1973. Immunological assessment of mice with chronic jaundice and runting induced by reovirus 3. Br. J. Exp. Pathol. 54:329-345.

Walzer, P. D., and M. J. Linke. 1987. A comparison of the antigenic characteristics of rat and human *Pneumocystis carinii* by immunoblotting. J. Immunol. 138:2257-2265.

Walzer, P. D., and M. E. Rutledge. 1981. Humoral immunity in experimental *Pneumocystis carinii* infection. I. Serum and bronchial lavage fluid antibody responses in rats. J. Lab. Clin. Med. 97:820-833.

Walzer, P. D., and M. E. Rutledge. 1982. Serum antibody responses to *Pneumocystis carinii* among different strains of normal and athymic mice. Infect. Immun. 35:620-626.

Walzer, P. D., V. Schnelle, D. Armstrong, and P. P. Rosen. 1977. Nude mouse: A new experimental model for *Pneumocystis carinii* infection. Science 197:177-197.

Walzer, P. D., R. Powell, and K. Yoneda. 1979. Experimental *Pneumocystis carinii* pneumonia in different strains of cortisonized mice. Infect. Immun. 24:939-947.

Walzer, P. D., R. Powell, Jr., K. Yoneda, M. E. Rutledge, and J. E. Milder. 1980. Growth characteristics and pathogenesis of experimental *Pneumocystis carinii* pneumonia. Infect. Immun. 27:928-937.

Walzer, P. D., M. E. Rutledge, and K. Yoneda. 1983. Experimental *Pneumocystis carinii* pneumonia in C3H/HeJ and C3HeB/FeJ mice. J. Reticuloendothel. Soc. 33:1-9.

Walzer, P. D., D. Stanforth, M. J. Linke, and M. T. Cushion. 1987. *Pneumocystis carinii*: immunoblotting and immunofluorescent analyses of serum antibodies during experimental rat infection and recovery. Exp. Parasitol. 63:319-328.

Walzer, P. D., C. K. Kim, J. Linke, C. L. Pogue, M. J. Huerkamp, C. E. Chrisp, A. V. Lerro, S. K. Wixson, E. Hall, and L. D. Shultz. 1989. Outbreaks of *Pneumocystis carinii* pneumonia in colonies of immunodeficient mice. Infect. Immun. 57:62-70.

Wang, S. P. 1971. A microimmunofluorescence method. Study of antibody response to TRIC organisms in mice. Pp. 273-288 in Trachoma and Related Disorders Caused by Chlamydial Agents. Amsterdam: Excerpta Medica.

Ward, D. C., and P. J. Tattersall. 1982. Minute virus of mice. Pp. 313-334 in The Mouse in Biomedical Research. Vol. II. Diseases, H. L. Foster, J. D., Small, and J. G. Fox, eds. New York: Academic Press.

Ward, G. E., R. Moffatt, and E. Olfert. 1978. Abortion in mice associated with *Pasteurella pneumotropica*. J. Clin. Microbiol. 8:177-180.

Ward, J. M. 1974. A naturally occurring Sendai virus disease of mice. Lab. Anim. Sci. 24:938-942.

Ward, J. M., and D. M. Young. 1976. Latent adenoviral infection of rats: Intranuclear inclusions induced by treatment with a cancer chemotherapeutic agent. J. Am. Vet. Med. Assoc. 169:952-953.

Ward, J. M., D. P. Houchens, M. J. Collins, D. M. Young, and R. L. Reagan. 1976. Naturally occurring Sendai virus infection of athymic nude mice. Vet. Pathol. 13:36-46.

Ward, J. M., M. J. Collins, and J. C. Parker. 1977. Naturally occurring mouse hepatitis virus infection in the nude mouse. Lab. Anim. Sci. 27:372-376.

Ward, J. R., and B. C. Cole. 1970. Mycoplasmal infections of laboratory animals. Pp. 212-239 in The Role of Mycoplasmas and L Forms of Bacteria in Disease, J. T. Sharp, ed. Springfield, Ill.: Charles C Thomas.

Ward, J. R., and R. S. Jones. 1962. The pathogenesis of mycoplasmal (PPLO) arthritis in rats. Arth. Rheum. 5:163-175.

Warnock, M. L. 1964. Isozymic patterns in organs of mice infected with LDH agent. Proc. Soc. Exp. Biol. Med. 115:448-452.

Warren, J., R. J. Mason, L. H. Barbosa, K. L. Gabbard, and M. Bucy. 1968. Increased susceptibility to murine hepatitis virus infection by treatment with iron salts. Proc. Soc. Exp. Biol. Med. 129:637-642.

Warren, K. S., M. S. Rosenthal, and E. O. Domingo. 1969. Mouse hepatitis virus (MHV3) infection in chronic murine *Schistosomiasis mansoni*. Bull. N.Y. Acad. Med. 45:211-224.

Watson, K. C. 1970. *Salmonella typhimurium* infection in mice treated with niridazole. J. Med. Microbiol. 3:361-365.

Wehner, R. W., and R. D. Smith. 1983. Progressive cytomegalovirus glomerulonephritis. Am. J. Pathol. 112:313-325.

Weinman, D. 1944. Infectious anemias due to *Bartonella* and related cell parasites. Trans. Am. Philos. Soc. 33:243-350.

Weir, E. C., D. G. Brownstein, and S. W. Barthold. 1986. Spontaneous wasting disease in nude mice associated with *Pneumocystis carinii* infection. Lab. Anim. Sci. 36:140-144.

Weir, E. C., P. N. Bhatt, S. W. Barthold, G. A. Cameron, and P. A. Simack. 1987. Elimination of mouse hepatitis virus from a breeding colony by temporary cessation of breeding. Lab. Anim. Sci. 37:455-458.

Weir, E. C., D. G. Brownstein, A. L. Smith, and E. A. Johnson. 1988. Respiratory disease and wasting in athymic mice infected with pneumonia virus of mice. Lab. Anim. Sci. 38:133-137.

Wilsnack, R. E., J. H. Blackwell, and J. C. Parker. 1969. Identification of an agent of epizootic diarrhea of infant mice by immunofluorescence and complement fixation tests. Am. J. Vet. Res. 30:1195-1204.

Weisbroth, S. H. 1972. Pathogen-free substrates for gerontologic research: Review, sources and comparison of barrier-sustained vs. conventional laboratory rats. Exp. Gerontol. 7:417-426.

Weisbroth, S. H. 1979. Bacterial and mycotic diseases. Pp. 193-241 in The Laboratory Rat. Vol. I, H. J. Baker, J. R. Lindsey and S. H. Weisbroth, eds. New York: Academic Press.

Weisbroth, S. H. 1982. Arthropods. Pp. 385-402 in The Mouse in Biomedical Research. Vol. II: Diseases, H. L. Foster, J. D. Small, and J. G. Fox, eds. New York: Academic Press.

Weisbroth, S. H., and E. H. Freimer. 1969. Laboratory rats from commercial breeders as carriers of pathogenic pneumococci. Lab. Anim. Care 19:473-478.

Weisbroth, S. H., and N. Peress. 1977. Ophthalmic lesions and dacryoadenitis: A naturally occurring aspect of sialodacryoadenitis of the laboratory rat. Lab. Anim. Sci. 27:466-473.

Weisbroth, S. H., and S. Scher. 1968a. *Corynebacterium kutscheri* infection in the mouse. I. Report of an outbreak, bacteriology, and pathology of spontaneous infections. Lab. Anim. Care 18:451-458.

Weisbroth, S. H., and S. Scher. 1968b. *Corynebacterium kutscheri* infection in the mouse. II. Diagnostic serology. Lab. Anim. Care 18:459-468.

Weisbroth, S. H., S. Scher, and I. Boman. 1969. *Pasteurella pneumotropica* abscess syndrome in a mouse colony. J. Am. Vet. Med. Assoc. 155:1206-1210.

Weisbroth, S. H., S. Friedman, and S. Scher. 1976. The parasitic ecology of the rodent mite *Myobia musculi*. III. Lesions in certain host strains. Lab. Anim. Sci. 26:725-735.

Weiser, J. 1965. *Nosema muris* n. sp., a new microsporidian parasite of the white mouse (*Mus musculus* L.). J. Protozool. 12:78-83.

Weiser, W. Y., and F. B. Bang. 1977. Blocking of in vitro and in vivo susceptibility to mouse hepatitis virus. J. Exp. Med. 146:1467-1472.

Weiss, E. 1949. The extracellular development of agents of the psittacocis-lymphogranuloma group (Chlamydozoaceae). J. Infect. Dis. 84:125-149.

Wells, A. B. 1970. The kinetics of cell proliferation in the tracheobronchial epithelia of rats with and without chronic respiratory disease. Cell Tissue Kinet. 3:185-206.

Welsh, R. M. 1978. Cytotoxic cells induced during lymphocytic choriomeningitis virus infection of mice. II. Characterization of natural killer cell induction. J. Exp. Med. 148:163-181.

Welsh, R. M., Jr., and W. F. Doe. 1980. Cytotoxic cells induced during lymphocytic choriomeningitis virus infection of mice. Natural killer cell activity in cultured spleen leukocytes concomitant with T-cell dependent immune interferon production. Infect. Immun. 30:473-483.

Wenner, H. A. 1948. Isolation of LCM virus in an effort to adapt poliomyelitis virus to rodents. J. Infect. Dis. 83:155-163.

Wensinck, F. D., D. W. Van Bekkum, and H. Renaud. 1957. The prevention of *Pseudomonas aeruginosa* infections in irradiated mice and rats. Radiat. Res. 7:491-499.

Werner, G. 1957. Infection of laboratory mice with *Salmonella kentucky*. Am. J. Vet. Res. 18:954-955.

Werner, R. M., A. M., Allen, J. D. Small, and A. E. New. 1981. Clinical manifestations of mousepox in an experimental animal holding room. Lab. Anim. Sci. 31:590-594.

Wescott, R. B. 1982. Helminths. Pp. 373-384 in The Mouse in Biomedical Research. Vol. II: Diseases, H. L. Foster, J. D. Small, and J. G. Fox, eds. New York: Academic Press.

Wescott, R. B., A. Malczewski, and G. L. Van Hoosier. 1976. The influence of filter top caging on the transmission of pinworm infections in mice. Lab. Anim. Sci. 26:742-745.

Westerberg, S. C., C. B. Smith, B. B. Wiley, and C. Jensen. 1972. Mycoplasma-virus interrelationships in mouse tracheal organ cultures. Infect. Immun. 5:840-846.

Wetmore, P. W., and W. G. Hoag. 1960. *Salmonella binza* and *Salmonella bredeney* from laboratory mice. J. Bacteriol. 80:283.

Wheater, D. F. W. 1967. The bacterial flora of an S.P.F. colony of mice, rats, and guinea pigs. Pp. 343-360 in Husbandry of Laboratory Animals, M. L. Conalty, ed. London: Academic Press.

Wheelock, E. F. 1966. The effects of nontumor viruses on virus-induced leukemia in mice: Reciprocal interference between Sendai virus and Friend leukemia virus in DBA/2 mice. Proc. Natl. Acad. Sci. USA 55:774-780.

Wheelock, E. F. 1967. Inhibitory effects of Sendai virus on Friend leukemia in mice. J. Natl. Cancer Inst. 38:771-778.

White, J. D., F. G. Shirey, G. R. French, J. W. Huggins, O. M. Brand, and H. W. Lee. 1982. Hantaan virus, aetiological agent of Korean hemorrhagic fever has Bunyaviridae-like morphology. Lancet i:768-771.

Whitney, Jr., R. A., J. D. Small, and A. E. New. 1981. Mousepox—National Institutes of Health experiences. Lab. Anim. Sci. 31:570-573.

Whittlestone, P., R. M. Lemcke, and R. J. Olds. 1972. Respiratory disease in a colony of rats. II. Isolation of *Mycoplasma pulmonis* from the natural disease, and the experimental disease induced with a cloned culture of this organism. J. Hyg. 70:387-407.

W.H.O. (World Health Organization). 1983 Hemorrhagic fever with renal syndrome: Memorandum from a WHO meeting. Bull. W.H.O. 61:269-275.

Wigand, R. 1980. Age and susceptibility of Swiss mice for mouse adenovirus, strain FL. Arch. Virol. 64:349-357.

Wigand, R., and T. Adrian. 1986. Classification and epidemiology of adenoviruses. Pp. 409-441 in Adenovirus DNA: The Viral Genome and Its Expression, W. Doerfler, ed. Boston: Martinus Nijhoff.

Wigand, R., H. Gelderblom, and M. Ozel. 1977. Biological and biophysical characteristics of mouse adenovirus, strain FL. Arch. Virol. 54:131-142.

Wightman, S. R., J. E. Wagner, and R. M. Corwin. 1978. *Syphacia obvelata* in the Mongolian gerbil (*Meriones unguiculatus*): Natural occurrence and experimental transmission. Lab. Anim. Sci. 28:51-54.

Wiktor, T. J., M. V. Fernandes, and H. Koprowski. 1965. Detection of a lymphocytic choriomeningitis component in rabies virus preparations. J. Bacteriol. 90:1494-1495.

Wildfeuer, A., B. Heymer, H. Schafer, and O. Haferkamp. 1978. The cervical lymph nodes in Streptococcus pyogenes, group A, type 50, infection in mice. Med. Microbiol. Immunol. 165:129-137.

Willenborg, D. O., K. V. Shah, and F. B. Bang. 1973. Effect to cyclophosphamide on the genetic resistance of C3H mice to mouse hepatitis virus. Proc. Soc. Exp. Biol. Med. 142:762-766.

Williams, D. L., and N. R. DiLuzzio. 1980. Glucan-induced modification of murine viral hepatitis. Science 108:67-69.

Williams, D. M., J. Schacter, D. J. Drutz, and C. V. Sumaya. 1981. Pneumonia due to *Chlamydia trachomatis* in the immunocompromised (nude) mouse. J. Infect. Dis. 143:238-241.

Williams, D. M., J. Schacter, B. Grubbs, and C. V. Sumaya. 1982. The role of antibody in host defense against the agent of mouse pneumonitis. J. Infect. Dis. 145:200-205.

Williams, D. M., J. Schacter, J. J. Coalson, and B. Grubbs. 1984. Cellular immunity to the mouse pneumonitis agent. J. Infect. Dis. 149:630-639.

Williams, S. 1941. An outbreak of infection due to *Streptobacillus moniliformis* among wild mice. Med. J. Aust. 28:357-359.

Williford, C. B., and J. E. Wagner. 1982. Mycotic diseases. Pp. 65-68 in The Mouse in Biomedical Research. Vol. II: Diseases, H. L. Foster, J. D. Small, and J. G. Fox, eds. New York: Academic Press.

Wilsnack, R. E., and W. P. Rowe. 1964. Immunofluorescent studies of the histopathogenesis of lymphocytic choriomeningitis virus infection. J. Exp. Med. 120:829-840.

Wilson, J. M. 1979. The biology of *Encephalitozoon cuniculi*. Med. Biol. 57:84-101.

Wilson, P. 1976. *Pasteurella pneumotropica* as the causal organism of abscesses in the masseter muscle of mice. Lab. Anim. 10:171-172.

Wimer, R. E., and J. L. Fuller. 1966. Patterns of behavior. Pp. 631-633 in Biology of the Laboratory Mouse, E. L. Greene, ed. New York: McGraw-Hill.

Winkelstein, J. A., and A. J. Swift. 1975. Host defense against the pneumococcus in T-lymphocyte deficient, nude mice. Infect. Immun. 12:1222-1223.

Winters, A. L., and H. K. Brown. 1980. Duodenal lesions associated with adenovirus infection in athymic "nude" mice. Proc. Soc. Exp. Biol. Med. 164:280-286.

Woglom, W. H., and J. Warren. 1938. A pyogenic agent in the albino rat. J. Exp. Med. 68:513-528.

Wojcinski, Z. W., and D. H. Percy. 1986. Sialodacryoadenitis virus-associated lesions in the lower respiratory tract of rats. Vet. Pathol. 23:278-286.

Wolf, J. L., G. Cukor, N. R. Blacklow, R. Dambrauskas, and J. S. Trier. 1981. Susceptibility of mice to rotavirus infection: Effect of age and administration of corticosteroids. Infect. Immun. 33:565-574.

Wolff, H. L. 1950. On some spontaneous infections observed in mice. I. *C. kutscheri* and *C. pseudo-tuberculosis*. Antonie van Leeuwenhoek 16:105-110.

Wongwiwat, M., S. Sukapanit, C. Triyanond, and W. D. Sawyer. 1972. Circadian rhythm of the resistance of mice to acute pneumococcal infection. Infect. Immun. 5:442-448.

Wood, B. A., W. Dutz, and S. S. Cross. 1981. Neonatal infection with mouse thymic virus: Spleen and lymph node necrosis. J. Gen. Virol. 57:139-147.

Wood, W. B., Jr. 1941. Studies on the mechanisms of recovery in pneumococcal pneumonia. I. The action of type specific antibody upon the pulmonary lesion of experimental pneumonia. J. Exp. Med. 73:201-222.

Wood, W. B., Jr., and M. R. Smith. 1950. Host-parasite relationships in experimental pneumonia due to pneumococcus type III. J. Exp. Med. 92:85-100.

Woode, G. N., J. C. Bridger, J. C., T. H. Flewett, A. S. Bryden, H. A. Davies, and G. B. B. White. 1976. Morphological and antigenic relationships between viruses (rotaviruses) from acute gastroenteritis of children, calves, piglets, mice, and foals. Infect. Immun. 14:804-810.

Woodland, R. M., A. P. Johnson, and M. Tuffery. 1983. Animal models of chlamydial infection. Br. Med. Bull. 39:175-180.

Woodrow, D., P. Ronco, Y. Riviere, J. Moss, I. Gresser, J. C. Guillon, L. Morel-Maroger, J. C. Sloper, and P. Verroust. 1982. Severity of glomerulonephritis induced in different strains of suckling mice by infection with lymphocytic choriomeningitis virus: Correlation with amounts of endogenous interferon and circulating immune complexes. J. Pathol. 138:325-326.

Woodward, J. M. 1963. *Pseudomonas aeruginosa* infection and its control in the radiobiological research program at Oak Ridge National Laboratory. Lab. Anim. Care 13:20-26.

Wosu, N. J., R. Olsen, J. A. Shadduck, A. Koestner, and S. A. Pakes. 1977. Diagnosis of experimental encephalitozoonosis in rabbits by complement fixation. J. Infect. Dis. 135:944-948.

Wozniak, J., and F. Hetrick. 1969. Persistent infection of a rat nephroma cell line with Kilham rat virus. J. Virol. 4:313-314.

Wu-Hsieh, B., D. H. Howard, and R. Ahmed. 1988. Virus-induced immunosuppression: a murine model of susceptibility to opportunistic infection. J. Infect. Dis. 158:232-235.

Wullenweber-Schmidt, M., B. Meyer, V. Kraft, and J. Kaspareit. 1988. An enzyme-linked immunosorbent assay (ELISA) for the detection of antibodies to *Pasteurella pneumotropica* in murine colonies. Lab. Anim. Sci. 38:37-41.

Wyand, D. S., and A. M. Jonas. 1967. *Pseudomonas aeruginosa* infection in rats following implantation of an indwelling jugular catheter. Lab. Anim. Care 17:261-267.

Wynder, E. L., K. T. Taguchi, V. Baden, and D. Hoffman. 1968. Tobacco carcinogenesis. IX. Effect of cigarette smoke on respiratory tract of mice after passive inhalation. Cancer 21:134-153.

Yager, R. H., W. S. Gochenour, Jr., A. D. Alexander, and P. W. Wetmore. 1953. Natural occurrence of *Leptospira ballum* in rural house mice and in an opposum. Proc. Soc. Exp. Biol. Med. 84:589-890.

Yamada, A., Y. Osada, S. Takayama, T. Akimoto, H. Ogawa, Y. Oshima, and K. Fujiwara. 1969. Tyzzer's disease syndrome in laboratory rats treated with adrenocorticotropic hormone. Jpn. J. Exp. Med. 39:505-518.

Yamanishi, K., J. R. Dantas, M. Takahashi, T. Yamanouchi, K. Domae, J. Kawamata, and T. Kurata. 1983. Isolation of hemorrhagic fever with renal syndrome (HFRS) virus from a tumor specimen in a rat. Biken J. 26:155-160.

Yamanouchi, T., K. Domae, O. Tanishita, Y. Takahashi, K . Yamanishi, M. Takahashi, and T. Kurata. 1984. Experimental infection in newborn mice and rats by hemorrhagic fever with renal syndrome (HFRS) virus. Microbiol. Immunol. 28:1345-1353.

Yanagihara, R., H. L. Amyx, and D. C. Gajdusek. 1985a. Experimental infection with Puumala virus, the etiologic agent of nephropathia epidemica, in bank voles (*Clethrionomys glareolus*). J. Virol. 55:34-38.

Yanagihara, R., C. T. Chin, M. B. Weiss, D. C. Gajdusek, A. R. Diwan, J. B. Poland, K. T. Kleeman, C. M. Wilfert, G. Meiklejohn, and W. P. Glezen. 1985b. Serological evidence of Hantaan virus infection in the United States. Am. J. Trop. Med. Hyg. 34:396-399.

Yang, Y. H., and J. S. Campbell. 1964. Crystalline excrements in bronchitis and cholecystitis of mice. Am. J. Pathol. 45:337- 345.

Yang, Y. H., C. Y. Yang, and H. C. Grice. 1966. Multifocal histiocytosis in the lungs of rats. J. Pathol. Bacteriol. 92:559-561.

Yokoiyama. S., and K. Fujiwara. 1971. Effect of antibiotics on Tyzzer's disease. Jpn. J. Exp. Med. 41:49-57.

Yoneda, K., and P. D. Walzer. 1980. Interaction of *Pneumocystis carinii* with host lungs: an ultrastructural study. Infect. Immun. 29:692-703.

Yoneda, K., and P. D. Walzer. 1981. Mechanism of pulmonary alveolar injury in experimental *Pneumocystis carinii* pneumonia in the rat. Br. J. Exp. Pathol. 62:339-346.

Yoneda, K., and P. D. Walzer. 1983. Attachment of *Pneumocystis carinii* to type I alveolar cells: Study by freeze fracture electron microscopy. Infect. Immun. 40:812-815.

Yoneda, K., P. D. Walzer, C. S. Richey, and M. G. Birk. 1982. *Pneumocystis carinii*: Freeze fracture study of stages of the organism. Exp. Parasitol. 53:68-76.

Yoshikura, H., and F. Taguchi. 1979. Induction of lytic plaques by murine leukemia virus in murine sarcoma virus-transformed nonproducer mouse cells persistently infected with mouse hepatitis virus MHV-S. Intervirology 11:69-73.

Yost, D. H. 1958. Encephalitozoon infection in laboratory animals. J. Natl. Cancer Inst. 20:957-960.

Youn, J. K., and G. Barski. 1966. Interference between lymphocytic choriomeningitis and Rauscher leukemia in mice. J. Natl. Cancer Inst. 37:381-388.

Young, C., and A. C. Hill. 1974. Conjunctivitis in a colony of rats. Lab. Anim. 8:301-304.

Zeman, D. H., and G. B. Baskin. 1985. Encephalitozoonosis in squirrel monkeys (*Saimiri sciureus*). Vet. Pathol. 22: 24-31.

Zinkernagel, R. M. 1976. Cell-mediated immune response to *Salmonella typhimurium* infection in mice: Development of nonspecific bactericidal activity against *Listeria monocytogenes*. Infect. Immun. 13:1069-1073.

Zinkernagel, R. M., and P. C. Doherty. 1973. Cytotoxic thymus-activated lymphocytes in cerebrospinal fluid of mice with LCM. J. Exp. Med. 138:1266-1269.

Zinkernagel, R. M., and P. C. Doherty. 1975. H-2 compatibility requirement for T-cell-mediated lysis of target cells infected with lymphocytic choromeningitis Virus. Different cytotoxic T-cell specificities are associated with structures coded for H-2K or H-2D. J. Exp. Med. 141:1427-1436.

Zinkernagel, R. M., and P. C. Doherty. 1979. MHC-restricted cytotoxic T cells: Studies on the biological role of polymorphic major transplantation antigens determining T-cell restriction-specificity function and responsiveness. Adv. Immunol. 27:51-177.

Zucker, T. F. 1954. Resistance of rats to inoculation with *Corynebacterium pathogenesis* in pantothenate deficiency. Proc. Soc. Exp. Biol. Med. 85:521-524.

Zucker, T. F. 1956. Thiamine, pyridoxine and pantothenic acid in the natural resistance of the rat to a Corynebacterium infection. J. Nutr. 59:287-298.

Zucker, T. F. 1957. Pantothenate deficiency in rats. Proc. Anim. Care Panel 7:193-202.

Zucker, T. F., and L. M. Zucker. 1956. Antibody formation and natural resistance in nutritional deficiencies. J. Nutr. 59:299-308.

Zurcher, C., J. D. Burek, M. C. J. van Nunen, and S. P. Meihuizen. 1977. A naturally occurring epizootic caused by Sendai virus in breeding and aging rodent colonies. I. Infection in the mouse. Lab. Anim. Sci. 27:955-962.

Zweerink, H. J., M. C. Gammon, C. F. Hutchison, J. J. Jackson, G. B. Pier, J. M. Pucket, T. J. Sewell, and N. H. Sigal. 1988. X-linked immunodeficient mice as a model for testing the protective efficacy of monoclonal antibodies against *Pseudomonas aeruginosa*. Infect. Immun. 56:1209-1214.

# Index

## B



## C

## D

## E

## I



## J



## K



## L

## R

## S